you can
breastfeed
your baby
...even in special situations

you can
breastfeed
your baby
...even in special situations

By Dorothy Patricia Brewster
Illustrations by Barbara Field
Photographs by
       Sandra C. Wallace
       Anne Chapman Tullar
       and The Rodale Press Photography Staff

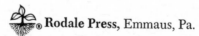® **Rodale Press**, Emmaus, Pa.

Printed in the United States of America on recycled paper containing a high percentage of de-inked fiber.

Library of Congress Cataloging in Publication Data

Brewster, Dorothy Patricia.

You can breastfeed your baby, even in special situations.

Bibliography: p.
Includes index.
1. Breast feeding.   I. Title.

RJ216.B86   649'.3   78-31241
ISBN 0-87857-256-2 hardcover
ISBN 0-87857-276-7 paperback

4   6   8   10   9   7   5   3   hardcover
4   6   8   10   9   7   5   3   paperback

Dedicated to my husband, Bob, and our children Susan, Sharon, Karen and David, without whose patience, cooperation and concern this book could never have been written.

Contents

Contents

Contents

Contents

Contents

Foreword

You Can Breastfeed Your Baby . . . Even in Special Situations will be extremely helpful to both the layperson and the medical community. Based on a wide range and variety of case histories, this very comprehensive book continues where other books stop, and indeed it does this very well. It makes a timely contribution to the knowledge regarding the management of breastfeeding in circumstances which were thought to be impossible a few years ago.

Scientific investigations reveal many physical and emotional advantages unique to breastfeeding—advantages which benefit babies in both normal and special situations. In 1973, the Pan-American Health Organization published results of a long-term Inter-American Investigation of Mortality in Childhood, undertaken in 10 countries of the Americas. Nutritional deficiency was found to be the most serious health problem; but breastfeeding provided substantial protection from both malnutrition and diarrheal disease, especially in the first year of life. In so-called developed, industrialized countries, severe forms of malnutrition were not as evident. However, new patterns of childhood and adult disease have emerged, including a rising tide of emotional and psychological problems and allergic disorders. Additionally, obesity, in infancy as well as in adult life, is becoming a problem in affluent westernized populations.

Research has proven beyond any doubt what the mothers in this book have discovered—that breast milk makes for healthier babies. It has unique properties for the human infant not possessed by the milk of any other mammal. It is now known that over 100 interacting constituents are present in breast milk in proportions and chemical composition that are quite different from the equally complex composition of milks of other mammals. Infant formulas are only approximate imitations of the main known ingredients of human milk. Producing a formula "just like human milk" is literally impossible.

At all ages of life, feeding is much more than the supplying of needed nutrients. Recent work, including the information presented in this valuable book, proves that in addition to the overwhelming accumulation of scientific data concerning specific nutritional and antiallergic properties in human milk, the whole process of breastfeeding has a special significance for both mother and baby, from both the emotional and economic points of view. Bonding of mother and baby after birth, for example, occurs more readily with the breastfed baby and his mother, who are in a more direct and intimate biological relationship with each other. The potentially harmful consequences of warped bonding (produced by the curious taboos of Western-style childbirth practices, such as bottlefeeding and separating mother and newborn) are only beginning to manifest themselves as one factor (among many others) that seems to be related to the rising tide of psychosocial emotional abnormalities such as child abuse and stress suicide in teen years.

Attention is being focused increasingly on the importance of interaction between mother and child. The mothers whose observations are recorded in this book augment our insight and they should be counted among the pioneers of health care and medical progress for their determination and courage in emphasizing the case for breastfeeding.

Until recently, procedures in many maternity units have often interfered with the management of breastfeeding. However, the more opportunities that physicians have had to observe breastfed babies, the more they have noted the advantages to baby and mother. Many physicians now strongly encourage mothers to breastfeed, and this has been emphasized by a 1978 Report by the American Academy of Pediatrics.

The trend is now back to breastfeeding. In 1976, the number of mothers commencing breastfeeding in the United States had increased to 38 percent, compared with only 18 percent in 1966; the number had more than doubled in 10 years. In 1978, over 50 percent of newborn babies were breast-fed. While this is an excellent trend with newborns, it is to be hoped that very soon similar statistics might be reported from all over the world and include older babies. In any part of the world, no single pediatric measure has such widespread potential for child health as the return to breastfeeding.

By breastfeeding their babies and encouraging others to do so, too, mothers can only enhance our environment. They are supplying, conveniently and at low cost, the correct dosage of nutrients, anti-infective agents and emotional support at the time when development of both brain and personality is most rapid and critical. In special situations, the very life of the child may depend on these advantages.

As significantly pointed out in the pages of this book, breastfeeding is not totally instinctive. Successful lactation is a confidence trick, and accomplishing it in difficult situations is best achieved with knowledge and emotional support. The enlightenment and encouragement offered in this work, through the shared experiences and the data collected, make *You Can Breastfeed Your Baby . . . Even in Special Situations* a valuable reference. It is hoped that in the years to come the author will accept the challenge to update and revise this unique volume and thus continue its great service for the child-caring professionals and for the benefit of mothers and babies.

Derrick B. Jelliffe, M.D.

Professor of Pediatrics and of Public Health, Head, Division of Population, Family and International Health
University of California at Los Angeles

Foreword

Recently a young mother phoned me in a state of desperation. Rose's two-month-old son, Billy, born with a number of medical problems, had been hospitalized from birth. Although she hadn't been allowed to breastfeed him, she continued to express her breast milk, waiting for the day when she could start nursing him as she had her other children. But the doctors weren't at all supportive of her breastfeeding Billy and, by this time, she was beginning to wonder if she were being selfish by her persistence, and was more than a little worried about carrying it off to the doctor's satisfaction when she was finally allowed to try. Her reason for calling was simply to find out if I knew of another mother, anywhere, who had breastfed a baby with the same kind of problem.

Today, for the first time in generations, more than half the babies born in the United States start off at their mother's breast. And some of those mothers, like Rose, will find themselves confronted with situations they are not prepared for. In the past such an occurrence usually also precluded the possibility of breastfeeding. But today, faced with undeniable evidence of the nutritional and immunological advantages of mother's milk and the special closeness of the nursing relationship, a mother is not apt to give up so easily.

Yet advice on breastfeeding when a baby has a specific medical problem or the mother is ill or has a handicap, to mention just a few of the situations she might encounter, is often hard to come by. That's what makes this book so useful and so unique. Gathered together in one volume we find advice from physicians who have had experience dealing with exceptional situations while keeping the baby at the breast, and inspirational as well as practical first-person stories from the mothers themselves.

This book should be useful not only to parents but to medical students, physicians, and nurses as well. While anecdotal information has never been given much credence by the scientific community, there is much to be learned from the real-life examples of women who committed themselves to giving their babies the best possible start in life no matter how severe the challenge.

In 1977 the theme of the XV International Congress of Pediatrics held in India was "Breastfeeding with Love Leads to Better Child Health." Scattered throughout the city were billboards carrying colorful pictures of babies and the slogan, Our Birthright Mothers' Milk. With this book Mrs. Brewster brings that right closer for all babies.

Marian Tompson

President of La Leche
League International

Acknowledgments

Many individuals have contributed to the development of this book over the past five years.

Jody Nathanson first focused my attention on the need for readily available breastfeeding information and kindled my interest in writing a book. She has been a tremendous source of inspiration, help and encouragement, many times urging me to continue when I was discouraged and thought of giving up. She shared with me a wide range of information and reference sources, read and commented on almost every chapter and patiently discussed various approaches to presenting material.

Marian Tompson, President of La Leche League International, Betty Wagner, Chief Executive Officer, and other board members of L.L.L.I. gave me encouragement by pointing out that the book would be valuable to mothers and La Leche League leaders. They offered help in many ways, including printing a request in *La Leche League News* and *Leaven* for mothers to share their experiences. I am especially grateful to the hundreds of mothers who responded to these requests.

Dr. Paul Fleiss and Dr. Margaret Davidson helped determine how the volume of material would be organized and were always available to answer my many questions.

This book is enhanced by the dedicated efforts of Regina Carlson, Justine Clegg, Nancy Cohen, Phyllis Dahl, R.N., Nancy Hieta, Margaret Howie, R.N., Jeanne Shaw, R.N., M.N., Karolyn Simon, R.N., and Rose Sodergren, and you can read more about these women at the end of the book. A special word of thanks goes to the late Linda Lehrer whose concern and desire to help others was truly inspiring. The motivation of these mothers to share their particular knowledge on specific topics will be appreciated by many mothers in the future.

I greatly appreciate the help of many knowledgeable mothers, nurses and doctors throughout the country, who reviewed and offered valuable suggestions on one or more chapters: La Leche League International Board Members Mary Ann Cahill, Betty Ann Countryman, R.N., M.N., Elizabeth Crofts, R.N., Jody Nathanson and Mary White. Also, Suzanne Bauer, Kathy Blanchard, Mayno Blanding, Ann Bodine, Alice Bricklin, Barbara Casey, Justine Clegg, Dr. Lewis A. Coffin, Nancy Cohen, Kay Coulson, R.N., Sandy Davis, Sandy Erikson, R.N., Dr. Paul Fleiss, Marti Fritz, Sharon Giboney, Sue Giobbi, Dr. Jerome Glaser, Dr. James Good, Sheri Hansen, Anne Hatcher, Kathie Hoch, Barbara Horan, Kathleen Huntsman, Dr. Charles J. Hyman, Dr. Derrick B. Jelliffe, Roberta Johnson, Glenda Keyser, Dr. C. Seybert Kinsell, Maureen Koestler, Lois Krensky, Marilyn Lap, Jenny Lee, Karen Lew, Linda Lehrer, Dr. George Lewis, Dr. Harold M. Maller, Dr. Vincent A. Marinkovich, Mary McIntyre, Dr. Robert Mendelsohn, Dr. John D. Michael, Mable O'Donnell, Marge O'Sullivan, Mary Orr, Skip Rapp, Dr. Alfred Scherzer, Jeanne Shaw, Dr. Gerald and Karolyn Simon, Rose Sodergren, Peggy Teeter, R.N., Dr. Mark Thoman, Sandy Wallace, Charles and Louise Wills, Dr. Raymond I. Wintroub, Lynne Endicott-Wismer, and Joan Zinda.

Throughout the writing of the book, it has helped immeasurably to be able to consult at any time and on any topic not only with Jody Nathanson, Dr. Paul Fleiss, and Dr. Margaret Davidson, but also with Liz Crofts, Sheri Hansen, Dr. Derrick B. Jelliffe, Dr. John D. Michael, Peggy Teeter, R.N., and Dr. Mark Thoman. Also, Dr. Harold M. Maller has driven to my home many times to spend a whole afternoon in discussion.

How can I adequately thank my husband and children who did housework and cooking, ignored the many piles of letters, research materials and papers standing about the house, and put up with the postponement of many projects until . . .

"After The Book"? They each helped with clerical work. My husband, Bob, devoted many hours to Xeroxing, proofreading, and acting as a sounding board. My sister, Marjie Sullivan, and my mother, Mrs. Elsie Meder, invited our children to visit so that I could work undisturbed at times.

Finally, I would like to thank all the mothers who loaned their personal photos; Rose Sodergren and Shirley Bedeski for assistance in reading letters; Mary Carson, Marybeth Doucette, Linda Imai, Peggy Mills, R.N., Mable O'Donnell, Gail Taylor, Judy Torgus and Lynne Endicott-Wismer for research; La Leche League Area Coordinators Kay Coulson, R.N., Ann Lillich, and Kay Williams for putting me in touch with many mothers who have experiences to share; Marilyn Cobb, Traci Gill, Marion Kibler, K. T. Lapham, Carol Potter, Rose Sodergren, Joanne Touchton, Neva Winn, and Grace Wright for extra typing; Mary Cuni, Brenda Fraser, Donna McAnear, Mary McIntyre, Susan Myers, Dr. Jennifer Sillence, Romalda Yamagisawa, and Joan Zinda for proofreading; and my editor, Carol Stoner, who was careful and considerate in editing this book.

One of the nicest things about writing this book has been the marvelous people I have come to know as the book has developed, mothers and specialists alike, who generously shared their time, experience, and knowledge. Space does not permit a listing of all who have shared, nonetheless, I am deeply appreciative of their contributions.

Pat Brewster

Introduction:
The Kindness of
Human Milk

This book has been written with the intention of sharing information about breastfeeding and in particular the experiences of mothers in different nursing situations. Until now, information about how to handle many of these situations has been minimal, lacking, or difficult to obtain.

My own interest in breastfeeding came as a result of nursing my four children. When minor difficulties arose while nursing my first child, I turned to La Leche League for answers and support. Out of this initial contact I became very involved with the organization and became a La Leche League leader, which I have been for the past 15 years. Being a leader gave me an opportunity to help hundreds of nursing mothers through both normal as well as special breastfeeding experiences.

Over the years I became especially interested in gathering and sharing information about breastfeeding in special circumstances. As a mother of twins, I found my acquaintance with another mother who had breastfed her twins to be a big inspiration and help to me. In addition, as editor of the California page of *La Leche League News*, some of my correspondence was with mothers who have encountered unusual situations. In some cases, little positive help was available. It seemed that it would be highly desirable to have information on a wide variety of nursing situations made easily accessible in one volume.

A request I put in *La Leche League News* for information about special breastfeeding experiences brought letters from hundreds of mothers in the United States and abroad. I was touched by the many ways these mothers have managed to help themselves, sometimes through serious crisis and tragedy. Many times they have received a great deal of help and encouragement from their husbands, doctors, and friends. However, occasionally problems have been caused or magnified by well-meaning but uninformed professionals and friends. The mothers themselves have shown tremendous amounts of patience, courage and determination, confident that breast-feeding was best for their babies. In practically every circumstance, mothers have been able to find a successful solution. And you will see that not only has breastfeeding been important, but the mothering inherent in nursing has been a significant factor as well.*

Why did these mothers choose to nurse their babies, at times under very difficult circumstances? The reasons given include many of the commonly stated advantages of breast milk such as better digestibility, superior nutrition, and the presence of antibodies which protect against infection.

Mother also benefits from breastfeeding; it speeds the return of the uterus to its normal size, and immediate and unrestricted nursing promotes early bonding of mother and baby. Hormones released during breastfeeding usually delay ovulation and menstruation for several months—provided breastfeeding is complete, successful and unrestricted. Furthermore, studies have shown that during lactation the hormone prolactin increases a mother's gentleness, loving emotions, and awareness of her baby's needs.

In addition to these benefits, there are further advantages to breastfeeding when a special situation occurs. For example, sick babies who are breastfed recover faster. If they are hospitalized, breastfeeding seems to relax them and give them a sense of security. Mothers who work, who are hospitalized, or who have special physical problems often emphasize that breastfeeding has significance to them because they are giving their babies something that no one else can give. Some babies,

---

* All anecdotes in this book are authentic case histories. In some cases, the names have been changed to avoid confusion or protect privacy.

such as those who are premature or allergic, derive special benefits from breastfeeding and breast milk. In some cases, breastfeeding is literally a lifesaver.

In various chapters of the book there is a certain amount of information which is applicable and useful in the normal nursing situation, as well as the unusual. This is true in particular of these chapters: "What's Normal?"; "Nursing Techniques"; "Nutrition for Mother and Baby"; "Working Together: Doctor, Hospital, Parents"; "Nursing during Stressful Times"; and "Traveling with a Nursing Baby."

All the chapters in the book are full of personal anecdotes sent by mothers who have experienced the particular nursing situation covered. Each chapter has been reviewed by several people whose expertise or educational background qualifies them to verify the accuracy of the information.

Because of the highly variable nature of breastfeeding—it is unique to each mother and baby—there can be no rigid set of standards for dealing with problems. Yet by blending your personal experience with the information and ideas presented in this book, you can determine for yourself the best approach to nursing. Both you and your baby can enjoy the emotional and physical bonus of breastfeeding—a bonus which can make your baby healthier and happier throughout his life.

Chapter 1

What's Normal?

My baby nurses every two hours, her baby every four,
Why does "Baby Perfect" have to live next door?
Hers plays happily, mine's in arms all the time,
But the doctor says both are "doing fine."

Her baby's an angel and loves to sleep,
But mine would rather learn how to creep.
Hers never fusses, but, oh, not mine,
Yet the doctor says both are "doing fine."

Hers has a bowel movement every day,
Once a week is my baby's way.
Mine's a picky eater, hers loves to dine,
But the doctor says both are "doing fine."

Her baby greets people with happy sighs,
My baby's shy and sometimes cries.
My baby is toothless, hers has nine!
But the doctor says both are "doing fine."

When her baby's sick, he never shows it,
When mine is sick, he lets everyone know it!
Her baby weaned first, and mine is much older,
I guess "normal" like "beauty" is in the eye of the beholder.

My Baby, Her Baby
by Rose A. Sodergren

When mothers of babies with problems are unsuccessful in breastfeeding it is oftentimes *not* because of the problems but because of a lack of general knowledge of breastfeeding and a lack of support. This chapter provides basic information that can help you attain a rich and satisfying breastfeeding relationship. It may also reassure you that even though your baby may have problems, his behavior is reasonable for a "normal" breastfed baby. Certain terms used throughout the book are defined in this chapter for those just learning about breastfeeding.

This chapter attempts to discuss only certain aspects of the breastfeeding situation. It touches on just a few topics—mainly points that have been mentioned by concerned mothers who have written to me about their unusual breastfeeding experiences. Entire books have been written about the normal course of breastfeeding. You may wish to read one or more of them, which are listed in the Bibliography under "General Recommended Reading," in addition to this book.

Milk Production and Release

The information in this section is basic to understanding your breastfeeding experience. Since it is more technical than the rest of the chapter, at this point you may wish to just read over the section to gain a general understanding of how the breasts function, and then come back to it for parts you may want to reread.

Breast Structure

The complex system provided for a woman to produce milk and feed her baby is truly an impressive feat of engineering.

Milk is manufactured within the breasts in grapelike clusters of tiny, rounded sacs called alveoli (see illustration). It is transported from the alveoli towards the nipple along small channels called ductules which, like tributaries of a river, empty into the main channels, the ducts. There are from 15

Structure of the Breast
Davol, Inc., Subsidiary of International Paper Co.

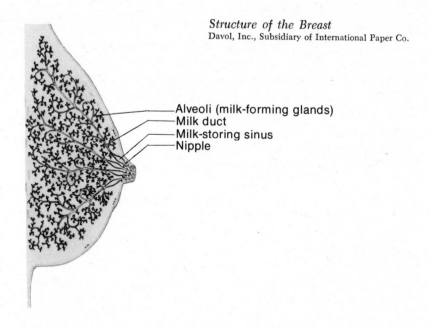

Alveoli (milk-forming glands)
Milk duct
Milk-storing sinus
Nipple

to 20 ducts, which empty into tiny openings in the nipple through which the milk flows. Directly behind the areola (the darker area which surrounds the nipple), each duct widens into a reservoir for the milk, called a sinus.

During pregnancy the milk ducts and alveoli increase in number and size. Usually about the fifth month of pregnancy the alveoli start producing colostrum.* This is the creamy yellowish fluid secreted before the milk comes in. It is rich in antibodies. During pregnancy some colostrum may drip occasionally from your nipples. Colostrum is somewhat sticky and may cause your skin to stick to your bra or clothing. If so, don't pull off your clothing, because it will hurt; rather, wet the clothing with some warm water first, then remove.

The areolar area itself has a large number of oil and sweat glands. It is the secretions from these glands which keep the skin of the nipple soft, pliable and protected from the baby's

---

* Onset of production of colostrum varies. Some women do not produce it before delivery, while in others it may be present quite early in their pregnancy. (1)

saliva and the friction of his sucking. The secretions also kill bacteria on the nipple. Breast milk itself also has antiseptic qualities. (2)

The size of the breast does not determine how much milk it can make. Much of its size is made up of nonfunctional fatty and connective tissue rather than milk-producing glands. (3) (4)

Let-Down Reflex

The skin covering the nipple contains many nerves which are stimulated when your baby sucks. This sucking stimulation causes the release of the hormone prolactin which in turn signals the alveoli to make milk. The sucking stimulation also causes the release of the hormone oxytocin which causes cells surrounding the alveoli and ducts to contract. The alveoli are compressed and the ducts are widened so that the milk is squeezed into and through the duct system. This ejection reflex, which may cause a momentary pressure or tightening or tingling sensation in the breasts, is often called "let-down." It is *not* necessary to feel this let-down. Many women don't, yet still produce ample supplies of milk. Even if you don't feel the let-down you may be able to notice its occurrence while nursing because you may hear the baby swallowing or you may leak milk from the other breast. The let-down sensation is usually more noticeable during the first few months of lactation and often causes leaking. It usually occurs simultaneously in both breasts, when the baby is nursing or when the mother's thoughts are centered on baby, such as when he is crying. Light pressure on the nipple area with the heel of your hand will usually prevent leaking when milk let-down occurs. If other people are around, casually clasping your hands together while pressing on the nipple area with your forearms will usually stop the milk without calling attention to what you are doing.

Mechanism of Sucking

Most infants have an instinctive "rooting reflex" which

causes them to turn their mouths towards the nipple when it touches their cheeks. When a baby sucks, he draws the nipple into the back of his mouth by suction so that the sinuses are between his upper and lower jaws. When your baby nurses, he does not actually remove milk by suction. The suction is simply to keep the nipple in place in the back of his mouth. Then with his tongue and jaws he compresses the areola and the large milk sinuses and presses the milk that is in the sinuses into his mouth. By this combination of pressure and suction he milks the breast.

The further back in the baby's mouth the nipple lies, the less it will be rubbed by his tongue as he sucks. The effect can be felt by sucking on your own thumb. The further back the thumb is in the mouth, the less rubbing there is on the end of it. (5) (6)

Nipple Preparation and Care

Nipple preparation during the last weeks of your pregnancy is a good idea. It's possible that without it you *may* have no difficulty with sore nipples once you start nursing. However, if this is the first baby you will be nursing, it is better to prepare than to take a chance.

In order to condition the nipples, rub them *gently* with a towel or washcloth each time you dress and undress. Bras protect our nipples from friction. Going without a bra for part of the day or at least wearing a nursing bra and leaving the "trap door" down is helpful. Nipples are exposed to the air and the gentle friction of your outer clothing, thereby hastening the "toughening" process.

Some mothers also regularly condition their nipples during the last few weeks of pregnancy by pulling them out firmly with their fingers and rolling them gently between the thumb and forefinger, once or twice daily. (It's a good idea to use a very small amount of lubricant, such as cold cream or baby oil, on your hands to lessen your grasp and prevent bruising.) Do any such rubbing or pulling only until it is slightly uncomfortable, never to the point of pain. (7)

It is possible to express (manually squeeze out) drops of

colostrum during pregnancy and some people recommend doing this daily from about the seventh month of pregnancy to clear the milk ducts. However, most women never express colostrum and don't have trouble with milk flow when they start nursing. If you do try expressing some colostrum during pregnancy, be gentle. It is possible to overdo and bruise the nipples and the surrounding area. Hand expression can be of great importance in case an emergency situation should arise. There are instructions for hand expression in chapter 2, "Nursing Techniques."

Inverted nipples (nipples that retract rather than protrude when stimulated) can cause a problem during nursing because the baby cannot grasp the nipple easily. Truly inverted nipples are rare, and some babies can grasp and pull out even truly inverted nipples. This, in itself, is corrective treatment. Other babies may not be so helpful! Ask your doctor to check for this condition during your pregnancy, or check your nipples yourself. (See Inverted Nipples in chapter 4, "Breast and Nipple Problems" for instructions on checking for inverted nipples and for an explanation of what to do about them. Be sure to test both nipples, since only one may be inverted.) Women with nipple irregularities are more prone to nipple soreness and should use preventive measures and/or treat soreness aggressively. Change nursing positions frequently. Use breast shields prenatally and during the first weeks of nursing. (See Shields Used during Pregnancy or between Nursings in chapter 2, "Nursing Techniques.")

To cleanse the nipples during pregnancy and nursing just rinse with water during your regular bath or shower. Avoid soap on the nipples because it removes the oil secreted by the skin glands and will dry the nipples. Dryness can lead to cracked, sore nipples.

When you are nursing, it is important to make sure there is no moisture remaining around the nipples because this, too, can contribute to the development of sore nipples. Change your bra and nursing pads whenever they are wet and avoid plastic-backed pads or bras as these prevent the circulation of air, retain moisture, and can encourage growth of bacteria.

Many mothers experience some degree of discomfort in their nipples, from mild irritation the first couple of days to more severe soreness. Prevention—by preparing the nipples beforehand—is the best cure. However, there are several standard treatments you can use should you have a problem. Sunlight and air are particularly beneficial in conditioning and in treating sore nipples. Be very careful, though, to avoid sunburn. Start with only two minutes once or twice a day and increase the time slowly. You can do this discreetly at home in front of an open window. (8) There also are mild ointments which are helpful in treating sore nipples. Pure (hydrous) lanolin and A and D Ointment can be obtained from your druggist and are not harmful to baby. If you use them sparingly, you can nurse your baby without removing them. Make sure that your baby has the whole nipple squarely in his mouth, so that he is not chewing on the tip or side. If he is impatient for the milk to start flowing and pulls or tugs on the nipple, express some milk to start the let-down before starting to nurse.

The First Days of Nursing

Birth, expulsion (or removal) of the placenta, and nursing your baby (plus, perhaps, other stimuli as yet undiscovered) signal your body to produce milk. When babies are kept on a schedule of nursing every 4 hours, the milk can be expected in about three to five days, but sometimes it takes a week or more. However, if you nurse your baby soon after birth and on demand thereafter, as with rooming-in or a home birth, your milk may "come in" about 24 to 48 hours after delivery.

Before the milk comes in, your newborn nursing baby will be getting colostrum. This is the perfect first food for him. Since it is almost devoid of fat and carbohydrates it is easier for him to digest than milk. It is extremely rich in immunity factors, too, and it has a slightly laxative effect which helps clear out the meconium (the dark green or blackish matter discharged from a newborn's bowels), preparing his digestive tract for the milk. The colostrum level decreases as the milk level increases.

Long intervals between feedings allow the breasts to fill and sometimes even overfill with milk when true milk production begins. This "engorgement" is a common problem when babies are only brought to their mothers for nursing every four hours. The overly full feeling is caused not only by the sudden presence of milk but also by an increased flow of blood to the breasts. If your baby has difficulty grasping the nipple properly while you are engorged, express some milk before nursing to soften the area around the nipple. Engorgement usually doesn't last more than a few days. The best treatment is very frequent nursing using both breasts at each feeding. (You don't have to wait for baby to wake or cry before starting to nurse.) Applying heat—a warm shower or even warm wet washcloths for 10 to 20 minutes before nursing—may also help. And cold packs applied *after* nursing can relieve the ache and slow circulation temporarily.

As your baby nurses during the first several days after birth he stimulates certain nerves in the nipples which cause oxytocin to be released, thereby stimulating uterine contractions. Your uterus will return to its normal size more rapidly than that of a mother who doesn't nurse. Contractions may be fairly uncomfortable for a few days; later on the contractions still occur but cannot be felt by most women.

What Will Your Milk Look Like?

Breast milk's appearance differs somewhat from that of cow's milk. This is to be expected since the ingredients vary; cow's milk is meant to meet the needs of growing calves and mother's milk to meet the needs of human babies. The first milk baby gets in a feeding, or fore milk, is low in fat content so it looks thin and slightly bluish. The later milk or hind milk has a higher fat content and looks thicker and creamier. Milk collected at different times of the day will look different because the fat content changes. When milk is put in a container, the cream will rise to the top.

Duration of
Each Feeding

Most successful nursing mothers do not limit nursing times, except perhaps in the first few days when nipples are unaccustomed to sucking. Nursing times vary greatly among babies; some seem to be satisfied with a 5-minute nursing, others want to nurse 40 minutes or more.

As your baby grows, his nursing pattern will probably change. Babies become quite efficient the more they develop, and can obtain more milk in a shorter period of time. Around three months many babies drastically cut down on the amount of time they nurse at each feeding. Actually a baby can obtain most of the milk in a breast in the first seven to ten minutes of vigorous nursing.

Weaning, when it is gradual baby-led weaning, sometimes involves shorter and shorter nursing periods so that the last nursings may be only a minute or two.

Illness, travel, and other unusual experiences can upset any baby and nursing babies often seek additional comfort and security through longer or more frequent breastfeeding during these stressful times.

Frequency of Nursing *

Frequent nursing is the best way to insure a good milk supply. This is more important than *length of time* at each feeding. Most newborns need to be fed about every two to three hours. Behavioral scientist Niles Newton says in an article about the normal course and management of lactation that:

---

* Frequency of nursing refers to the length of time from the beginning of one feeding to the beginning of the next.

The advice given by Southworth in Carr's *Practice of Pediatrics,* published in 1906, is still worth remembering, since at that time successful breastfeeding was the rule rather than the exception. He advised four nursings on the first day, six on the second, ten a day for the rest of the first month, eight a day for the second and third months, seven a day for the fourth and fifth months, and six a day for the sixth through eleventh months. He also approved of night feedings up through the fifth month.*(9)

Carr's advice gives a general idea of what *might* be expected during successful nursing. However, such "regimentation" is not necessary. You and your baby will probably establish your own pattern of nursing.

Some infants, such as premature babies or babies born with heart defects, may need to be fed more frequently than others because they tire easily, and also because their suck is not usually as strong.

Three of my four babies nursed about every three hours as newborns. Suzy, our first baby and our biggest (9½ pounds at birth), nursed every four hours, even as a newborn. This is quite unusual for a breastfed infant but was a normal pattern for Suzy, and she gained well. Some breastfed babies do seem to be inclined to nurse only once every four, five, or six hours, *and do not gain well.* In such a case, you should encourage your baby to nurse more often.

As your baby grows older he will probably want to nurse less often. Exceptions might be when he is hurt, frightened, or sick. Also, babies go through "growth spurts" when they want to nurse more frequently for a few days. This is part of nature's wonderful "supply-and-demand" arrangement for building up your milk supply when baby needs more. Babies grow irregularly. During periods of particularly rapid growth, a baby's appetite can temporarily get ahead of the milk supply. Such growth spurts commonly occur around the ages of four to

---

* Night feedings for much longer are now considered desirable.

six weeks and three months, but anytime can be normal for
your particular baby.

Sucking and Suckling

In their original meanings, the baby "sucks" and the
mother "suckles." Today the term "suckling" is used when
referring to both *deriving* and *providing* nourishment at the
breast. Both a mother's role in giving and a baby's role in
taking are important for the mutual enjoyment and success of
breastfeeding. Because of this beautiful interrelationship between nursing mother and baby, they are often referred to as
a "nursing couple."

Some babies need a lot more sucking than others. Babies
often need more sucking in the early weeks and months, it
seems, and many need lots of sucking throughout the early
years. Some become very discriminating about their sucking.
Sharon, one of our twins, loved to nurse and would have
nothing to do with anything else in her mouth—bottles,
pacifier, or thumb. By comparison, Karen, her twin, put
everything in her mouth. Karen loved to nurse, but she also
happily took an occasional bottle, found pacifiers, toys, and
furniture good to chew on, and sucked her thumb until she was
six years old.

"Nursing" versus "Breastfeeding"

Marge, a mother of six, explains how she discovered for
herself the real difference between breastfeeding and nursing:

> Breastfeeding sounds like a-way-to-get-milk-into-a-baby,
> and nursing is a whole, complete experience, a nurturing,
> a way of life. I breastfed my first two sons, in the same
> way my mother and many aunts bottlefed. The only
> difference was that I used the breast instead of the bottle.
> From my third baby on they were nursed without regard
> to how recently they "ate" or what time it was or what
> the reason for nursing was. I relaxed and really enjoyed
> them.

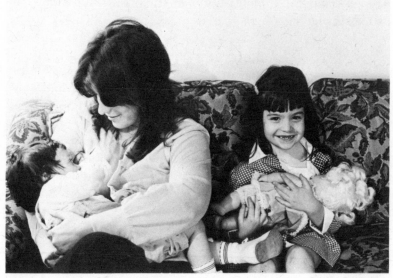

Sandra C. Wallace

Nursing is more than just a source of physical nourishment—it fulfills baby's emotional needs, too.

Dr. John D. Michael, a pediatrician at the Ross Valley Medical Clinic in Greenbrae, California, puts it this way:

> Breastfeeding is a specific act of feeding, of giving and receiving food. Nursing is a holistic experience and way of life, the ability to give and receive that extra psychological, emotional and physical warmth and support so desperately necessary for total human development.

"Spoiling?"

It used to be thought, and still is by some people, that if your baby is seemingly well-fed and comfortable, if you pick him up when he cries (either to offer more nursing or just to hold him), you will be "spoiling" him. Actually, you are likely to be satisfying what has come to be recognized as a primary need of infants, the need for affectionate tactile stimulation— the need for fondling and rhythmic motion. (10) You can't spoil a tiny baby. Dr. Carl A. Holmes explains that until some months after birth, nerve fibers are not yet connected to the thinking, remembering part of the baby's brain. (He has to be able to remember that it is nice to be picked up before he can cry to be picked up.) He operates, instead, on a reflex level—without voluntary control. (11)

An infant's emotional needs are just as strong and just as important as his physical needs. Dr. Michael expressed it this way when he wrote to me about the premature babies he cares for (but his remarks apply also to full-term babies):

> My personal philosophy is that a child cannot be held "too much," especially a premature baby (unless the premie is *so fragile* that the doctors feel he needs to use *all* his energy to live and breathe but *even then he should be touched if not held*). If a baby believes that he is able to get his needs satisfied when he wishes them to be so, such as being fed when he is hungry, being changed when he is wet, or being burped and gently caressed when he needs a change of position, then I believe a child grows up feeling that the world is a responsive place in which to live; even though there are frustrations and inconveniences along the way, the child believes the world is a good world, and that child has a very positive attitude toward what he can accomplish in his environment.
>
> On the other hand, I believe that if a baby is made to adjust to outside requirements which do not fit his needs, then the child will grow up with the feeling that the world does not seem to respond to his needs and that the inconveniences and frustrations which he meets as he gets older are more proof that the world is hostile and that an individual is at the mercy of his environment rather than being able to influence it.

In describing how all too often we try to fit our babies into patterns we do not expect of ourselves, Ellen Bingham of Edmonton, Alberta, Canada, says in an article in *La Leche League News* (12):

Why is so much made of keeping our babies to a strict three- or four-hour feeding schedule when we as adults feel free to snack at every twinge of hunger and seldom go more than two hours without a meal or a "coffee-break"?

Why is it considered indulging a baby to allow him to go back to the breast when he had "finished" 15 minutes earlier, while we may enjoy an additional cup of tea after breakfast as we start the morning projects?

Why is it "spoiling" a baby to give comfort if he cries "when there is nothing wrong," while it is showing love and affection when our husbands take us in their arms when we feel depressed or out of sorts?

Why do we fear becoming a slave to our babies when we rock them back to sleep, while we give our older children a few moments of conversation or prayers in the dark cosiness of their beds, or while we as parents lie close and talk quietly before dropping off?

Why do we feel compelled to leap at the first buzz of the doorbell or jangle of the telephone, when we willingly put our children off with "just a minute" when they want something?

Why are we surprised when our children are irritable or throw tantrums on the slightest provocation right before mealtimes, when it is a well-known business technique never to make a request of someone just before lunch if one wants a positive response?

Again and again I catch myself demanding something of our young son that I do not expect of myself.

Further thoughts about spoiling are mentioned in an article entitled, "What Makes a Spoiled Baby?" (13) Author Eileen Eldridge says:

Professionals in the field of infant care tell us that an infant whose needs are satisfied gradually becomes less demanding, happier, more good-natured, independent; a baby who doesn't get enough satisfaction becomes more shrill in his demands, less tolerant of frustrations, and has a harder time outgrowing full dependence on mother.

Inborn temperament as well as physical characteristics play a part in a baby's behavior. One infant is complacent, easily satisfied, another is highstrung and demanding; one eats and sleeps, another eats and cries. The point to keep in mind is that no baby can help being just as he is when he is born. If life is hard for him at first, and consequently hard on you, this is not his fault or yours. You can't change these circumstances overnight, but you can make things more tolerable for him. And when you do—when you hold, feel, rock, entertain and soothe him—you're not being weak-willed and foolish, and you're not spoiling your infant. You are being strong and sensible and kind. You are insuring your baby against hurts and fears and loneliness. You are teaching him, very gradually, to trust you and to want to please you.

You can, of course, drive yourself beyond what's good for either you or the baby. If loss of sleep and aching bones play havoc with your disposition, baby will sense the change. Then he may pick up nervous tension rather than the comfort from your handling and your voice. That's why parents of a "difficult" infant should spell one another and occasionally get someone to help out—someone who believes that a crying baby has genuine needs and requires attention and comfort.

Crying

Babies cry for many reasons. If it isn't hunger, what might it be? Dr. Niles Newton suggests three possible answers and what a mother can do to quiet her baby. (14)

Physical Discomforts

• Some babies fuss while they are having a bowel movement. It sometimes helps to give an infant's feet something firm to push on. Try holding him up over your shoulder as you walk back and forth, and place your second hand under the soles of his feet so he can push against it.

• To get rid of an uncomfortable air bubble, lay your baby across your crossed knees, holding his abdomen with one hand while his head rests against your arm. With the other hand gently rub his back with an upward motion.

• Dirty and wet diapers do not bother babies unless they have sore bottoms. If diaper rash develops, try leaving off diapers and plastic pants. Free circulation of air helps skin heal, and a baby usually loves it.

Missing the Womb

• Baby may miss the rhythmic sound of your heart. Lullabies are used the world over to supply these sounds after birth, as are radios, record players and cassette tape recorders.

• The warmth and snugness of the womb can be recreated by wrapping blankets tightly around your baby. If you are placing him on his side, put a rolled blanket behind his back, since he cannot at first control his own wiggling and gets upset by his unrestrained sprawling.

Boredom

• Since baby can't move around on his own, yet is intrigued by new sights and sounds, a good solution is a baby carrier.

• Another way of giving variety and stimulation is to take a bath with your baby.

• Babies sometimes like to look at the floor instead of being held upright. Place baby lying face downward on your knees, looking at the floor. Gentle rocking can be accomplished by lifting one heel and then the other.

Teething

Crying during a feeding may be caused by teething. Your baby may begin a feeding as usual, then after a few minutes, pull away crying. The pressure on his gums from his vigorous sucking seems to cause discomfort. The answer to his distress may be small, frequent nursings.

Your baby may enjoy having you rub your finger on his gums between feedings. An ice cold teething ring, cold, peeled apple, a cold, hard vegetable, chewing toys or a pacifier to bite on can also help. Some babies like a washcloth with an ice cube in it. Moisten the washcloth before giving it to your baby so he won't have to wait for the ice to start melting before getting something to "slurp" on. A wet washcloth placed in the freezer for an hour is nice, too. Once the tooth has worked through the gum, your baby will probably enjoy nursing for longer periods again.

Bowel Movements

The stools of breastfed babies vary greatly. Some babies start with one bowel movement with every diaper change, and some start with one to three a day and cut down to once a week. All are normal.

The breastfed baby's stool is usually quite loose and unformed, often of soupy consistency with cottage cheese-type curds in it. Colors range from yellow to yellow green to brown. Even an occasional green, watery stool is okay in an otherwise healthy baby. The more frequent the bowel movements are, the more likely they'll just be a stain in the diaper.

A breastfed baby has less waste to excrete than a formula-fed baby. Not only are the stools different in color, consistency and possibly frequency, but also the odor of the stools of the breastfed baby is usually mild and not unpleasant (unlike the stools of the formula-fed baby!). This is because breast milk is more totally assimilated by the baby than cow's milk. There is less carbohydrate left in the intestines for the bacteria to ferment, so the unpleasant odor of milk fermentation usually is not present.

Weight Gain

Adults come in many different shapes and sizes, but when it comes to babies, all too often a baby is expected to gain a set amount, regardless of the size and bone structure of his parents or siblings. This can cause a breastfeeding mother a great deal of unnecessary concern and contribute to loss of confidence about her ability to adequately nourish her baby. (15)

If you're nursing your baby as often as he wants, if he has frequent wet diapers, and if he appears healthy, then whatever he is gaining is probably just right for him. Some babies gain rapidly at first, then stabilize; others gain slowly but steadily.

One mother who was successfully nursing her fourth baby, after bottlefeeding the other three, brought the baby to the doctor for her monthly checkup. When the scales showed a weight gain of less than a pound in a month, the doctor began to show some signs of concern. But the mother had had the foresight to check the doctor's weight records of her other babies, and was able to point out to him that her second daughter had only gained a total of four pounds in seven months, despite early feedings of solids, plus her formula. This child, now at the age of five, was a fine, healthy child. Perhaps, suggested the mother, the three-month-old was merely following a family pattern. The doctor agreed that this might be the case, and since the baby looked and acted well, the mother continued to nurse her without solids or supplements. Needless to say, the baby thrived. (16)

Even within the same family there can be variations in weight gains among the children. A mother of completely breastfed twins said that one twin doubled her birth weight around three months, while her twin brother doubled his at

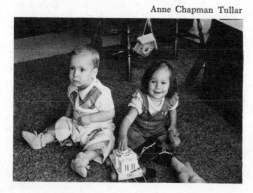

Anne Chapman Tullar

*Variations
in Weight Gain*

Amy and Robby, both 12 months old. Amy weighs 19 pounds, has gained 12 pounds since birth (full term). Robby weighs 23½ pounds, has gained 17 pounds since birth (1 month premature).

six weeks. The boy tripled his weight at six months, while the girl hadn't quite tripled at a year.

All this is not to say that weight gain should *never* be a concern for a breastfeeding mother, just that babies having vastly different weights can be perfectly normal and healthy. There are unusual situations in which babies are not gaining as well as they should. (See Slow Weight Gain and Rapid Weight Gain in chapter 7, "Newborn and Infant Problems.")

Solid Foods

Breast milk contains all the nutritional requirements for most babies for about six months, or longer. In the second half of the first year of life, a baby's digestive system has developed so that it can more effectively digest additional food. There are some good reasons for waiting to offer solid foods. Besides breast milk being the perfect food for your baby, delaying introduction of solids helps you maintain a good milk supply, and it lessens the possibility of allergies and obesity for your child. The younger the baby, the more likely that other foods and liquids will cause allergies. (17)

In the second half of the first year, the stored iron supply that a full-term baby has at birth begins to run out if he has been fed early on food that doesn't contain iron or fed cow's milk (which causes intestinal loss of blood). Breast milk, however, is a good source of iron because the iron in human milk is more completely absorbed than the iron in cow's milk. In fact, studies have suggested that breastfed infants without supplements generally do not become anemic, and that they receive adequate iron throughout nursing. (18)

Starting solids very selectively at six months gives you lots of time to determine your baby's preferences and tolerances. Moreover, most babies begin wanting food from your plate when they can sit up, and will chew instinctively between six and nine months.

Why is it that some babies are started on solid foods after just a few weeks, or a few months? Sheri, one mother I spoke with, says:

My doctor said I could start solids with my baby, Molly, at three months. I think this is one of the reasons Molly simply stopped nursing about six months. With a tummy full of food she was less interested in nursing, and my breasts were less stimulated to produce milk.

When I asked my doctor later, "What would you have said if I'd said I didn't want to start solids at three months?" he answered, "I would have said 'Bravo.'" "Then why did you suggest I start at three months?" I asked. "Because I get so much pressure from other mothers."

Molly was a healthy baby, had been gaining well, and didn't need those solids at three months.

Early weaning does not always occur when solids are introduced early. But it happens often enough to add it to the list of reasons to wait until your baby really needs the solids and is ready for them.

My own personal reason for delaying introduction of solids as long as possible was that they're so messy, especially with a baby who can't handle them well!

The contraceptive effect of breastfeeding should also be mentioned. While your baby is being *completely* breastfed (no solids or other supplements), you are much less likely to ovulate. The hormones of lactation, stimulated by nursing, usually hold back ovulation and menstruation for several months. When you do resume menstruation, the first and often several menstrual periods may be sterile, without ovulation. (19) However, though the percentage is small, it *is* possible to ovulate and conceive before the first menstruation, while nursing. If you do *not* wish to conceive it is very important to choose an additional method of contraception. *The Art of Natural Family Planning* (20) and *Breastfeeding and Natural Child Spacing: The Ecology of Natural Mothering* (21), by Sheila Kippley, are good books to read on this subject.

Weaning

When I was pregnant with my first child, my obstetrician suggested I consider breastfeeding—for six months. It seemed reasonable. I started attending La Leche League meetings and found out some mothers nursed longer. I was curious and still had my doubts about nursing when teeth came in, and what it would be like to let the baby wean herself, as the six-month limit approached. I didn't wean at six months, but decided to continue for a few more days or perhaps a few more weeks. Then one morning when Suzy was several months older, as I offered to nurse her she turned away, uninterested, struggling in fact, as though she didn't know what I was doing. I continued to offer to nurse her for several days after that. She'd only been nursing for a minute or two each day before the day she lost interest, but now she declined all offers except on the third day which was, by a happy coincidence, the only day I felt any fullness at all. It was a lovely way to wean.

With our next babies I had a better understanding of the needs of babies and more confidence in myself. I remember asking our pediatrician when the twins had their two-year checkup (and were still interested in nursing), "Is there any reason why I shouldn't continue to nurse them—other than it's just not done by many mothers?" He replied, "Not at all. In some cultures babies nurse for four or five years or longer."

When you consider that even in our society it's not uncommon for a two- or three-year-old to have a bottle, why should there be any question about the acceptability of a child of the same age breastfeeding?

Edwina Froehlich, a founding mother of La Leche League International, says:

> If we consider nursing only as a means of nourishing the infant, then we can readily see why it might be feasible to bring nursing to an end at an early date. There would be no reason why this date could not be as early as the baby could handle a variety of solid foods and milk

from a cup—about six to eight months of age. But if we view the nursing experience as a whole, if we see it as a vital part of motherhood, if we understand that baby has emotional needs which for many months can best be satisfied through this important, intimate relationship, then it is hard to understand why we should set a specific time when this relationship *must* be ended. (22)

Baby-led weaning is the very best for the baby. Growing from infancy to childhood can be a hard adjustment for a child. It's nice to know he can come back to that safe, familiar nestling point.

Baby-led weaning often proceeds gradually, with baby nursing less and less frequently and for shorter periods of time. As Penny said of her nursing experience, "We continued until 17 months (if you call two sips, six pinches and four giggles each side once a day 'nursing'). Then one day Caroline inspected my nipples and said 'bye, bye nur.' !"

Weaning isn't always this gradual. Occasionally, for various explained and unexplained reasons, a baby weans suddenly. Then mother is left high and not-so-dry. Expressing your milk whenever you feel full will help you through the next few days as your milk is gradually reabsorbed by your body. (You may want to consider whether this is a "nursing strike," rather than true weaning, by reading chapter 20, "Nursing Strikes and One-Sided Nursing.")

Babies who nurse into toddlerhood sometimes go on a "nursing binge." This can include a lot of night waking. Sometimes they drop off this binge drastically even to the point of weaning within a month or so. The more mother worries about this increased nursing, the longer it takes the baby to get it over with. Her anxiety causes him to be anxious, which increases his need for the security of nursing.

Mothers have decided to wean their babies for various reasons, among them hospitalization of mother or baby, return to work, pressure from the father or relatives, or pregnancy. However, many times there are ways of overcoming what can seem to be obstacles to continued nursing, if you just look for them, as you will see in the following chapters.

If you do initiate weaning, do so gradually if at all possible. Wean to a bottle rather than a cup if the need to suck is still great. Eliminate one feeding from the breast at a time, with at least a week in between, and plan to spend more time with your baby in other ways to compensate. You are ending this special relationship and beginning other special experiences.

Individual Differences

Just as adults are individuals in all things, so are babies. No two are just alike, not even identical twins. Some are fast gainers, some are slow; some are active, some aren't. There are all sorts of variations. Some are friendly with everyone and others are quite choosy about whom they'll smile at. Some are very sensitive to how people feel towards them and others don't seem to notice a difference.

"Normal" is obviously not "average."

"Normal" can be a very wide range of acceptable behavior.

In the letters mothers have written to me there are some very good examples of individual variations among normal babies. Differences seem the most striking when they are within the same family, involving siblings who are offered the same feedings and being cared for in the same way, especially twins who receive feeding and care at the same time in the family's life. Having two such babies certainly gives an especially deep understanding and appreciation of "individual differences." Here are some quotes from mothers.

Siblings

Sandy wrote me:

I have two children who are often as different as night and day in needs and temperament. One nursed for an hour every two hours around the clock for several months, continued to nurse often and long until 2 years, began solids at 6 months, fed himself, liked only finger foods and weaned completely at 2¾ years, a week or so after the second child arrived. He never sucked his thumb, potty-trained himself at 22 months, and regularly "slept" through the night at 3½ years.

The second one nursed for five minutes at each breast every three to five hours, fussed herself to sleep at night, sucked her thumb with a peak around 3 to 4 months, started solids at 8 months, preferred nonfinger foods, but very little of anything. At 14 months she still nurses irregularly, after sleeping through the first 6½ months. She seems to enjoy nursing more as she grows older (as a new-born we thought she might be one of those early weaners at 9 months). She no longer sucks her thumb. Even as a newborn, she was often easily distracted and had to be nursed in a quiet place. If we were out somewhere, she preferred to fuss instead of nursing when tired. Her brother could nurse anywhere, anytime as a baby and was very quiet nursing.

Twins

I received some interesting replies to a questionnaire I sent to 23 mothers of twins. As might be expected, many times there were differences between the twins. Identical twins seemed to be more similar than fraternal twins. The following selections are from some of the questionnaires.

Karolyn had fraternal twin boys, Joshua and Gabriel:

Joshua was a voracious nurser. He would sometimes nurse every hour, but more often every two hours. His fraternal twin, Gabriel, has always been more placid and would nurse for a long time, dawdle, then not want to feed for three or four hours.

When sick, Joshua screamed a lot and Gabriel wanted a lot of cuddling. Nothing seemed to make Joshua feel better. I would usually put him in the Happy Baby Carrier and just endure the screaming—there was no way to stop it. Gabriel would be happy, no matter how miserable he felt, as long as I held him and cuddled him.

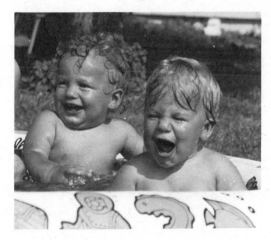

*Different
Feeding Patterns*

*Joshua (left) and
Gabriel on their
first birthday.*

Kathy's fraternal twin boys, Nels and Jared, both nursed about every 2½ hours until well after solids were started at eight and nine months. Kathy says:

> Nels always required a longer time at the breast. He would nurse for 40 minutes while Jared nursed for 20 minutes. Jared had daily bowel movements. Nels went very infrequently. The longest was 14 days and then it had the appearance of yellow toothpaste—not constipated but firmer than usual. He never had a stool more often than every 4 days until after a year of age.

Some people may tell you that giving your baby solids will help him sleep through the night. Actually, the solids are more likely to have the opposite effect, especially if the baby's digestive system is not yet mature enough to handle them. Marion tried a double experiment with her twins. She says:

> Peggy and Patty were six weeks old when I tried the solids. Peggy slept *all* the time. I had to wake her up to feed her or she would sleep through a feeding. Patty had colic for three full months and slept little and cried a lot. One night, just to see what would happen, I gave Peggy cereal, but not Patty. That night *Patty* happened to sleep all night for the first time and Peggy was up all night

fussing and crying (for the first time). I stopped solids and they went back to their previous sleep habits. Patty started sleeping through the night after her three-month stint with colic.

They are 13½ years old now and Peg still sleeps a lot and eats little, and Patty eats a lot and sleeps little. There are about 2 inches in height and 30 pounds difference between them.

At birth, both of Edith's fraternal twin girls were eager to nurse:

Even with Andrea's cleft palate she kept trying at my breast as much as Kendal did. In the weeks following their birth Kendal was what you might call an "easy baby." She would sleep and eat and play quietly. Andrea wanted and needed a lot of nursing and got it. She slept about as well as Kendal did, but when she was awake she had to be nursing or carried. When Andrea was about four months old and had doubled her birth weight she eased up on the continual nursing somewhat.

Katie's fraternal twins, Kacie and Betsy, had different temperaments:

Betsy knew how to nurse right away. Kacie was very hard to get to take the breast, had a weak suck and was a gourmet, taking a few sips at a time. Differences in dis-

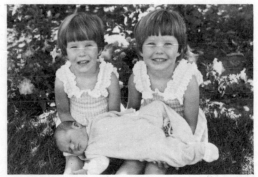

Different Temperaments

Kacie (left), and Betsy at 4 years of age.

position and temperament—very, very different. Betsy is much more easy-going and able to cope. Kacie is more tense and easily frustrated and doesn't cope well with new situations. Weaning—not good! I didn't intend to wean them but left them for a vacation thinking they'd nurse when I returned. I expressed my milk while gone to keep up my supply. However, Kacie, who'd missed me most, refused to have anything to do with me. Betsy nursed once a day for two more months. Kacie weaned at 11 months, Betsy at 13.

Jeanne's twins, Sheila and Joseph, exhibited different behaviors:

For the first three weeks Joseph choked at let-down, while Sheila, who sucked less vigorously, didn't. Joseph would nurse as long as I'd let him or until he fell asleep. Sheila would nurse until she was finished and let go herself. Sheila barely burped after feeds, but Joseph threw up "gallons" (and gained faster). Sheila was delicate, blue-eyed, blonde. Joseph was *fat*, with brown eyes and dark hair. Sheila bit me when she began teething, but Joseph never bit.

Sheila crawled and walked two months ahead of Joseph. Joseph went off with a friend first. Sheila cut teeth at five months, Joseph at nine months. Sheila, now six years old, loves milk and cheese. Joseph hasn't drunk milk since he weaned. He also hates cheese. (And he's big-boned, husky, energetic.)

What's normal? Whatever fills the needs of a child at the given moment. There seem to be patterns of temperament for each child, but babies grow and change so fast that schedules and "normal" behavior can change even from day to day. Simply appreciating each child for his own unique characteristics makes parenting a joy.

Chapter 2

Nursing Techniques

The purpose of this chapter is to give additional information which you may be able to use at certain times, especially if you have a special nursing situation.

Certain techniques, such as hand expression, are good to learn, or at least be aware of, in case an emergency should arise. Leaking milk can be bothersome to any mother even if she is able to stay home most of the time with her baby. It may especially be a problem if your situation requires many trips to a doctor's office or hospital, or necessitates separation from your baby for a while.

Several mechanical aids to *nursing* are discussed. However, keep in mind when using one of these that in general such aids should be considered temporary and used only as necessary. Baby carriers, however, are a desirable aid to *mothering*.

Some items may be available from many sources. Although I have described only two or three, you may find others. By sending to the address given at the end of the chapter, you may obtain current information.

Expressing Your Milk

Hand Expression

The ability to easily hand express your milk is a technique that can be extremely helpful in certain situations, such as when your baby's suck is not yet well developed, when your baby is premature, when you are separated from your baby due to hospitalization, when you are inducing lactation for an adopted baby, or when you are nursing and working. The technique can also be used to give you relief if you are engorged (overly full with milk), or have extremely sore, cracked or bleeding nipples. If you want to increase your milk supply, expressing in addition to nursing will enable you to produce more milk.

Some women find it easy to express milk, but I have had letters from many other women who say they just haven't been able to hand express at all.* For most women it does take practice. For these reasons I suggest that you reread the section on Milk Production and Release in chapter 1, "What's Normal?" and then consider the following facts.

As a baby nurses, certain things happen. The closer you can approximate these when you are hand expressing, the more efficient you are likely to be. Usually during nursing, there is: the warmth of your child's face touching the skin of your breast; nipple stimulation from your baby's sucking; external massage and gentle pressure on the sinuses (reservoirs for the milk); and suction on the breast ductules by your nursing baby.†

Dr. John D. Michael, a pediatrician who has helped many mothers of premature babies learn to express their milk, suggests that the four steps of normal nursing just described be approximated in the following ways, in order to get maximum expression of available milk:

1. Apply warmth to your breasts: use a moist towel wrapped around a heating pad or hot water bottle, or any other method to *gently* warm the skin of your breasts, but not the nipple area itself. The heat may be applied several times during the day, ideally for half an hour prior to nursing.

---

* The "test" of a breastfeeding woman is not how much she can express but how she nurses. Some women feel that if they can't express then they must not be producing milk. *This is false.*

† See illustration of breast structure in chapter 1, "What's Normal?" for location of sinuses and breast ductules.

The warmth seems to increase the blood supply reaching the milk production cells.

2. Stimulate your nipples by physical rolling (like rolling a marble between your fingers), or any other gentle rhythmic stimulation, just prior to expression. (Be sure your hands are clean before touching nipple or areola area.)

3. Massage your breasts with your hands, starting back at the chest wall and moving down toward the areola. Smooth, strong, compressive strokes should be used, two or three times at each position. Rotate your hands so that you are massaging from different points all around the breast. The purpose is to compress the milk glands and to push milk down the ducts to the sinuses.

4. Next, place the tips of your thumb and first finger or fingers on opposite sides of the areola, then squeeze them rhythmically together. Rotate around the nipple, trying to empty all the sinuses which surround the nipple.

NOTE: Steps 1, 2, and 3 are especially helpful when using either an electric or manual breast pump. Step 3 can be done (with help) during the pumping itself to accomplish both suction and pressure at the same time.

Here are some further suggestions for hand expression, from mothers who have done it successfully:

• One good way to learn how to hand express is to see someone else do it.

• Open and close your fingers and thumb rapidly in a scissors motion. Your fingers should not slip forward on the breast, as this may cause your skin to become irritated.

• Don't worry if nothing comes out the first few times you try it. Keep trying, in different positions. Different mothers find they need to press at different places—anywhere from the outer edge of the areola to up fairly close to the nipple. Some find that pressing gently inwards, towards the ribs, is helpful.

• Try to relax. Think about the baby. This helps you to get the let-down reflex and then the milk just flows out. When

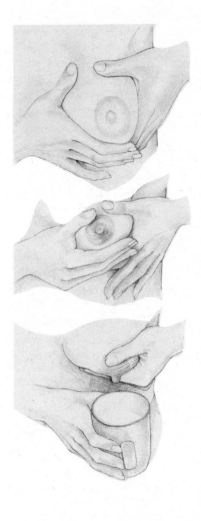

*Hand Expression with
Breast Massage*

A. Enclose the whole breast with
your hands, starting against
the chest wall.

B. Move your hands down towards
the areola, exerting pressure
from above, below, and from
sides.

C. Squeeze thumb and fingers together, rotating around breast.
If you're not holding a container you can support your
breast with your free hand.

NOTE: Steps A and B may not be
necessary if step C alone produces
good results.

you're just learning, it's easier if you can practice while you're
having a let-down.

• A warm washcloth or hot steaming towel on your breast
helps you get the let-down quickly.

• A hot bath or shower just before expressing helps you to
relax.

• Massage your breast (from the chest towards your nipple) *while you are expressing,* to encourage your milk to flow down the ducts.

• Have something to drink within reach as you are expressing.

• Your expressed breast milk will not look like cow's milk, although it is normal for your milk to separate into two layers with the cream coming to the top.

• If at first you can only express one tablespoon of colostrum, for a premature baby this may be more than enough for a feeding.

• As you practice and get better at expressing, your supply will increase. It's good to stay ahead of your baby's needs because it's far easier to *decrease* your milk supply than it is to *increase* it. Express regularly, every two to three hours.

• You can express from each breast with either hand. Alternate your hands if they get tired. (They will get stronger with practice.) Alternate breasts frequently, to give the sinuses a chance to refill.

• You can express from both breasts at the same time. Or, you can nurse your baby on one breast and express from the other at the same time. (This can be very effective since your baby's sucking will probably cause you to let down in *both breasts.*) *

• If baby wants to nurse soon after you have expressed, *do not panic:* you'll find there's always some milk being produced.

• If you have had no trouble expressing, but suddenly, during an upsetting situation, you can't get anything, you haven't "lost

---

* In *rare* circumstances, some women find the let-down response on one side diminished or absent due to disease, disuse, or other reasons. It is more common to have the let-down in both breasts while nursing, but the let-down may be less pronounced in the side not being nursed and therefore go unnoticed.

your milk." Try to rest. Drink extra fluids—wine or tea or whatever appeals to you. Turn on some music you like. Then start expressing.

• If you know far enough in advance that you will be away from your baby during one of his feeding times, start 24 hours before going out and express your milk after each nursing. Keep a sterile bottle in the refrigerator or freezer and keep adding the milk you express. (Cool the new milk first, before adding.) The amount you get in 24 hours probably will be just about right for one feeding.

• If you are only expressing to relieve fullness or to empty the breast, you can collect the milk in a cup or bowl and then throw it away. If you want to freeze the milk for future use, or to donate to a local milk bank, see the section in this chapter, Storing Expressed Breast Milk.

• If your baby is hospitalized, ask how much milk your baby is given at each feeding. That's all you should put in each container. Any extra milk will probably be thrown away.

Storing Expressed Breast Milk

Your milk should be expressed and stored in sterile containers if it is to be used at home, taken to the hospital, or donated to a milk bank. One-time disposable bottles shouldn't be used for storage, since the milk can be contaminated by leeching out certain chemicals.

If you have a dishwasher that uses 180°F. water, this will sterilize your equipment well enough. Before putting baby equipment in the dishwasher or sterilizing it, be sure it is clean and free from any milk scum. Use a bottle brush on the inside of the bottle and a nipple brush in the inside of the nipple.

To sterilize just a few things, fill a pot with enough water to completely cover the items you are sterilizing (bottles, cups, bottle caps, nipples, funnels). Bring the water to a boil over high heat, then turn down the heat just enough so that the water continues to boil gently. After 5 minutes of boiling, remove the nipples with sterile tongs. Place them on a clean towel. Allow the other items to boil 15 minutes longer. Do not touch the rims of the bottles or the insides of the caps.

If your baby will be given your milk at home, within 24 hours after it is expressed, you can keep it in the refrigerator. According to La Leche League, if you're planning on storing milk any longer, it *must* be quick-frozen and kept at 0°F. Milk stored under these conditions may be kept up to two years. NOTE: Unless your refrigerator has a dual-temperature freezer section, the milk will probably keep for only two weeks. (1)

How to Freeze Your Milk

Place containers (with lids on) in the refrigerator to cool. When cold, place the milk in the coldest part of the freezer.

The next time you express, place the milk in the refrigerator for about half an hour to cool, then it can be added to the storage container already in the freezer. Do *not* add warm milk to frozen milk as this will cause the milk on top to thaw and expressed breast milk must never be refrozen. Any liquid, including milk, will expand as it freezes, so fill containers only three-quarters full to prevent them from bursting. (2)

When transporting frozen milk, use dry ice or an ice chest to prevent thawing.

Thawing and Warming Your Milk

Do not let frozen milk stand at room temperature to thaw. It is much better to thaw it more quickly by putting the container under running water which is first cold, but gradually becomes warmer, until the milk has liquefied. Then it can be heated in a pan of water on the stove.

Thawed milk must be used within three hours of thawing to prevent bacterial buildup. If it has remained thawed longer, discard it.

Feeding Your Milk to Your Baby

Your baby can receive your expressed milk in several ways: with a small spoon, small cup, eyedropper, nursing supplementer, or a bottle.

A fussy baby may take the milk more happily from a babysitter if she sits where you often sit while feeding the baby. Also, though it may appear ludicrous, it may help if your sitter wears something you often wear. I heard of one mother who worked two hours twice a week teaching at a local junior college. Her husband stayed with the baby while she taught, but he often had trouble because the baby fussed so much while he fed her. In his frustration he put on some of his wife's clothing, and it worked. His wife came home from school to find her husband sitting in the rocking chair, wearing her frilly bathrobe. Their contented baby was well fed and sleeping blissfully.

Breast Pumps

Like hand expression, using a breast pump can be valuable in special circumstances. Some mothers believe they do better expressing their milk with a breast pump, rather than by hand. Other mothers, who have become adept at hand expression, find that method far preferable for them. However, even though you can hand express, there may be a time when a breast pump is far more feasible, for instance, if you are hospitalized and are receiving intravenous feedings. Other uses for breast pumps include relieving engorgement, drawing out inverted nipples, and bringing in milk for an adopted baby. When a mother and baby must be separated, a breast pump can be valuable for building and maintaining the milk supply. For long separations, or if you must be hospitalized, an electric pump is usually preferable, since it takes less effort on the mother's part. However, electric pumps are expensive. Most mothers rent them. Your insurance plan may pay at least part of the rental cost, especially with a doctor's prescription. If money is a problem or for short separations, the Loyd-B hand pump, the ORA-LAC pump, or the Breast Milking/Feeding Unit are satisfactory.

Before going into further detail on the use and the kinds of breast pumps let me emphasize that breast pumps should be used only when absolutely necessary: hospitalization of the mother when the child cannot be admitted, too; hospitalization of your child if you cannot be in attendance; if your baby is a very small premie being fed by naso-gastric tube. Even the most efficient breast pump is not as good as a baby's sucking. Remember, breastfeeding is much more than milk being supplied to a baby and a bottle full of breast milk is *not* breastfeeding.

How to Use a Breast Pump

Inexpensive hand breast pumps are available in drug-stores. However, many mothers have found they are not easy to use. If you *do* decide to use one, here's how: Moisten the inside of the pump's cone with warm water. Compress the bulb *halfway,* slip the cone over your breast so that the nipple points toward the bulb, then gently and rhythmically apply and release pressure on the bulb. Milk will collect in the bubble at the flared end. Be sure to sterilize the pump after every use.

Electric breast pumps come with some directions for use

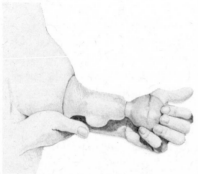

Hand Breast Pump

With the cone fitted over your breast, rhythmic squeezing on the bulb causes milk to collect at the flared end.

and for regulating the degree of sucking action to your own comfort. Before starting the breast pump, read over the suggestions in the Hand Expression section earlier in this chapter. In particular, Dr. Michael's suggestions for applying heat, stimulating the nipple, and massaging the breast can make the pumping more effective.

Hand expression before using a breast pump helps to soften the areola and minimize irritation to a too-full nipple when the pump is started. As the breast pump is working, you can nurse your baby or hand express from the other breast at the same time. This can produce a let-down reflex on the breast being pumped as well as the one where you are nursing or hand expressing.

Switch the pump from one breast to the other every few minutes if you are not simultaneously nursing or hand expressing. This allows more milk to flow down the ducts into the sinuses in the breast not being pumped, to be available when you switch back to that breast. Also, for maximum milk expression, have someone else hold the breast shield-cup which collects the milk so that you can use both hands to compress and massage your breasts.

Be cautious when you first use the pump, since its action may irritate the nipples. Limit your time at first to five minutes on each breast, and increase the time gradually. If your nipples begin to get sore or tender, reduce the time again.

Frequent, regular pumping during the day (every two to three hours) is advisable to maintain or increase your supply. Nighttime pumping depends on your situation. Frequent feedings stimulate your breasts to produce more milk.

It's not easy to feel maternal towards a machine. Some mothers, though, find they can get a let-down if they think about the baby. You might sit in a comfortable chair or rocker, hold a pillow in your arms, close your eyes and imagine your baby at your breast. Privacy helps a great deal.

Drink a glass of fluid 15 minutes before pumping. You should also be eating well, especially if you are under a great deal of stress.

Types of Breast Pumps

As already mentioned, there are inexpensive hand breast pumps, available in drugstores. There are also three other nonelectric pumps now available. While they cost more than the hand operated types, many mothers find them easier and more comfortable to use.

The Loyd-B Pump was designed by a La Leche League father. It is hand operated with a trigger action similar to that found in spray attachments sold for some household cleaning products. It is a very efficient pump if used correctly. It helps if the shield is moistened first with comfortably warm water. The pump is small enough to be carried in a purse and all parts that come in contact with the milk can be sterilized. The price of this pump is currently around $30.

The ORA-LAC breast pump was designed by a nursing mother who spent several years perfecting the design with the cooperation of several interested doctors. Suction is obtained by means of a tube which the mother puts into her mouth. The milk goes directly into the collection bottle. This pump is also small enough to fit in a purse and has been found to be successful by the mothers who have used it. The current price is less than $20.

The newly available Breast Milking/Feeding Unit from Happy Family Products is a combination of a comfortable,

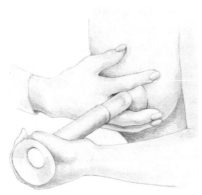

The Breast Milking/Feeding Unit

Make sure your nipple is placed exactly in the center of the flared part of the outside cylinder. Keeping this flared end pressed against your breast, gently pull the outer cylinder back and forth, creating suction to draw the milk out.

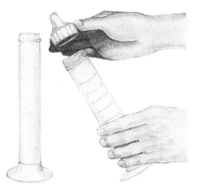

Once the milk has been collected, the outer cylinder is transformed into a nursing bottle by attaching a nipple. A scale on the side makes it easy to determine the amount expressed.

easy-to-use pump and an infant feeder. The two main parts are telescoping cylinders, with the outer one shaped to fit your nipple area. It comes with two adapters for your comfort. Gentle suction is initiated by moving the outer cylinder back and forth in a pistonlike manner. The inner cylinder is removed after the desired amount of milk is collected and the outer cylinder can be converted into a feeding bottle by attaching the ordinary nipple that comes with the pump. Avoiding the need to transfer milk also makes it possible to keep the oxidation and loss of nutrients to a minimum. Nipples designed for babies with special needs can be used. The pump is all plastic and is easily cleaned in the dishwasher or it can be boiled. Cost is currently about $20.

Electric breast pumps are usually much more efficient than

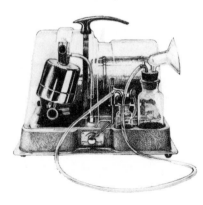

Egnell Breast Pump

This electric breast pump is especially effective if you massage the surrounding breast tissue with your free hand, as you are using it.

hand breast pumps. The hospital may have one you can use, or you may be able to rent one. There are two types available.

The Egnell Breast Pump is about the size of a four-slice toaster. It is available for rent through some La Leche League groups, drugstores, and hospital supply companies. The current fee is around $15 for five days' rental plus a necessary kit of accessories which you keep. The cost to purchase an Egnell Breast Pump is about $685.

A less expensive electric pump is an adaptation of an aspirator pump with certain Gomco parts. This Gomco suction machine presently costs about $385 and is available from medical supply dealers. It is used in some hospitals, where it is cleverly adapted to be used as a suction pump for breast milk. The suction is continuous (in the Egnell it is more rhythmic, more like a baby's sucking) and is regulated by placing your thumb or finger over a hole in the tubing.

The Egnell pump with its variable suction strength is considered superior, but the Gomco can do a good job also. Gomco pumps can also be rented from some La Leche League groups.

Milk Banks

If a crisis situation should arise where you are unable to meet your allergic, premature, or ill infant's need for breast milk, there are milk banks from which your physician can request extra milk. Milk banks are usually affiliated with a hospital but there are independent organizations. (3)

Most milk banks are small and are run on a completely voluntary basis. Approved mothers in the community are asked to donate milk. Sometimes they are paid (from 5 to 25 cents an ounce), but more often they are voluntary donors. The milk is picked up, tested, and frozen (either raw or pasteurized) for storage. Because of the small size and voluntary nature of these milk banks their breast milk is primarily for in-hospital use. Only rarely do they have any surplus milk; however, if they did have some to spare they would come to the assistance of another local hospital or a critically ill infant in the area. Some milk banks will ship milk, others will not. A doctor's prescription is always required. If there is a cost involved it can be from 30 to 75 cents an ounce, or the cost of shipping, when applicable. You might receive aid to cover the cost of the milk from your hospitalization insurance, or in some states The March of Dimes or Department of Welfare.

Milk banks fulfill an important need in the community. They are a service and depend on nursing mothers who wish to help. There are many operational costs. Part of the cost may be borne by an organization such as United Way, but most milk banks rely completely on donations.

Milk banks are an invaluable resource in an emergency situation. Through the efforts of many, you can be assured of the help you need until you are able to completely fulfill your baby's breast milk requirements yourself.

See Appendix: Organizations to Help the Nursing Mother for a list of milk banks.

Clothing for Discreet Nursing

Being able to nurse discreetly is a good trick for any nursing mother, but it is especially desirable if you're in a situation where attention may be focused on you. Discreet nursing is amazingly simple if you wear clothes that help. Instead of unbuttoning your blouse from the top down so that your breast is completely exposed, simply pull your blouse up from the bottom or unbutton the bottom buttons so that the top of your breast remains covered. The baby's body will cover any bare midriff and your nipple will be in his mouth, so that it appears that you're holding a sleeping baby, not a nursing one. A sweater or knit top is even easier: just pull it up as far as you need to nurse. La Leche League meetings are a good place to observe nursing techniques and you may pick up some ideas from those mothers who are nursing most discreetly. Practice at home in front of the mirror, and with your family and friends.

Some mothers who can nurse very discreetly this way have difficulty when it comes time to hook their bra flaps. They find that they can comfortably wear regular bras which have elastic under the cups and still have proper support. Here's how to do it: at nursing time, slip your thumb under the elastic and slip the cup up over your breast. When the nursing is over, again slip your thumb under the elastic and pull the cup back down into place. Be careful that whatever kind of bra you wear is not binding and does not suppress the free flow of milk as this can cause a plugged milk duct.

Today's fashions are wonderful for the nursing mother. At home, slacks and a blouse, jeans and a T-shirt, or shorts and a top are comfortable and work very well for nursing. For dressier occasions, suits with a jacket or vest are nice, because when you nurse you can pull part of the jacket around the baby, providing you both with a little more privacy.

On cooler days the "layered look"—a blouse with a sweater and perhaps a jacket—works well, too. With so many layers of clothing it may appear difficult, if not impossible, to nurse, but it's really quite simple. All you need to do is leave the middle buttons of your blouse unbuttoned. The sweater or sweater vest will cover the blouse, so it won't show. At nursing time, pull the sweater up a little just as you would if you were wearing a single top.

Dresses that have seams under the bust can be easily adapted for discreet nursing. You can do this by opening the appropriate seams and inserting invisible zippers, Velcro, or snaps. Invisible zippers do not show except for the zipper pull, and that can be hidden under a little trim.

A poncho or shawl makes a nice wrap for cooler weather because you can hold the baby underneath it to nurse while you remain completely covered and both of you stay nice and warm. On hot summer days when you go to the beach or the pool, take along a loose-fitting T-shirt or similar type of top to be worn over your swimsuit at nursing time.

For further what-to-wear information for nursing mothers, send for La Leche League's "Nursing Fashions Packet." (4)

Leaking

Leaking between feedings can be a problem in the early weeks but often disappears within a couple of months as the breasts become adjusted to a regular nursing routine. Leaking *at* feeding time can continue longer since the let-down causes milk to flow from both breasts at the same time.

To take care of leaking milk, slip some kind of absorbent lining inside your bra. Disposable nursing pads are sold in drugstores. They are comfortable and convenient. Reusable pads available in department stores are less expensive than disposable ones. Be sure they don't have plastic covers. The contoured ones are nicest.

If you don't want to go to the expense of buying nursing pads, you can easily make your own. You can use clean folded handkerchiefs, or you can cut out four-inch circles from diapers or old T-shirts and stitch three or four thicknesses together. You can use disposable diapers cut into nine sections (remove the plastic lining since plastic traps moisture around the nipple and can cause soreness). Be sure that reusable pads bought or homemade are laundered and rinsed with special care to remove all detergent residue which may be irritating to the nipples.

Whenever you feel the tingle of the let-down reflex, you can prevent leaking by pressing against the nipple with the heel of your hand or your forearm for a few seconds. However, it is best to do this after baby is about six weeks old and your milk supply is more established. You can also catch leaking milk in cups. See the section, Shields Used during Pregnancy or between Nursings, for a further discussion.

Special Feeders and Feeding Techniques

What do you do if your baby does not suck well at the breast? Perhaps he was premature and has not yet developed a strong enough suck or perhaps you have little or no milk, as is often the case with adoptive mothers. Brain injured babies often have a poor sucking ability at birth though it tends to improve with time. Cleft palate babies may not be able to maintain suction to get enough milk from the breast. Medication taken during childbirth often affects baby's sucking ability at first.

For these babies and others who need assistance in obtaining milk from the breast, there are certain techniques and artificial devices to assist in feeding a baby supplemental breast milk or formula. These alternate methods of feeding may need to be used only temporarily until your baby is able to breastfeed normally.

If your baby was born with a feeding problem, your doctor and the maternity nurses may help you by suggesting which feeding technique or special nipple to try first.

One way to give your baby extra milk if he is not yet sucking well is to feed him the milk from a spoon. This way he will need to rely on *you* to fulfill his sucking needs, and the additional sucking will help increase your milk supply.

If you can drip milk from an eyedropper into your baby's mouth as he nurses at the breast, he will be encouraged to nurse longer, and this longer nursing will also stimulate your breasts to make more milk.

You may also consider using the Lact-Aid nursing supplementer to feed additional milk to your baby as you nurse. For further explanation of how this device works, see *Supplementing at the Breast,* in the section on Supplemental Food, chapter 15, "Inducing or Reestablishing Your Milk Supply."

Cleft Palate Babies

Before resorting to any special feeding devices you should try nursing your baby directly from the breast. The feeding technique that Edith found to be very successful with her cleft palate daughter is described in the Cleft Palate section in chapter 8, "Malformations of Baby's Nose, Mouth and Digestive Tract."

Many mothers of cleft palate babies have had success

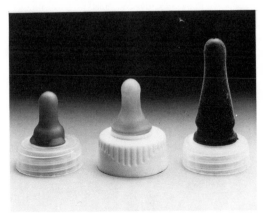

From left to right:

Premie nipple

Regular nipple

Lamb's nipple with adapter

Rodale Press Photography Staff

using a premie nipple, usually shaped like a regular bottle nipple but red in color and much softer than the regular nipple. In many cases the premie nipple hole has to be enlarged by making either a cross-cut opening or large hole or many small holes (similar to the breast nipple) so that the milk will flow with very little effort. (Don't make the hole too large until you can determine that baby can handle a greater flow without choking.) Premie nipples are readily available in most drugstores and are inexpensive and less conspicuous than some other feeding devices.

For some cleft palate babies a lamb's nipple may be used when feeding breast milk. Lamb's nipples are long black nipples (about twice as long as normal), which are used for feeding baby lambs. They are made by Davol and may be obtained from some animal feed stores, hospital pharmacies, and other pharmacies where they have been special-ordered. This nipple will not fit a regular baby bottle so you must either use a special bottle designed for this nipple or get an adapter that enables you to use the lamb's nipple on a regular baby bottle. Ask your doctor where lamb's nipples, special bottles, and adapters can be obtained in your area.

A Beniflex Nurser can also be used with cleft palate babies. The top part of this six-ounce nurser is hard-formed

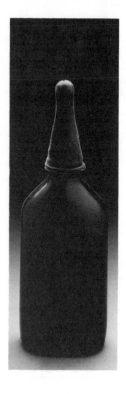 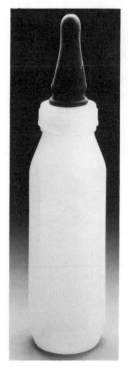 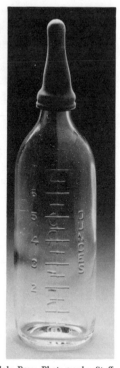

Special glass bottle and lamb's nipple.

Regular bottle with lamb's nipple and adapter.

Special glass bottle and lamb's nipple.

plastic, and the bottom section is a soft plastic pouch that resembles a plastic bag. Pressing the soft plastic section creates pressure that helps to force the milk into the baby's mouth. If you don't want to use a Beniflex Nurser you can create similar pressure by using nurser bottles with disposable plastic bags.

Babies without Sucking Problems

With a baby who has an adequate suck but who is occasionally fed from a bottle you can use a Nuk Orthodontic Nipple with a regular bottle. This nipple was designed to

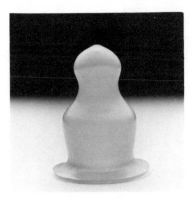

Nuk Orthodontic Nipple

The shape and texture encourage a sucking motion that duplicates breastfeeding. The nipple can be fitted on a regular bottle.

Rodale Press Photography Staff

resemble the shape and texture of a mother's nipple when it is inside a baby's mouth during breastfeeding. It encourages oral exercise and allows a slow intake of milk, like breastfeeding.

Time and Energy Savers

"Eat well, rest a lot, relax," is good advice for any mother. But it may be harder to do if yours is an "unusual situation." Here are some thoughts from other mothers that you may find useful.

Simplify Your Life

Consider priorities. When running a house at top efficiency conflicts with full-time attention to the needs of one of the family members, let the housework go, or at least find shortcuts for getting the bare minimum done.

Alternate your jobs so that a standing one is followed by a sit-down one. Let dishes drain dry. Rest when you can. Lie down as you nurse, when possible.

One mother wrote, "I have found that letting the baby nurse as much as he wants without rush gives me extra time. The unhurried, leisurely nursing produces a calm, relaxed baby who will let me accomplish more than if I were tense and anxious and trying to hurry it."

Meal preparation can be simplified. (See Quick Meal Planning in chapter 3, "Nutrition for Mother and Baby.") With a baby food grinder you can grind up nutritious table foods for your older baby. It saves money and space in the refrigerator, because you need to prepare only the small amount your baby eats. You can grind foods wherever you are, at home, on a trip, in a restaurant, or at a hospital. Cost of the grinders at time of publication is less than ten dollars. At least one brand comes with a Baby Feeding Chart which gives a lot of good nutritional information.

If the housecleaning doesn't get done, it's not the end of the world. Maybe there's one thing (sinks) or one room (living room) that must be clean or you feel miserable. Concentrate on that and give other areas a "lick and a promise" as time permits. Laundry is more urgent than cleaning. Maybe you can have someone help you with it. Disposable diapers or a diaper service save time. Accept all the help that is offered to assist you with housework, cooking and laundry, so that *you* can take care of the baby.

Baby Carriers

Many mothers use a baby carrier at home, as well as when they go out with baby. You can give your baby lots of extra cuddling this way, and get some of your housework done at the same time. Then, when the baby's ready for a nap, you can take a nap, too.

The Happy Baby Carrier is economical as well as useful. I used it with our twins from the time they were two weeks old. In the morning our babies especially liked it when I leaned over to make a bed, or jiggled a lot as I brushed my teeth. Vacuuming, while riding on Mommy's back, no longer seemed to be a frightening experience. Some nights, when dinner was late and both twins were fussing, I had both in carriers—one in front and one in back!

When a baby has a cold, a carrier can be especially helpful. Because of a stuffed-up nose baby may find it impossible to nurse himself to sleep for his nap as he is used to doing. You'll

Snugli Baby Carrier

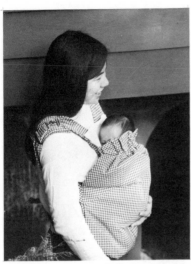

With a baby carrier, baby is comfortably and safely supported, while mother's hands are free to do other things. A carrier allows mother more freedom of movement, both inside and outside of the home.

Snugli Cottage Industries

find that he will often fall asleep comfortably without nursing while in the carrier. In order to get a few winks yourself without disturbing the baby you can turn a chair sideways at the kitchen table, put a pillow on the table and lay your head on it, and catch a nap yourself while baby is comfortably upright getting some needed sleep.

Mothers have written to me about using baby carriers in many special situations. If your baby has to be held upright all the time, a baby carrier is indispensable. A brain injured baby is stimulated more by always being where things are going on (as all infants are). Babies recovering from cleft lip or cleft palate surgery should be kept from crying as much as possible. In a baby carrier they can feel close and loved. Even babies with I.V.'s in their arms or heads can sometimes be held in carriers while the I.V.'s are in place.

There are many kinds of baby carriers. Besides the Happy Baby Carrier there is the Snugli Carrier, pictured in chapter 6, "Nursing a Premature Baby" and chapter 14, "Working Together." Another popular one is the Gerry Carrier; baby needs to be old enough to sit up to use this one, or at least be propped with a pillow or blanket and strapped in. Most carriers range from $15 to $45.

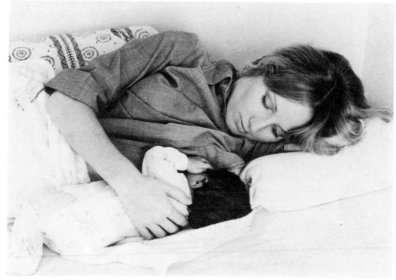

Sandra C. Wallace

Nursing Lying Down

Lie on your side facing baby with your arm under his head. He may begin by nursing the lower breast (one closest to him). To switch breasts, shift your body to bring the nipple of the upper breast against baby's cheek. He will then turn towards it and resume nursing.

Comfortable Nursing Positions

Lying down to nurse at least once a day can be a great way to help you get enough rest. It is also good to learn to nurse comfortably while lying down so that night nursings can be accomplished easily with a minimum of interruption to your sleep.

Lie down facing the baby with your arm either above the baby or under his head. With your other arm move your baby close enough so that his cheek is touching your breast. He will turn his head towards the nipple and start to nurse. If you pull his legs close to you, it will probably angle his body enough to keep his nose free. A pillow behind your back may help you relax. And you may want to place a pillow between

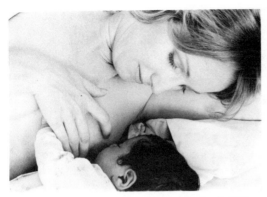

Mother's left arm is extended above baby while right hand is pressing her full breast away from baby's nose, to allow him ample room to breathe.

Sandra C. Wallace

your baby and the edge of the bed so you don't have to worry about his rolling off.

When removing the baby from the breast, be sure to first gently press the breast away from the corner of his mouth with your finger until the suction is broken. Just pulling him off the breast can be hard on the nipple.

If your breast is very full, as it may be at the early morn-

Sandra C. Wallace

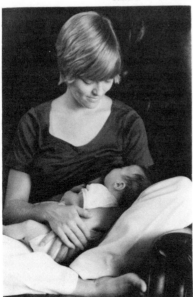

Try different nursing positions until you find the one that suits you. Here, the mother has settled in a comfortable chair, feet tucked up, with left knee propped on the chair arm. This helps support the baby.

51

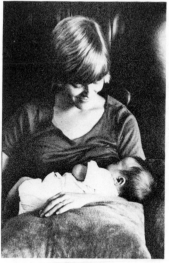

Nursing following a cesarean birth can be made easier by sitting up, with baby lying on a pillow placed across mother's lap. Also, it may help to hold baby in the "football hold" position (see illustration in chapter 18, "Nursing Twins") to keep him off your healing incision.

Sandra C. Wallace

ing feeding, your baby may find it difficult to grasp the nipple. If he cries and acts frustrated, hand express a little milk to get the flow started and to make the breast less full so your baby can grasp the nipple more easily. You may also need to press your breast away from his nose a bit so he can breathe as he nurses. If your milk is coming out too fast at first so that your baby is gulping or choking, try letting some of it run into a cup or diaper and then let your baby take over when the flow has slowed down.

When sitting up to nurse, you may find you're most relaxed in a certain chair, with pillows at your back, elbow, or under the baby, and your feet up on a footstool. If you're sitting on a flat surface such as the floor or a bed, raising a knee can be helpful.

If you have sore nipples or a plugged duct, change nursing positions at each feeding. Varying the pressure points on a sore nipple will hasten the healing and toughening process. A different position may allow the baby to exert more effective suction on a duct that is plugged—and free it. Sit up for one feeding, lie down for the next. Sometimes use the football hold. Even try *unusual* positions such as lying flat on your back and nursing your baby with his body by your shoulder and his legs by your head.

How to Insure a Good Milk Supply

One of the advantages of breastfeeding is that it is so flexible and suited to a baby's needs. Operating on the law of "supply and demand," the more milk that is removed from the breasts, the more milk they produce. You may be wondering though, especially if this is your first baby, how you can tell that you have enough milk.

You Do Have Enough Milk If:

• Your baby has regained his birth weight by about two weeks of age; *or*

• Your baby gains several ounces per week (after the first two weeks); *or*

• Your baby's weight and height are in the proper proportion on the doctor's growth chart, regardless of weight gain alone.

You Also Have Enough Milk If:

• Your baby nurses vigorously, then calms down and is contented or dozes off to sleep.

• Your baby has a lot of wet diapers (six or more a day).

• Your baby calms down when picked up and held in your arms.

• Your breasts feel softer after nursing than just prior to nursing.

Minor fluctuations of milk supply occur in most nursing mothers. Some days you will seem to have more or less milk than other days. The following list gives some common causes of a lowered supply. If, after increasing the frequency of nursing for a couple of days, your supply still seems low, you might consider whether or not one or more of these causes could be contributing to your problem.

Some Conditions That Can Adversely Affect Milk Supply

- Low thyroid hormone secretion

- Excessive cigarette or marijuana smoking

- Pregnancy

- Use of a pacifier. This can confuse a baby since the artificial nipple requires different mouth and tongue positions. Baby might begin to prefer the rubber nipple to mother's. Using a pacifier every day for periods of more than five or ten minutes might seriously affect your milk supply because of decreased breast stimulation.

- Birth control pills. The Food and Drug Administration has warned that they are not to be taken by breastfeeding mothers. They may reduce a mother's milk supply as well as have harmful effects on the milk and on the baby.

- General anesthetic. This can cause a temporary drop in a mother's milk supply.

- High fever in mother can cause milk supply to be reduced temporarily.

- Mother's let-down inhibited because she is upset, worried, tired, or in pain.

- Feeding baby unnecessary liquids (water, juice, or formula) or unnecessary solids. These can interfere with an ample milk supply by diminishing your baby's need to nurse for nourishment. Less sucking stimulation leads to a decreased milk supply. Most breastfed babies don't need solids until about the middle of the first year. If for some reason your baby must have solids earlier, nurse first before offering the solids.

• Baby with an initially weak suck, such as a premature or brain injured baby, or one with a cleft palate.

Ways to Maintain Your Milk Supply

• Give your baby both breasts at each feeding. It is generally considered best if the baby nurses from the first breast for about ten minutes. Before he gets too tired, he should be switched to the second (full) breast, and be allowed to nurse there for as long as he likes. At the next feeding use the "second side" first. (A safety pin attached to your bra is a handy way to remember which breast you'll offer first at the next nursing.)

• Feed your baby frequently. Breastfed infants usually need to nurse about every two to three hours. Remember the baby in utero receives nourishment through the umbilical cord with every beat of mother's heart. (Formula-fed babies can "last" longer because the curds in cow's milk are harder to digest.)

• "Demand feeding" usually works best. Though your baby may be nursing about every two to three hours, he may have one longer stretch, perhaps during the night. Also, you may find that there are some days when he seems to need to nurse more frequently than usual. This is likely to happen during a "growth spurt." He suddenly needs more milk, and nature's way of providing this is by his stimulating more milk production through more frequent nursing. Such growth spurts usually last only a few days. They often seem to occur at about four to six weeks and three months, but could occur at any other time, too.

• Drink a lot of liquids—water, juice, milk or soup—to replace the fluids used in making milk, as well as for your own needs. One to two quarts a day is usually a good amount. Drink more if you're nursing twins or siblings, or if you are feverish or vomiting. *Moderate* intake of coffee, tea, soft drinks, beer or wine usually causes no problems in the breastfed baby.

• Eat healthful food. A good basic diet is essential while you are nourishing a baby.

• Make a special point to relax before and during nursing. Try some of these suggestions:

Take a hot bath or shower before a feeding.

If nipples are sore, some doctors recommend taking a pain-killer 30 minutes before a feeding. (Don't exceed the recommended daily dose for the painkiller.) Touch your nipple with ice just before nursing. Also, see if expressing a little milk before feeding will cause a let-down. It will be easier on your nipples if you start nursing as the milk lets down. Eat a nutritious snack, have something to drink just before or during a feeding. Some mothers have an occasional glass of beer or wine to aid in relaxing.

Remove distractions. Take the phone off the hook. Ignore the doorbell. Nurse in a quiet room.

Breathe deeply before nursing. Use relaxation techniques you may have learned in childbirth preparation classes.

Nurse in a comfortable position and in a comfortable chair or rocker. Lie down if that's the most relaxing position. If you're sitting in a chair, put your feet up. Use pillows for added comfort.

As you nurse, let your shoulders sag, your jaw droop. Listen to soothing music before and during a nursing.

Read something enjoyable.

Ways to Increase Your Milk Supply

The following methods have been used by other mothers who have experienced a temporary drop in their milk supply. For the most part the ideas are not necessary in the normal nursing situation. However, you may still find one or more suggestions that you wish to follow even though you are only concerned about *maintaining* your milk supply, not *increasing* it.

• Nurse frequently. The quickest and most successful way to boost your milk supply is to let your baby feed more frequently. Also keep in mind that your breasts are continuously producing milk and if your baby doesn't settle after a feeding, another little nursing—a little "dessert"—maybe 15 to 30 minutes later, will often satisfy him.

• Switch breasts several times during a feeding. Nurse five minutes from the first breast, then five minutes from the second breast, then repeat the process.

• Gently massage your breasts before feeding to move more milk down the ducts. As you are nursing you might massage again, with your free hand, especially after your baby seems to have obtained most of the readily available milk in a breast. (If you notice his nursing pattern changes from long, slow, rhythmic mouth movements to rapid, shallow mouth movements, that's a good time to massage.)

• Express milk after feedings and/or between feedings. Again operating on the law of supply and demand, the more milk that is removed from the breasts, the more they will produce. (For expressing milk, see suggestions at the beginning of this chapter.)

• Check your activities. If you feel your milk supply is low, you may be trying to do too much. Can you cut down? Can you get help? Consider the following:
   How active are you in carpooling, P.T.A., other school activities, church activities, and organized social groups? Do you hold offices or specific responsibilities for these groups?

• Are you doing too much housework? Does a messy house bother you, make you tense?

• Are you decorating or remodeling your house? Do you have noisy workmen coming in daily?

• Are you moving or anticipating a move or a change of employment?

• Holidays and birthday parties—are you celebrating and preparing for them elaborately or simply?

• How busy are you with the needs of other children?

• Remember your first concern is to enjoy and care for your baby. Other jobs should be taken on by other people, at least for a while. Rest is important. If you can't manage a long nap each day, at least lie down as you nurse. Appeal to your husband, your relatives, your friends and neighbors for help with housework, shopping, meals, care of your other children. People are often glad to help. You can always return the favor later on.

• Ask your doctor about using oxytocin temporarily if you are anxious and your let-down is slow. Oxytocin comes as a nasal spray or in tablet form and is used just before each feeding. It can cause the milk to let down in spite of worries a mother may have.

• Have your baby in your bedroom at night, either in a bed next to you or in your own. The instinctive security of closeness will make you less anxious about him, and it's easy to nurse with baby nearby.

• Find someone understanding to discuss any problems which seem to be affecting your general disposition. Your husband is very important, of course. Others may include a close friend, an understanding doctor, or a member of a group that helps parents. (See Appendix: Organizations to Help the Nursing Mother.) Try to associate mostly with those people who understand your desire to nurse and recognize its benefits.

Shields Used during Pregnancy or between Nursings

The plastic breast shields illustrated here help correct inverted nipples, relieve engorgement, help treat sore or cracked nipples, and protect clothes from excessive milk leakage. They fit inside your bra, with the nipples projecting through the

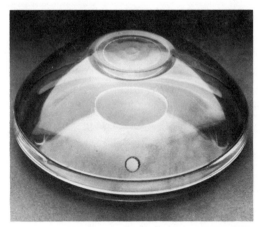

*Two-Piece Plastic
Breast Shield*

Rodale Press Photography Staff

center holes and the small airholes placed uppermost. Wear a bra at least one size larger than usual when using these shields. The shields come apart for easy cleaning with soap and

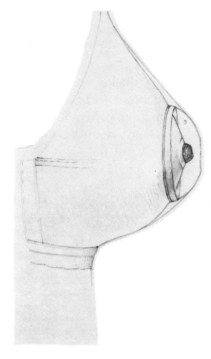

Plastic breast shield fits inside bra. Nipple passes through center hole, but does not come in contact with outer shell. Small opening allows for air circulation. This hole is also used for pouring out excess milk between feedings.

Comes apart for easy cleaning.

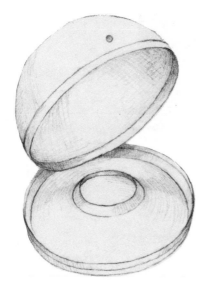

water. The "Netsy" Swedish Milk Cup and Breast Shield and the La Leche League International Breast Shield can be sterilized in boiling water (two to three minutes), if necessary. If you are experiencing milk leakage, periodically pour out the excess milk which collects in the cups.

When used prenatally, these breast shields help correct inverted nipples by exerting an even, continuous but painless pressure which eventually causes the nipple to project from the breast. After your baby is born, you can wear the shields between feedings for several days to draw out the nipple.* It may take longer to correct a true inverted nipple which was not treated during pregnancy.

The shields also prevent irritation to sore nipples by holding the bra away from nipples and allowing air to circulate. Engorgement can be relieved by the continuous, gentle pressure exerted around the nipple which pushes milk out of the overly full milk ducts. There is a slight chance they can make your breasts sore; if they do, use only occasionally.

---

* Meredith Breast Shields, available from the Nursing Mothers' Association of Australia, are for use only during pregnancy.

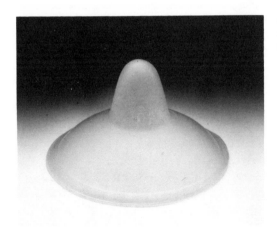

All-rubber breast shield, used over the nipple while nursing.

Rodale Press Photography Staff

Cost of these breast shields ranges from $4 to $8 a pair. They can be obtained from La Leche League International, Nursing Mothers' Association of Australia, or The Netsy Company. Addresses can be found in Appendix: Organizations to Help the Nursing Mother.

Rodale Press Photography Staff

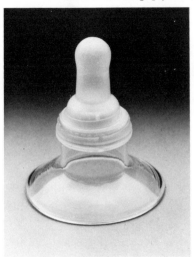

Nipple shield, used while nursing, has changeable rubber nipple, with glass or plastic base.

Shields Used during Nursings

There are two types of shields which can be used over the nipple, during nursing. Many problems are created by these shields, however, so it is generally recommended that you try other means to encourage your baby at the breast and use the shields only as a last resort. The following is not meant as a recommendation of these shields, but simply as a description of how some mothers have found them useful.

One of these shields is all rubber and is called a breast shield, although it bears no resemblance to the plastic breast shields described in the previous section. The other shield has a plastic base and removable rubber nipple and is called a nipple shield.

These shields are sometimes recommended to protect sore nipples or relieve engorgement, but many mothers find that they prevent proper sucking and even create more nipple soreness.

The nipple shields are meant to serve as an aid in drawing out flat or inverted nipples so that the baby can easily grasp them. First lubricate the shield with water, then place it over your nipple and encourage your baby to suck. After a minute or so your nipple may be more pronounced, so you can remove the nipple shield and have the baby suck directly from your breast. You may have to try a number of times before you can manage to switch your baby from nipple shield to breast. Many mothers with inverted nipples find that the nipple shields don't help at all. Some mothers find that nursing through the shield does pull out the nipple but they have to remove it several times during a feeding.

I know of one unusual situation in which an all-rubber breast shield helped a mother of a baby with Down's syndrome who had no sucking instinct at all. Once she got her baby to suck, she spent three weeks trying to nurse him. Finally, with the help of a breast shield, the baby nursed and eventually his mother was able to dispense with the shield.

Use these shields for as brief a time as possible. Babies

can become confused by sucking from different nipples, and some babies become dependent on them. Also, with the plastic base nipple shield, the baby must get the milk by suction alone (not by pressure directly on the milk ducts), so he may get very little milk, which affects your milk supply. You may be better off using the plastic breast shields (described in previous section) between feedings or using one of the other methods described in chapter 4, "Breast and Nipple Problems."

The shields described in this section are available in many drugstores.

For Up-to-Date Information

If you'd like current information about availability, prices and where to order breast pumps, reusable nursing pads, special feeders, baby food grinders, baby carriers, or breast shields, enclose 50 cents to cover handling costs and send to:

Nursing Techniques—RP
28221 Lomo Drive
Rancho Palos Verdes, CA 90274

Chapter 3

Nutrition for Mother and Baby

Sound Nutrition

We have all heard that good nutrition is the foundation of good physical and mental health. How and where to begin building this foundation is a big question. With your time at a premium it may not be easy to remember to eat well and get the extra nutrients you need to avoid becoming fatigued or irritable.

The basic suggestions for good nutrition and ways to simplify meal preparation included in this chapter will help you have the energy to deal with both pregnancy and lactation. However, there are many wonderful publications that cover the subject of nutrition more thoroughly than this book can. A good way to expand your understanding of the principles and values of nutrition would be to follow up on some of the references listed in the Bibliography.

The Four Basic Food Groups

Good health hinges on exercise, adequate rest, and a diet that includes a variety of nutritious foods. Building a foundation for fitness means choosing carefully from the four basic food categories each day.

The *protein group* provides iron and B vitamins as well as being the primary source of protein. Included in this group are eggs, fish, poultry, beef, and protein plants like peas, beans and nuts. Your protein requirements can be met meatlessly if you learn to use extra milk products, eggs and "complementary plant proteins." Each plant protein contains only *some* of the essential amino acids needed for proper nutrition. Combining these proteins assures you of a complete protein. Pea soup with cornbread or beans with rice are good examples of complementary proteins.

The *fruit and vegetable group* contributes vitamins C and A and the roughage that is often lacking in American diets. This roughage prevents constipation. Among foods highest in vitamins A and C are dark green vegetables such as broccoli and spinach; dark yellow vegetables such as squash, carrots and sweet potatoes; and citrus fruits. Eating them raw or lightly steamed until tender provides more nutrients. Root vegetables and certain fruits should be scrubbed but not peeled, as there is an abundance of vitamins right under the skin. Cooking water, which contains many soluble nutrients, can be saved for soups, gravies or making bread.

The *milk group* includes cheeses, yogurt and ice cream in addition to milk. These milk products are high in good quality protein, and provide calcium (necessary for your milk production) and vitamins A and D. Nonfat dried milk can be added to many foods to boost nutrition, with no change in taste. Yogurt and buttermilk are occasionally better tolerated by milk-sensitive people because the fermentation process breaks down some of the protein.

Whole grain breads and cereals provide roughage and contain many valuable nutrients, especially B vitamins and vitamin E. Natural whole grains can't be matched nutritionally by enriched white flour.* In addition, they offer different textures and flavors.

Nutritious Snacks

Nutritious snacks are important for mothers before, dur-

---

* Commercial white flour is flour with all its wheat germ and bran milled out, taking with it most of the vitamin E, sixteen B vitamins, and minerals. The bread manufacturers then restore B_1, niacin and iron—in lesser amounts than were originally present—and call the resulting bread "enriched."

ing and after pregnancy, and especially in special circumstances. You may not have time to prepare or sit down to a meal or you may be too nervous or tense to eat full meals. Snacking can keep energy levels high and prevent fatigue.

Here are a few nutritious and delicious between-meal snacks. By planning ahead, you can have them ready and waiting when the "hungries" strike:

A bowl of cut-up vegetables or fruit and a yogurt dip

Bananas dipped in wheat germ

Celery or apple slices spread with peanut butter

Cheese cubes

Popsicles made from juices or yogurt

Frozen bananas

High-protein almond drink made by liquefying 1 cup of water or apple juice, ¼ cup almonds, 1 or 2 ripe bananas, 1 teaspoon brewer's yeast (1)

Foods high in sugar provide quick energy which is soon gone, while foods high in protein are digested more slowly and provide sustained energy. An eggnog, cheese and an apple, or a peanut butter sandwich are good energy choices. Fruits like bananas, grapes, and apples are high in natural carbohydrates and give quick energy without any refined sugar.

Quick Meal Planning

Meal planning for a mother under stress *can* be made easier. If people ask what they can do for you, say, "Help with meals would be nice." Someone helping you prepare meals will appreciate a week's menu of foods that are familiar and well liked and perhaps specific recipes also.

Making double recipes saves time. Freeze half for the future or use the other half the next night in another form ("planned-overs"—a large pot of beans can be served with cornbread one night, then as enchiladas).

Start meals early in the day while baby naps. Meatloaf

can be made and refrigerated until an hour before dinner. "Slow cooker" meals, which need six to eight hours, are another smart, economical choice. Plan *simple* meals—roast beef with unpeeled vegetables placed in the same pan, baked whole chicken. Avoid recipes with a long list of ingredients or many cooking steps when your time is at a premium. Recipes that eliminate cooking can save preparation and clean-up time, too. Shirley Boie's *Cookless Recipes* (2) has many to choose from.

Mother's Nutrition

Diet during Pregnancy and Lactation

At no other time in your adult life is nutrition more important than during pregnancy and lactation. Good nutrition plays a critical role in your baby's fetal growth and development. It has been shown that an inadequate maternal diet can affect a baby's brain development and his mental and physical potential after birth. In addition, Michael and Niles Newton, authors of *The Normal Course and Management of Lactation* (3), have found that you are better able to nurse your baby for as long as you like if your diet is good during the latter half of your pregnancy. However, it should be emphasized that even a starving mother can and does lactate in cultures where breastfeeding is necessary to ensure the survival of the baby.

By striving for optimal nutrition during pregnancy you will be in the best condition should an emergency arise. Cesarean births, for example, are often unexpected. Nancy Cohen, co-founder of C/SEC (Cesareans/Support, Education and Concern) says:

> After a cesarean, some mothers are left on an I.V. for two or three days. Because of the surgery and perhaps a long labor prior to that (with nothing to eat during that time), the mother is in a weakened physical condition. The Jello water and ginger ale she often receives once off the I.V. aren't the best, either. This is less than an optimal way to

begin breastfeeding from a nutritional standpoint. Women whose nutrition and exercise regimen are good have less difficulty recuperating.

The nutritional requirements during pregnancy are higher than at other times. You especially have an increased need for protein, calcium and iron. Extra milk and the selection of iron-rich foods (liver, dried apricots, egg yolk) will help you meet these needs. Iron is utilized more efficiently when eaten at the same meal with citrus fruits or juices. It may be difficult to meet the recommended daily allowance for iron during pregnancy through your diet, so your doctor may prescribe a supplement. He may, as "insurance," also prescribe a multivitamin preparation.

During pregnancy, it's generally best to increase your intake of milk or cheese, fruit and fruit juices, yellow and green vegetables, whole wheat bread and whole grain cereals, fish and lean meats. Cut down on sugar and large amounts of unnecessary fats. If there is a strong family history of severe food allergies, you may be advised to limit the amounts of highly allergenic foods in your diet during pregnancy and lactation. Salt generally need not be restricted during pregnancy. There is no proof that using salt in moderation causes toxemia.

For too long, exaggerated fears about "excessive" weight gain during pregnancy have dominated many obstetricians and have made the joy of pregnancy a chore for women. It has been found, however, that women who gain about 20 to 35 pounds during pregnancy have a better chance of having full-term, good-sized, healthy babies, if the weight gained is due to eating nutritious foods. An increase of about 3 pounds a month permits the baby (and the maternal tissues which feed and protect it) to develop normally and provides a small reserve to help you start producing milk.

Nausea associated with early pregnancy can often be relieved by eating smaller, more frequent, protein-rich meals, such as cheese cubes, yogurt, or eggs. Vitamin B_6, or foods rich in B_6, such as bananas and wheat germ, have been known to be of some help.

If you are nursing a toddler while you are pregnant, you will need additional calories and protein. The amount needed will depend on how much your older child is nursing. If you are fully nursing him, it is recommended that you increase your caloric intake by about 500 calories and your protein intake by about 20 grams, over and above the recommended increases for pregnancy. (4) If you are not providing the entire nourishment for your nursling, the increases could be proportionately less. Make certain that you're getting an adequate supply of calcium, and be sure that your doctor is aware that you are nursing.

A breastfeeding mother has an increased daily need for protein and calories. The extra 20 grams of protein and additional 500 calories can be supplied as simply as adding a peanut butter sandwich and a glass of milk to your daily diet. You may find your appetite has increased during breastfeeding, but be careful not to add nutritionally empty foods, like candy bars. There are plenty of foods to choose from, with high nutritional value, that are also economical.

Sometimes a new nursing mother neglects her fluid intake. You need plenty of water—either "straight" or in the form of fruit and vegetable juices, milk, or soup. Make it a habit to have a drink beside you each time you sit down to nurse. Coffee and tea are all right in moderation (less than half of your fluid intake). Soft drinks which contain sugar and caffeine have no food value, are expensive and are not a good example for your children.

Most mothers report that no particular foods pose problems for nursing. If you are allergic to any foods, you may find your baby is allergic to those foods also, either when he is fed them directly or if he receives them through your milk. Foods which most commonly seem to cause allergic reactions in susceptible babies are milk products, eggs, wheat products, and citrus fruits. Learning to recognize the troublesome foods and avoiding them is far better for your baby than switching to formula. More information on nursing an allergic child is found in chapter 11, "Dealing with Allergies."

Lose Weight While Nursing?

Additional weight put on during pregnancy is frequently nature's way of providing the extra energy needed to keep up with a baby during its first year. A pound or two may be associated with the increase in your breast size and body fluids needed for nursing.

If you are overweight by more than ten pounds, a little extra effort to diet sensibly will do no harm to you or your baby.

Fad diets, especially those that emphasize one kind of food (grapefruit diet, all-protein diet) don't provide the proper variety and amounts of nutrients needed to maintain good health.

If you've decided that you must lose weight, first eliminate all nonessential, high-calorie "junk" foods. Look for sugar in your diet and eliminate or reduce it. Drink water in place of sugared ice tea, colas, or low value fruit drinks. Switch to skim milk and skim milk products. Give this regimen—and your nursing—time to help you lose weight before you change your basic diet. Don't sacrifice the recommended amounts of protein or a balanced diet to achieve speed in losing weight. Usually a breastfeeding mother should begin to lose when her baby is three to four months old.

Increasing Your Milk Supply

If you find your milk supply dwindling below your baby's need, it does not mean you need to wean. It is not at all unusual for a mother's supply to fluctuate. With a little effort, you can build it up again. Refer to chapter 2, "Nursing Techniques" and chapter 15, "Inducing or Reestablishing Your Milk Supply."

While you are building up your milk supply, pay careful attention to your diet. Make sure to drink extra fluids. It may be helpful to drink even more liquids if you find you can't eat. I know of one mother who was so upset she couldn't eat for several days. By heating soup and concocting egg, milk and chocolate drinks, she kept up her strength and her milk supply.

Some mothers have reported an increase in their milk supply when taking brewer's yeast, which is high in B vitamins, iron and protein. Start with ¼ teaspoon of brewer's yeast and increase gradually.* Remember the basics for good nursing: diet, liquids, rest, and frequent nursing.

Eating for Three

Nursing twins, or triplets, will obviously put more of a demand on your body. You probably will be much hungrier and thirstier than you expected.

Have a nourishing snack whenever you're hungry, not just when it's mealtime. You may need to eat one or even two extra meals a day with special emphasis on protein. A filling breakfast will help you get going and keep going all morning. Additional B vitamins in the form of brewer's yeast and wheat germ can help keep you from feeling tired and irritable.

Keep in mind that extra fluids are especially important for your double milk production. Have one or more glasses of some liquid each time you nurse, even if it's just water. And drink between nursings, too.

If You Are Sick or Hospitalized

When mother is ill, the responsibility of caring for herself is added to that of caring for her child. It's important for both you and your baby that you take steps to insure a prompt recovery; paying special attention to your diet can help.

Fever can affect your milk supply because it uses up body

---

* Large amounts of brewer's yeast in a mother's diet can cause the baby to have gas and abdominal discomfort. Reduce the amount you take if your baby seems to be having this problem. You can try to increase the amount gradually as your baby gets older. Also, brewer's yeast taken before a meal (not after) is less likely to cause gas for you.

fluids. If you are running a fever, you should increase the amount of fluids you are drinking.

When you are recovering from an illness, you need even more nutrients than when you are healthy. You need a variety of foods, with plenty of fruits and vegetables, to be sure you are getting all the different elements needed for healing. B vitamins are especially good. Citrus fruits (vitamin C) and dark green and yellow vegetables (vitamin A) help prevent infection and are good for healing.

When you are hospitalized, your diet will depend on the nature of your illness and what foods you can tolerate at that time. What foods should you ask for, to get optimal nutrition? Most hospitals have a standard diet and will not vary much. Choose foods high in protein, low in sugar, two vegetables (if possible, different colors for different vitamins) and fruit for dessert. Ask for whole wheat bread instead of white. Avoid stimulants, especially coffee.

Baby's Nutrition

Nutritional Advantages of Breastfeeding

The nutritional advantages of breastfeeding can sometimes be very persuasive in convincing an otherwise uncooperative doctor to allow you to continue nursing your baby in an unusual situation.

The change to cow's milk formula often causes problems. Cow's milk is not always well tolerated by humans. Many babies have serious allergic reactions, while a great many more only tolerate it, having vague problems such as stomach discomfort, constipation, and rashes. The more serious reactions include gastrointestinal disturbances, respiratory illness, stomach bleeding, growth retardation, or central nervous system damage. (5)

Breast milk is ideally suited for the human baby. It is easily digested, used more efficiently and contains the right kinds of nutrients in the proper amounts for your baby.

Formulas superficially simulate mature human milk but

not the colostrum, which gives the baby certain immunities. Breast milk itself provides protection from various illnesses such as diarrhea and respiratory infections in two ways. It is not contaminated by handling and storage and it also contains antibodies and special disease-fighting white cells that destroy harmful bacteria in your baby's digestive tract.

Breastfeeding may prevent your baby from becoming overweight. This is significant in light of studies that repeatedly show that obesity is more stubborn when it has occurred early in life. (6) Breast milk meets the caloric requirements for infants (20 calories per ounce of body weight) with no added starches or refined sugars. The fat in breast milk is readily assimilated by your baby's body and is not stored as excess fat and weight.

Dr. Lewis A. Coffin, author of *The Grandmother Conspiracy Exposed* (7), says:

> It has been found that babies who become fat while being breastfed do not develop the same problems as do babies who are getting solid food or formula. Fat babies who are breastfed only don't apparently add on abnormal fat cells, they just enlarge or fill those they normally have.

Conversely, a bottlefed baby who is encouraged to finish what's left in the bottle or is introduced early to foods with a higher caloric count can develop *more* fat cells.

Introduction of Solids

The Basic Concepts of La Leche League (8) states:

> For the healthy full-term baby, breast milk is the only food necessary until baby shows signs of needing solids, about the middle of the first year after birth.

Breast milk is the perfect and complete food for your baby for many months. In a family with a history of allergies, it may be wisest to hold off beginning solids for as long as possible: the younger the baby, the more likely it is that foods other than breast milk will cause allergic reactions. (9)

There is usually no reason to add anything else to your baby's diet during this period. You would be substituting inferior nutrition for the superior nutrition of breast milk. According to David M. Paige, researcher from Johns Hopkins School of Hygiene and Public Health, "Premature introduction of infant foods appears to be a critical factor in excessive nutrient intake" in babies, and may be contributing to obesity and degenerative diseases later in life. "It is important," says Dr. Paige, "that mothers do not yield to the strong commercial and peer pressures to introduce baby foods too soon." (10)

Another good reason to avoid introducing solids before your baby needs them is to maintain a good milk supply. Solids could leave him so full that he would nurse less vigorously and take less milk. The less milk he takes from the breast, the less there will be. Many babies who don't start solids until the second half of their first year continue to nurse happily for months or years longer, along with eating their solid foods.

Incidentally, while baby continues to nurse often you are much less likely to menstruate or ovulate. (11)

Since all babies develop at their own individual rates, how do you know when to start your baby on solids? He may suddenly increase his demand to be nursed and this increased demand may continue for several days. If you offer more frequent nursings, (making sure you have plenty of liquids yourself) and your baby doesn't seem to be satisfied, you may suspect the time has come to introduce solids. However, don't be completely convinced by these first signs—increased demand might be due to a growth spurt or a cold coming on or some unusual activity or tension in the family. The average age for introducing solids is around six months, but each baby is unique, so go along with the increased nursings at first to make sure that it is *hunger* that is responsible.

Why Wait until Your Baby Is Ready?

At times you may feel pressure to start solids from friends, relatives, or even the doctor, although your baby hasn't shown any signs of readiness. Their comments can make you doubt your own ability to judge what's best for your baby. It's helpful to examine the questions people may have so that you can respond more confidently.

"How much did your baby gain this month?"   This question is asked quite frequently, and suggests competitive thinking. Comparing babies' growth is not a reliable way to determine health. Obesity is a health problem in this country, and a fat baby is not necessarily a healthy baby. Babies, just like adults, come in all sizes and shapes. A happy, healthy baby is more important than a fast-gaining one.

"How can you be sure that your baby is getting enough milk?"   Check if his diapers are wet most of the time. Frequent wet diapers, provided that you aren't bothering with water or juice between feedings, are a good sign that your baby is getting enough breast milk. An alert baby with bright eyes and a good skin color and tone signals an adequate milk supply. See also *You Do Have Enough Milk If* . . . in the section on How to Insure a Good Milk Supply, chapter 2, "Nursing Techniques."

"My baby started sleeping through the night when I started solids. Has yours?"   Some babies sleep through and some babies don't, regardless of whether solids are started. Solids *can* create digestive discomfort for the baby not yet able to handle new foods. Some babies start waking up again when solids are introduced. With a breastfed baby, it's very easy to snuggle up and doze, so the issue of when your baby starts sleeping through the night won't be of such importance, anyway.

"Won't your baby become anemic if he doesn't get additional iron from solid foods?"   Human milk does contain a surprisingly low concentration of iron, about 0.5 mgm per liter. Iron-fortified formulas contain 12 to 18 mgm per liter. Yet

your breastfed infant, if full-term, doesn't begin to run the risk of developing iron-deficiency anemia until six to nine months, the same as bottlefed babies.

The major reason for this remarkable fact, first reported as early as 1928, is a protein called lactoferrin, contained in human milk. (12) A breastfed baby, thanks to lactoferrin, is able to digest the tiny amount of iron very efficiently while the bottlefed baby loses almost all his iron.

Lactoferrin has another important role. By binding iron in the intestine, it keeps disease-producing bacteria from utilizing the iron for their own metabolism. In other words, overloading the baby's formula with iron to make up for his less efficient digestion can be harmful because it may encourage the growth of dangerous bacteria.

Babies fed cow's milk become anemic for another reason. Their intestinal tracts can become damaged by the foreign proteins in cow's milk and tiny amounts of blood may be lost every day, eventually exhausting their iron supplies.

Studies have shown that babies fed only human milk may have sufficient iron intake until they triple their birth weights, usually at one year. (13)

Introduction of Solids—How and What

No special tools are necessary to prepare your own baby food, but some are handy to have. A portable food grinder is inexpensive and can be used both at home and while traveling. A blender is also useful at home.

The idea is to transform table food into a finer consistency, suitable for your baby. In many cases, you can mash food with a fork or scrape with a spoon to achieve this consistency. The food needn't always be lump-free, just reasonably smooth.

The food that you serve your baby should be nutritious and not salted, overly spiced or have added sugar. You can remove the baby's portion before you season the food for the other members of the family. Steam vegetables lightly to preserve vitamins and use the cooking liquid as added moisture to make blending easier.

Baby food can be prepared in large portions and frozen. *Confessions of a Sneaky Organic Cook* (14) suggests *dab cookery*—baby meals made in the form of dabs and frozen. Just drop the pureed food, like pancake batter, by the tablespoon onto a plate. The size of the dab is determined by your baby's appetite. Cover, then put the plate in the freezer for several hours. When the dabs are frozen solid, remove from the plate and store them in a plastic bag or a covered container. When you are ready to use the dabs, heat them on a warming tray, or in a pan of hot water. This procedure can also be followed using an ice cube tray. Fill the compartments half full and cover while freezing. When they are solid, empty the tray into a plastic bag and then take out as many cubes as you think your baby will eat.

Your baby will begin by eating very small quantities of food. Your goal, at the beginning, is to introduce him to tastes other than breast milk, not to fill him up with food. Nurse him first to take the edge off his hunger and to help maintain a good milk supply. Mashed ripe banana is a good first food.

Foods high in iron content are introduced next. Liver, meat and egg yolk (not the white, which may be more likely to cause allergies) are good choices.

Foods such as vegetables, breads and cereals can then slowly be introduced. Allow at least a week between each new variety of food to be sure that your baby has no allergic reaction.

Around seven or eight months you might start offering juice from a cup once or twice a day. Cow's milk could be started much later. Since it is a highly allergenic food, many parents prefer to wait until baby is a year old before introducing it. Other known allergenic foods are mentioned in *How to Start Solid Foods* in the section on Starting Solids, chapter 11, "Dealing with Allergies."

Once you have introduced your baby to new tastes, you can encourage eating by serving finger foods, such as dried bread slices in finger-sized pieces, bits of soft meat, cooked string beans, or cooked potato pieces. Table manners will come much later! If you have been using a blender you can gradually blend the food for shorter periods. This leaves some lumps and encourages chewing.

Avoid sweets, refined starches, and fatty foods which are high in calories but have little nutritional content. Dangerous foods include nuts, popcorn, and raisins. They are healthful but can cause choking if baby doesn't have the molars to chew them properly.

Commercial baby foods, in some cases, contain additives unsuitable for babies. Reading the labels can help you decide. Cost comparisons should convince you that the time spent in baby food preparation is well worth it.

Slow Weight Gain

Babies gain at different rates; even twins being fed by the same mother in the same way may vary. These individual differences should be recognized and accepted.

The baby who is slow in gaining weight is probably just following his own particular growth pattern. However, a baby who is sleeping excessively, not nursing well, and not gaining weight may need help and encouragement to nurse better. He should be watched carefully by a physician as these symptoms could indicate a very sick baby.

Various medical problems can account for slow weight gain, but if a baby is otherwise healthy, sometimes the introduction of mashed ripe bananas can help solve the weight gain problem. The added calories seem to boost the baby's vigor, enabling him to nurse more vigorously and stimulate mother's supply. The bananas can be stopped when he is nursing more eagerly and regularly, and gaining weight.

See Slow Weight Gain in chapter 7, "Newborn and Infant Problems," for additional discussion.

Food Supplements: Are They Necessary?
For Baby

Since human milk has evolved to specifically satisfy the nutritional needs of human infants, all the vitamins and minerals necessary for proper nutrition are present. Iron, in particular, is present in a form used more efficiently by babies.

In *Nursing Your Baby* (15), Karen Pryor points out that ". . . human milk contains 2-10 times as much of the essential vitamins as does (unfortified) cow's milk." This difference is doubled when cow's milk is diluted, as it must be for human infants. The vitamin content of formula is reduced further when subjected to the high heat needed to sterilize it. Breast milk is raw and fresh.

Many children's vitamin preparations contain sugar and artificial colorings and flavorings. Your doctor may prefer to give *you* a vitamin supplement to replace the vitamins that you are providing the baby in your milk. Your milk will have a good supply of vitamins in the proper proportions for your baby.

For Mother

Many mothers worry needlessly about their milk being deficient in vitamins and minerals. It has been found that the milk varies very little from mother to mother. If your diet is not adequate in vitamins and minerals, the baby will get first choice of the nutrients stored in your body and you can be left with a deficiency. It's best to eat a well-balanced diet, with as many natural, unprocessed foods as possible. Vitamins obtained from natural sources are better than synthesized vitamin pills.

Vitamin D can be added to your diet and your baby's without pills by the addition of approximately a half-hour of sunshine daily. Cod liver oil is a good source of vitamin D for you to take (not your baby) if the climate doesn't permit daily exposure to sunshine.

There is a great deal of controversy centering around fluoride. The chemical fluoride added to vitamins and water supplies is not the same compound that occurs naturally in some water. Occasionally, a mother will report that her baby seems to be affected by vitamins she is taking, especially those with fluoride. An article in *La Leche League News* tells of a baby who developed a severe rash and diarrhea, evidently from the fluoride in his mother's particular brand of vitamin. (16)

Premature Baby, Iron and Introduction of Solids

Since most of a baby's iron reserve is stored up during the eighth and ninth months of pregnancy, a premature baby may find his iron supply running out earlier than a full-term baby's. This does not mean that solids should be introduced earlier. In fact, premature babies often start solids later than many full-term babies because their digestive systems are not ready to handle them.

An average hemoglobin count for infants 6 to 12 months of age is 11. If the count is borderline, the use of iron-rich foods, such as meat, egg yolk, and iron-fortified baby cereal is suggested. If the count is below 9 it is important to build up the hemoglobin count quickly. This is where iron supplements are used, together with iron-rich foods if appropriate for the baby's age and development.

Nourishment for Your Baby during Illness

Breastfeeding for nourishment is more necessary than usual when a baby is ill. Some illnesses traditionally require special diets. A general rule is that if the baby can have any food, breast milk is best. The younger the baby, the more important it is for him to receive his mother's milk. Even though animal milk may aggravate certain illnesses, breast milk is usually well tolerated. You may need to remind the doctor that your baby is receiving only breast milk and that this is not the time to add new foods to his diet. Skim milk, though often recommended, can upset a child's body chemistry; commercial gelatins and carbonated drinks contain sugar, which can add to a sick baby's problems.

Special attention to fluids is important during an illness,

since dehydration can set in quickly if your baby is not nursing often. Your doctor may suggest giving water or juices. If your baby is not yet using a cup, try a spoon or dropper to give frequent small amounts of liquid.

Keep a close watch on your baby during an illness. Sleep is needed for recovery but your baby needs regular feedings, too. As your baby recovers, he may want to nurse frequently, both for comfort and nourishment.

When your baby is ready to take more than breast milk, serve only those foods that are easy to digest. A piece of dry toast, some clear soup or a small serving of homemade gelatin are easy-to-handle foods. To make the gelatin, dissolve a package of unflavored gelatin in a little fruit juice, heat it, and add more juice.

When a baby has been on an antibiotic, the beneficial intestinal bacteria are also destroyed along with the illness-causing bacteria. Some yogurt will help to reestablish the beneficial bacteria, as well as provide a source of protein. Many hospitals are now serving yogurt along with medication to prevent the diarrhea frequently associated with antibiotic treatment. There are some antibiotics for which milk or milk products are antagonistic. Make sure your infant is not taking one of those by checking with your pharmacist.

Nourishment for Your Hospitalized Baby

When a baby is sick, he often will not eat well, but you may find that no matter how ill he is, he will nearly always nurse a little. This not only comforts him but provides nutrition and fluids necessary for recovery.

Ask the dietician for your child's preferred foods, or choose what he likes from the daily menu. A portable food grinder can make many foods more palatable.

Plan on sharing mealtime with your child, even if you eat your own meals elsewhere. Your presence can make these times more pleasant and if your child is happy, he will eat better.

Breast Milk and Breastfeeding: Alternatives

Special circumstances sometimes necessitate finding alternatives to breast milk or the normal breastfeeding situation. Briefly, here is a list of possibilities, all of which are covered in more depth throughout the book:

- Express your milk by hand or by breast pump.

- Feed expressed milk by tube, spoon, eyedropper or nursing supplementer.

- Freeze expressed milk for later use.

- Milk banks or other nursing mothers may furnish a short-term supply.

- If breast milk is not available and baby is allergic to cow's milk formulas, other possibilities are soybean, goat's milk, meat base or other specialized formulas.

- "Nursing strikes" can be offset by offering various liquids, yogurt, homemade gelatin.

- As the situation improves, consider returning to breast-feeding.

Chapter 4

Breast and Nipple Problems

In the past, breast and nipple problems frequently resulted in weaning. Today's medical authorities agree that most problems can be treated while nursing continues. Some conditions clear quickly. Occasionally, a problem may be severe enough to advise temporary weaning from one or both breasts for a few days. You can pump or hand express milk during this time and breastfeeding can be safely resumed as nipples or breasts improve.

In this chapter, you will read how many mothers have dealt with breast and nipple problems. The various ideas and solutions presented may help you with your problem. Before trying any, discuss them with your doctor.

Inverted Nipples

An article in *La Leche League News* tells about a mother who ran into difficulties nursing her first baby. Her first attempts to breastfeed were fruitless, but she remained optimistic and felt things would improve when she got home from the hospital. To her dismay and frustration, they didn't. She decided to contact a La Leche League leader, who visited her and discovered that her difficulties were being caused by nipples that retracted when the areola (the dark area around the nipples) was squeezed. Upon discovering this she began wearing breast shields (see Shields Used during Pregnancy or between Nursings in chapter 2, "Nursing Techniques") and exercising the nipples so that they would protrude. Engorgement aggravated the problem and made hand expression difficult and painful. With an electric breast pump, she was able to relieve the engorgement and her baby soon could grasp the nipple and begin sucking on his own.

What to Do While Pregnant

There are several things that you should do if you suspect that you have inverted nipples. First, try this simple test to

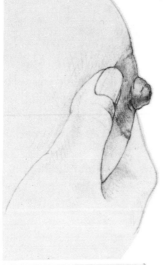

Test for Inverted Nipples

Normal nipple protrudes if areola is pinched.

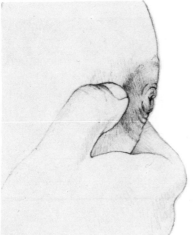

Inverted nipple retracts if areola is pinched.

determine if your nipples really are inverted. Using the illustrations to guide you, pinch the areola just behind the base of the nipple with your forefinger and thumb. As you press, the nipple should project away from the breast. If, instead, it shrinks or folds back when pressure is applied, it is inverted.

Completely inverted nipples are quite rare. The best treatment is the use of plastic breast shields. These exert a constant, even, and painless pressure which gradually forces the nipple further through the central opening of the breast shield. The length of time for which the shield should be worn depends upon the severity of the problem. If your nipples retract deeply or completely invert, you should begin wearing the shields in your third month of pregnancy. If the nipples are depressed only slightly, you should start no later than the thirtieth week of pregnancy. Begin by wearing the shields an hour or two, twice a day. You may steadily increase the time until they are kept on all day.

If you have flat, slightly retracted, or inverted nipples, you may try exercising the nipples several times a day by pulling them out quite firmly but gently with your fingers. This breaks any adhesions that lie at the base of the nipples and helps them protrude more as childbirth approaches. (1)

Michael and Niles Newton, in *The Normal Course and Management of Lactation* (2), state that "the nipple which is flat or even slightly inverted in early pregnancy will usually become protractile by the time of delivery." The hormones of pregnancy tend to prepare the shape of the nipples for breastfeeding without any other help.

According to the pamphlet, "Inverted Nipples," published by the Nursing Mothers' Association of Australia (3), the best treatment for inverted nipples is your baby's suckling; mothers who have successfully breastfed one baby rarely have any further trouble with inverted nipples.

It may be that the tender attentions of a man to a woman's breasts are part of nature's way of preparing them for the task of nursing a baby. Some couples find that the breasts play an important part in their lovemaking. If this appeals to both you and your husband, his gentle oral and manual stimulation of your breasts and nipples could be a most enjoyable and effective part of your prenatal nipple care.

What to Do after Baby's Arrival

If, after the baby's arrival, you discover a retracted or inverted nipple that you never suspected, then what? There are some simple measures that you can try at first if the baby is having difficulty grasping your nipples. If they are temporarily retracted because of engorgement, try hand expressing a little milk. You might express some directly into your baby's mouth to give him a taste and get him started. If your nipples are quite soft and flat and the baby is having trouble locating them, try applying a very cold cloth to the nipple area for a few seconds. This is often all that is needed to cause the areola to shrivel and the nipple to protrude and become firm. Sometimes a little honey applied to the nipples encourages the baby to grasp them. One mother used a pliable plastic cup to build up a vacuum and suction that forced the nipple out.

Occasionally with this type of nipple problem, the hospital staff will suggest that you place a nipple shield or premie nipple over your nipple. (See section, Shields Used during Nursings, chapter 2, "Nursing Techniques.") This does help the baby get milk, but it usually does not encourage the nipple to protrude and it may even confuse the baby as he tries to learn how to suck.

The plastic shields mentioned earlier may help you over this initial difficulty. They are worn between feedings in the same way that they are worn during pregnancy. A few minutes just before each feeding or just between two feedings is sufficient. But if the nipple is truly inverted improvement may take several weeks.

Zena found that nipple preparation pays off when you have an inverted nipple:

> I have only one inverted nipple, the other is perfectly normal. Actually, when the inverted nipple comes out it also is a well-formed, good-sized nipple, but most of the time it is tucked away inside.

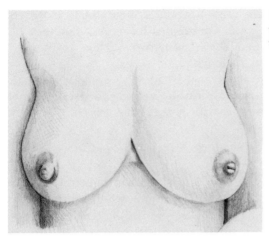

Nipple on left is normal. Nipple on right is inverted.

I have four children. When the first was born eight years ago I was aware of the problem, but although it was suggested at the time by a La Leche League leader that I should wear a breast shield for a while before the birth, I never bothered. Like many first-time mothers-to-be I was concentrating mainly on the childbirth and didn't really think too much about the breastfeeding part. Anyway, the baby turned out to be a pretty good sucker and soon got the knack of pulling out the nipple. However, the nipple got excruciatingly sore, having always been protected from the elements before the birth.

The next two children followed fairly quickly, and I simply didn't have the time to bother with nipple preparation before the second child, so again I became terribly sore. I managed to heal it with A and D Ointment well rubbed in every hour or so, but I didn't learn my lesson and went through agony again with the third. She was not a strong sucker and I found the little horn-type breast pump very helpful in drawing out the nipple so that she could get hold of it. And I was very sore again.

However, the third was 4½ when the last one was born so I had plenty of time for preparation. I began wearing a breast shield all day during the last month of pregnancy. I didn't wear it in bed. Once I'd pulled the nipple out myself the breast shield kept it out for the rest of the day. Since I didn't wear the shield in bed, the nipple popped right back in again as soon as I took the shield off but at least it was exposed for most of the time. I also applied A and D Ointment two or three times a day, and massaged thoroughly.

I am happy to report that I had only very mild soreness this time and would heartily recommend the use of breast shields to anyone with inverted nipples.

"Dimpled Nipples"

Michele wrote of a difficult problem she encountered due to an anatomical abnormality of her nipple where *only* the very tip folds back in like a dimple. She nursed her first baby and when the baby was around eight months old and still nursing

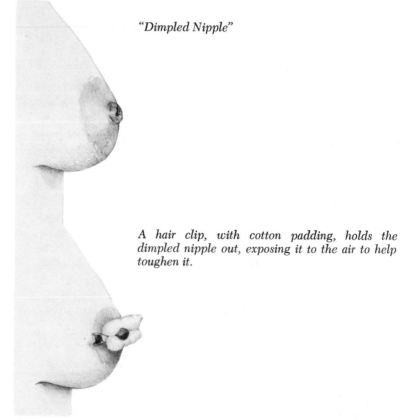

"Dimpled Nipple"

A *hair clip, with cotton padding, holds the dimpled nipple out, exposing it to the air to help toughen it.*

Michele had a little bleeding from her right nipple. She did not realize the cause of it and the baby weaned herself shortly thereafter.

The bleeding began again soon after Michele's second baby was born. Michele consulted doctors and followed their suggestions, including changing the baby's position at the breast, using lanolin on the nipples, starting each nursing period on the left side, and using a sunlamp. Nothing helped and the bleeding continued. She then began nursing from her left breast only and did so until her baby weaned himself several months later.

However, with her third child, Michele had a certain amount of success with nursing from both breasts. She realized that with the nipple tip folded back in, the nipple was always damp and unable to toughen or heal. She tried several methods to get air to her nipple, including using her hair dryer after each nursing, and sleeping at night without a top.

She learned to hand express for some feedings on the abnormal breast, sometimes expressing all day to give the sore breast a rest and a chance to heal. In this way, she paced herself and managed to successfully nurse from the right breast.

Treatment for Sore Nipples

If your nipples become extremely tender and sore, or in very rare cases, even cracked and bleeding, there are a number of things you can try to remedy the situation (in addition to other suggestions in chapter 1, "What's Normal?"). However, don't try all of these at the same time! Stick with one remedy until you're convinced it isn't working for you before trying another. I have heard of mothers who have tried three or four of the following suggestions at a time, and their lack of success was probably caused by overdoing the remedies.

Wine, Breathing Exercises and Hand Expression

Karyn found that taking a sip or two of a mild wine before nursing the baby and using her childbirth breathing exercises helped her to relax, then she used hand expression to get the milk flowing freely before putting the baby to the breast.

Tea Strainers and Breast Shields

Exposing the nipples to the air by going braless is helpful. Or you might remove the handles from two tea strainers and insert the strainers inside your bra to keep your clothing off the nipples. Some mothers have found the Netsy milk cups or breast shields which are worn inside the nursing bra also helpful in keeping clothing off the nipples.

Ointment

Lubricating the sore, cracked nipples before nursing can help prevent the healing skin from being pulled open again, and also prevents the wet milk from contacting the tissue. Use a mild ointment such as hydrous lanolin. If you are sensitive to lanolin, try A and D Ointment.

Avoidance of Plastic-Coated Bra Pads or Synthetic Clothing

Plastic-coated bra pads should be avoided because they hold moisture in and do not allow air to circulate. One mother suggests avoiding all nylon or synthetic material. Even a nylon blouse on top of a cotton bra can keep air from reaching the nipples.

Avoidance of Detergent Irritation

One mother who developed sore nipples tried several of the usual remedies to no avail. She finally suspected the detergent residue in her bra and in the handkerchiefs she used as nursing pads as the source of irritation to her moist nipples. She tried store-bought nursing pads and had no more sore nipples.

Ice

Another method of alleviating sore nipples is to apply crushed ice or ice water to them. The cold anesthetizes the sore nipples and has no effect on the milk supply. Wrap the ice in a washcloth and apply to the nipple area. Or wet small squares of cotton and put them in plastic bags in the freezer. One of these frozen cotton squares can be placed inside the bra when you can't use the ice bag. If it sticks to the cracked nipple, gently remove it with ice water.

Light and Heat Treatments

The use of an ultraviolet sunlamp or sunlight for healing sore nipples is often recommended. *The Womanly Art of Breastfeeding* (4) says:

> An expensive lamp is not necessary; you can buy an ultraviolet bulb and put it in any lamp stand or socket you find convenient to use. Sitting four feet from the lamp, expose yourself no more than one-half minute the first day, one minute the second and third days, two minutes the fourth and fifth days. If there is no indication of skin reddening by this time, you may increase to three minutes on the sixth day and keep it at that level once a day until the soreness is gone. If you do notice a redness at two minutes, then cut down to one minute and continue at that level for several days. Then try gradually increasing, one-half minute at a time, to see if you can tolerate a longer period. If not, keep it at the level that is best for you.

While using the lamp, protect your eyes with a towel or small protective plastic goggles. Use a timer. Keep babies and young children whose skin is very sensitive away from the light.

One mother found that using just the heat from a reading lamp, with the shade directing the light to the nipple area, for ten minutes on each side after nursing relieved the discomfort and promoted fast healing. After about two days of this heat treatment her cracked and bleeding nipples healed. The light bulb should be 60 to 80 watts—no more—and it should be kept 12 to 18 inches from the breasts. Some breastfeeding mothers feel that this type of heat is too drying to the nipples, but for this mother it seemed to do the trick. It may be especially helpful after bathing or showering, when the nipples have gotten thoroughly wet, or after prolonged nursing.

Nursing Position at Breast

In *Infant Feeding* by Mavis Gunther, M.A., M.D. (5), a problem called "positional sore nipples" is described. If the baby is not properly positioned he cannot grasp the nipple easily. This causes soreness. The problem is especially common with premature babies and generally results in a red stripe across the area of the mother's nipple that is not covered by the baby's tongue or palate. While nursing in a sitting position, place the infant on a pillow and hold his buttocks in your hand while his head is cradled on your elbow. Sometimes two pillows are necessary so that the baby's body is almost horizontal at the level of your nipples. The baby's head should tilt slightly backwards so that the nipple touches the roof of his mouth and so that his lower jaw has plenty of room for "milking action." The baby should be supported with his face and mouth facing towards your breast. Another helpful hint for your comfort and baby's is to use a step stool or chair rung to elevate your foot on the side on which baby is nursing. This will raise your corresponding knee and support your elbow which is cradling baby's head. This method prevents abrasions of the nipple by allowing the baby to get more of the nipple into his mouth as he sucks.

It may also be helpful to change your nursing position at each feeding. Sit up and nurse at one feeding and lie down at the next. This distributes the greatest pressure to different places.

Baby's Tongue Position

Andrea had a problem with her premie involving sore nipples and his way of sucking with his tongue against the roof of his mouth. To encourage him to nurse correctly, she propped him with pillows so that her hands were free. Then she opened his mouth and depressed his tongue with the fingers of one hand as she placed the nipple in his mouth with the other hand. At times it was very frustrating, because it took five minutes before they had it right. Eventually, by the end of seven weeks, he had learned to latch on by himself.

Short but Frequent Nursings

Nursing the baby more often for shorter periods of time often helps. The baby does not get ravenously hungry, so he nurses less vigorously. You can also begin on the less sore side first.

If your nipples are very sore, it may be necessary to limit your baby's sucking time to ten minutes on each side. He will get all the nourishment he needs during this time but this may not satisfy his sucking needs. You could try a pacifier to let him satisfy this need. If this is done, hold him at least as long as he would have nursed in order to satisfy his need for closeness to you also. When the nipples heal, go back to his full nursing period.

Expressing instead of Nursing

One mother who had a crack on only one nipple nursed primarily on the good side until it healed. If you do this, it will be necessary to express milk to keep the sore side from becoming engorged.

Relaxation Hints

Sometimes there seems to be a relationship between apprehension on the part of the mother and sore nipples. The nipple tenderness causes enough tension to hold back the let-down reflex. This frustrates the baby, and he pulls and tugs at the nipple, causing it to become sore. If this happens, you can try hand expressing a little milk to start the flow. A hot shower will help you relax and let the milk down also. Childbirth breathing exercises and total body relaxation can help, too. Another suggestion some mothers have used is to immerse the breasts in comfortably hot water. Sometimes a doctor will prescribe oxytocin nasal spray to help the milk let down. You can check with your doctor about the use of an analgesic such as Tylenol while your nipples are painfully tender. There are additional relaxation suggestions in How to Insure a Good Milk Supply in chapter 2, "Nursing Techniques."

Tea Bags

Some mothers have found some rather unusual solutions for healing their sore nipples. Melissa reported she had tried everything she'd heard of to heal her cracked and bleeding nipples. "I finally found that tea bags soaked in warm water and applied to the nipples for about 30 minutes after each nursing helped to relieve the pain," she said.

Vitamin E

Sara, who is red-headed and fair, said her nipples became very tender and sore. She had tried lanolin and the "usual remedies," but to no avail. Then she tried putting the oil from vitamin E capsules on them and they healed after just a couple of applications.

Temporary Weaning

Only in very rare cases of extremely sore nipples may it be necessary to *temporarily* discontinue breastfeeding. Sally's experience involved such temporary weaning:

For several months before delivery, I had prepared the nipples by rubbing them with a wet washcloth and exposing them to the sun for a few minutes at a time. However, a few days after our son Danny was born, the nipples became cracked and bleeding. I continued nursing and waited for them to heal by themselves as the books said they would. Finally I used lanolin, light bulb treatment, and tea strainers and I was determined to continue nursing no matter how it felt. But, after 12 days of severe discomfort, the let-down reflex stopped. I tried many methods of relaxing, but the reflex was so badly deconditioned that nothing worked, and I had to give Danny bottles.

After two weeks without nursing, the scabs fell off and I offered Danny the less injured nipple. It bled after only two minutes of nursing. I waited another week and tried the other nipple. It also bled after two minutes. By the fourth week, both nipples could take two minutes of nursing, and I increased the time gradually until Danny could nurse as long as he wanted. This process of toughening the nipples without opening the partially healed areas took about a month. By that time Danny had cut his formula intake in half. Then I concentrated on building up the milk supply.

Danny is now 14 months old and still nurses a great deal. It certainly was worthwhile putting in the extra effort to make nursing a success.

If your sore nipples are such that you too must temporarily wean, you can hand express your milk or use a breast pump (see Breast Pumps in chapter 2, "Nursing Techniques"), and then give the milk to the baby in a bottle, or with a spoon or eyedropper. If you use a "Nuk" nipple (pictured in chapter 2) while you are feeding from the bottle, the transition to the bottle and then back to the breast will be much easier. This nipple is shaped more like a breast nipple than are regular commercial nipples. As soon as your nipples respond to treatment, you can resume breastfeeding.

Thrush

Thrush is a common fungus infection which may occur in the baby's mouth or around the diaper area. Occasionally the organism causes vaginitis in the mother. If you have been nursing without any discomfort and suddenly develop sore nipples, you should check baby's gums and tongue for the milky white scum of thrush and call your doctor's attention to the situation. Of course, don't check right after your baby has nursed because milk in the mouth will look just like thrush. The infected mouth may be sore and the baby may have difficulty in feeding, but usually it doesn't seem to bother him.

Some mothers have found an ointment prescribed for yeast infections of this sort helpful in treating the nipples. Others have benefited from a baking soda treatment. Dissolve a level teaspoon of baking soda in a cup of water. After each nursing, swab the baby's mouth firmly and thoroughly, under the tongue, inside the cheeks, and on the gums, with this solution. Use a fresh cotton swab each time. This removes the milk from baby's mouth and gives the thrush fungus less to live on. Also, after each nursing, wash your nipples with this solution and apply a light coating of lanolin or petroleum jelly to counteract dryness. A fresh solution should be made each day and stirred before applying. If the soreness persists, you could try the lamp treatment as described in a previous section. If these remedies do not clear it up, check with your doctor.

Psoriasis

Psoriasis is a chronic recurrent skin disease of unknown origin characterized by dry, scaling patches. Terry described her experience with psoriasis:

When our second son Matthew was nine months old, I developed red rings encircling the nipple on the areola. My GP examined my breasts, took a culture, but found no fungus. Accompanying the rings was a distinct soreness which neither lanolin nor air seemed to help. The rings disappeared within a few months but then the nipples began to bleed. With each feeding the severity of the abrasion and pain increased slowly, crescendoed to the point where I was nursing, crying, and doing my childbirth breathing at the same time, and then finally subsided. This pain lasted for about a week at a time. I usually had about three to six weeks between bouts. Each time my nipples healed, I thought, "Well, thank goodness, that's that." But, "that never was that," and the cracking and bleeding always returned.

Finally, I visited a dermatologist. He immediately diagnosed the cracked condition as psoriasis. I had begun to suspect that the red blotches on my cheeks could no longer be attributed to the flush of pregnancy and nursing and that my flaky scalp might somehow be related. Indeed, the dermatologist diagnosed my scalp as psoriasis and my face as its cousin, seborrhea. He explained that when a person has a tendency towards these skin conditions, the "continued trauma" to the nipples during nursing is enough to cause psoriasis on the nipple area.

With the specific diagnosis of psoriasis, my GP was able to prescribe a medication that clears up the cracks in one to two days. The medication is to be used very sparingly on the cracked area after each nursing, and should be wiped off before each subsequent nursing, but I found that there was never medication left to wipe.

Growths on Nipples: Papillomas

Papillomas are benign wartlike growths with fingerlike extensions.

If you have had papillomas surgically removed from your nipples, rest assured that you can breastfeed your baby. La Leche League International's Professional Advisory Board has found that mothers who have had this surgery have managed quite well with nursing their babies.

If Baby Bites

It's natural for your baby to try out his gums or new teeth by biting everything, including *you*. But it's important to teach him immediately that biting is *not* allowed.

Babies who are teething can be given other things to bite on (see Teething section in chapter 1, "What's Normal?").

Don't delay teaching your baby not to bite. It's in his best interest to learn. Repeated biting may make you anxious anticipating a bite, and your let-down could be affected.

Even very young babies can be taught not to bite. Brigid was planning to nurse her second son who was born with a fully grown bottom middle tooth. She says that the main reaction she received from hospital staff members was, "Too bad you were counting on nursing him—if you want to nurse, have the tooth pulled!" She just could not see doing that because it might cause future dental problems. "He did bite, and though I had no problem teaching an eight-month-old not to bite, saying 'No' over and over to a baby twenty-four hours old seemed useless. However, in about two weeks Paul was nursing beautifully and never, ever biting—he had 'learned' and I was amazed at how much a newborn can grasp, mentally that is!"

Accessory Nipples

Having one or two accessory nipples is a rather common occurrence. These nipples, most often located in front of the armpits, are usually hardly noticeable. One mother told me that it took her 26 years and two babies to know what they were!

When your milk comes in, the area around the extra nipples may become engorged and tender. If you have just one accessory nipple the amount of milk in the area of the extra nipple will be related to the amount in the breast closest to it. Accessory nipples cause no problems after a few days of nursing. The amount of engorgement depends on the amount of mammary tissue beneath the nipples, which is quite variable.

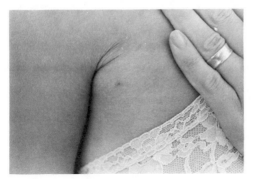

Extra nipples, often located in front of the armpits, can be painful for a few days, as well as annoying because of leaking milk.

Sandra C. Wallace

If the swelling around accessory nipples becomes great enough to be uncomfortable and makes it difficult to lower your arms, you might try wrapping Ace bandages around your chest just under your arms to compress the nipples for a few days, until the engorgement subsides permanently. Or try applying ice to relieve discomfort. Nursing frequently for the first few days after birth helps keep the engorgement to a minimum and ease the pressure on accessory nipples. Do not express any milk from them; just leave them alone and nurse from the regular set of nipples. The underarm breast tissue will then shrink to its pre-pregnant state, causing no further problem.

Eczema on Nipples

Occasionally a mother discovers dry skin and itching on the nipple and areola. Carole experienced this when her daughter was ten months old. She says:

> I continued to nurse Jocelyn although the skin on my nipple broke open and the pain was considerable when she latched on. My obstetrician diagnosed it as a breast infection and recommended that I continue nursing. He gave me penicillin. After that failed, I tried vitamin E applied to the nipple. The skin continued to break open, heal, and reopen. Finally an internist recognized the condition as eczema and prescribed steroids to clear it up.

Maureen had eczema on her hands and developed it on her nipple and areola area. Her doctor prescribed cortisone cream (a steroid) which relieved the symptoms somewhat, but not completely. The condition at times worsened and became severe with itching, cracking and bleeding. During these times, she used the Netsy milk cup to provide air drying and heat from the bedroom lamp for dry heat. She found that by lubricating her nipples before nursing, initial pain was lessened and so was the trauma of the dry, healing skin being pulled open again by baby's sucking.

Finally, she heard of someone with a fungus infection who had the same symptoms as she. Her doctor then ordered topical and oral antifungal medications for her. "This cleared up the infection and life became much more comfortable for me, although the eczema continued until the baby weaned," she said. (Cortisone cream was used as needed until all symptoms disappeared after weaning.) Fungal infections seem to be something that can recur and may be related to the mother having had a fungal or yeast infection such as vaginitis in the past.

Plugged Ducts

Plugged ducts usually result from inadequate emptying of one or more of the milk ducts. You will probably notice a reddened area on the breast and feel a small lump there which is painful to the touch.

A plugged duct can be the start of a breast infection, so be sure to treat it promptly. First, be sure your bra is not pressing too tightly on a milk duct. If dried secretions are covering some of the nipple openings, wash them off (soaking first if necessary) after each nursing. Keep the milk flowing and the breast fairly empty. Nurse often and longer from that breast, starting the feedings with the sore breast first. Massage during feedings and hand express afterwards and change nursing positions frequently.

Soaking the affected breast in very warm water for 20 minutes just before every feeding may help. Continue this routine until all soreness is gone.

Breast Infections

If, when nursing your baby, you develop any or all of the following symptoms you probably have mastitis, more commonly known as a breast infection: swelling, usually painful, and/or a painful lump in your breast; redness or localized soreness and tenderness; fever and a general sick feeling—tired, rundown, and aching.

Dr. Carolyn Rawlins, M.D., of La Leche League International's Professional Advisory Board says, " 'Flu' in the nursing mother is a breast infection until proven otherwise."

If infection occurs in the early weeks after your baby is born, it could be due to the breast remaining too full as a result of a sluggish let-down reflex. During the first few weeks, the let-down reflex is sometimes slow, especially with first-time mothers. Tension and discomfort can inhibit it. Too long a rest between nursings could be a contributory cause. Cracked nipples may give the infection a point of entrance. A bra that is too tight could plug a milk duct, stop milk flow, and allow infection to begin. Tensions, social pressures, the stress of adjusting to a new baby, and conflicts with relatives could inhibit the let-down reflex and be contributing factors.

Start all nursings on the affected side. Nursing the baby on the infected breast may be painful but the breast will hurt much less afterward. There is nothing in the milk that could hurt your baby.

Besides continuing to nurse, apply heat, wet or dry, to the affected area. If ice is more comfortable for you, try that. The heat can be provided by a warm shower, hot tub, hot wet towel, heating pad, or immersing the breast in comfortably hot water for five to ten minutes before nursing. Slow down and rest more. Go to bed if possible and take the baby with you. If your condition shows no definite improvement within 24 hours, call the doctor. He may want to prescribe a medication to be taken *in addition to* the above measures. Most such medications have no harmful effects on the nursing infant.

Remember, the three most important factors in the treatment of breast infections are: frequent nursing, hot wet soaks (or ice), and bed rest.

Occasionally a mother is troubled by repeated breast infections. What can be done for this disconcerting situation? One mother wrote to La Leche League International:

> I need help. I've had three breast infections and my baby is only two months old. Why? I eat well, I sleep well and take several naps a day. I take vitamin pills and drink plenty of fluids. I wear the proper size bra—not too tight. I nurse from each breast every two or three hours during the day (less frequently at night). And I nurse in different positions.
>
> When I had the breast infections the doctor prescribed an antibiotic called ampicillin and told me not to nurse from the affected side. I nursed on one side for three days. I took hot showers, used a heating pad, and stayed in bed.
>
> Why do the infections keep coming back? What can I do to prevent this problem?

In the reply to her letter the following suggestions were made:

> If you have another recurrence, a culture of your milk might be performed at the doctor's request to identify the infecting organism. Once the organism is identified appropriate therapy can be started. If it's a yeast infection (possibly this would be indicated by the baby having had thrush or your having had a problem with vaginitis), then the antibiotic wouldn't control it. How long did you take the antibiotic? We have found that many doctors only prescribe it for five days. It seems to take ten days for long-term effect. It would be best not to wear a bra to bed—use a towel under you for leaking. Leave your bra off as much as possible during the day for a while. Also check that the detergent is well rinsed out. Snack between meals on high-protein foods. It has been found that many people taking antibiotics benefit from eating some yogurt each day. The yogurt helps restore the normal intestinal bacteria and helps prevent diarrhea. Also, continue to treat yourself carefully for about ten days after the infec-

tion subsides so that your body can recover from the effects of an infection. Keep nursing.

The mother wrote back several months later:

You were correct about the five-day supply of antibiotic. I got repeated breast infections until given a ten-day supply. I have had *no* breast infections since then. . . . Your suggestion about high-protein snacks worked. And yogurt did help restore my system after the antibiotic.

If you repeatedly come down with breast infections, check the following questionnaire which is based on a list from Mary White, a founding mother of La Leche League International (6):

1. Does the baby nurse often? (At least 10 to 12 times in 24 hours.)
2. Does the baby nurse at night, too?
3. Does he nurse both sides at each feeding?
4. Are you taking your prenatal vitamins and iron?
5. Are you anemic? Have you had your hemoglobin checked?
6. Do you nurse even more often at the first sign of an infection?
7. Do you really get rest, off your feet, and use heat on the affected area?
8. Are you getting plenty of vitamin C? According to some doctors, taking extra vitamin C, at least for the duration of the illness, and probably a week or so after, is a good idea.
9. Are you perhaps taking too much antibiotic? This tends to prevent the body from building up its own immune system and strengths. We find that nearly all breast infections, if caught in time, can be cured without resorting to antibiotics. But *do* check with the doctor if the symptoms do not disappear within 24 hours.
10. Are you a heavy milk drinker? (Milk is higher in salt than most people realize, and this can influence susceptibility to infections.)
11. Have your menstrual periods resumed? The few days before each period are susceptible days (for the reason stated in Item 10—salt retention).

12. Do you enjoy nursing and caring for your infant?
13. Are you getting static from your husband or relatives about nursing?
14. Are you doing too much? Parties? Cleaning house?
15. Are you getting enough sleep? Napping off and on during the day? Taking baby to bed with you at night so as not to lose sleep?
16. Do you give your baby a pacifier? If so, throw it out!
17. Do you treat sore nipples thoroughly and carefully?
18. Can you rule out anything the baby is eating or being given other than nursing? Most babies under six months need be on breast milk only. The less to interfere with mother-baby relationship, the better.

Sometimes what seems to be two or three separate infections is really the same one which has begun to disappear and then pops up again because the mother hasn't continued to take care of herself.

Breast Abscess

On rare occasions, a breast infection will develop into an abscess. This is much less likely to happen if the infection is treated promptly. An abscess is a localized infection which requires incision and drainage of the surrounding pus. If the incision is outside the part of the breast which comes into contact with baby's mouth while he is nursing, and there is no drainage, he may be able to continue nursing on the infected side. Otherwise, you can keep nursing on the "good" side and hand expressing on the affected side while it's draining, to keep it empty. If you're hand expressing the milk, it will probably be only a few days until you can resume nursing on that side.

Mothers' experiences with breast abscesses vary. Some doctors place the patient under local anesthetic and incise and drain the abscess in their offices or in the emergency room of a hospital, while others hospitalize the woman and operate under general anesthetic. Sometimes, if the abscess is large, a small tube is inserted to drain the infected material from inside the breast. Sometimes the incision and drainage must be done several times. The time of healing varies, but it tends to be a long process.

Lumps in Breast

Fibrocystic Disease

In fibrocystic disease, cysts (lumps) and/or fibrous or hard benign growths form within the breast tissue.

Many mothers wondering whether they can breastfeed with fibrocystic disease of the breasts have turned to La Leche League International's Professional Advisory Board for advice. The board feels that breastfeeding is beneficial and that it will give relief from the symptoms. The symptoms mothers report are tenderness and soreness of the breasts that increases before or during menstruation and the presence of small pea-sized cysts. There is none of the redness, fever, or "sick" feeling that sometimes accompanies a breast infection. If you have this condition, you can plan to nurse for as long as you and the baby wish. The longer the better, the advisory board feels.

Benign Tumors

Many mothers have successfully breastfed after undergoing surgery to remove benign tumors. When Nancy discovered a large lump in her right breast near the armpit, surgery was decided upon to confirm that the tumor was benign. Nancy wrote:

> I did not want to be separated from four-month-old Bonnie, so the doctor suggested I have the surgery done under a local anesthetic. Three and a half hours later, when I returned home, Bonnie nursed. She was too young to grab the breast or pull at the bandage and was fairly still. The doctor had bandaged the entire breast for the first 24 hours which made it impossible to nurse her on that side unless I pulled the bandage back. I asked the doctor how he expected me to nurse this way and he in-

formed me that he preferred I did not nurse on that side until the drainage tube was taken out. I told him I felt that not emptying the breast might lead to engorgement which would lead to plugged ducts, possible breast infection and torn stitches. He gave me permission to pull back the bandage from the breastbone as long as I didn't interfere with the stitches. I did this and everything went very well. The baby's face got stuck in the tape a few times, but all the problems were minor.

Shari discovered a tumor in her right breast when her daughter was 17 months old and still nursing. She says:

The surgeon wanted to dry me right up—because he had never cut on a productive breast. Well, nothing doing! The doctor soon saw that I would not wean my daughter and not only agreed to the operation, but admitted me late Friday and arranged for the baby to come in for nursings. Saturday at 9:00 A.M. a benign tumor the size of a walnut was removed and a drain put in. At 11:00 A.M. I nursed my baby on that side. The doctor released me Sunday morning.

Bleeding from Breasts

The most common cause of bleeding from the nipples is a little crack in the nipple itself. This is usually sore and can be easily treated. (See Treatment for Sore Nipples, earlier in this chapter.)

Bleeding from within the breast is much less common and is usually painless. It is most often due to bleeding from a benign tumor called an intraductal papilloma and the bleeding usually ceases soon after lactation is established. Much rarer causes include other tumors (benign and malignant) and a variety of inflammatory conditions. In all cases, since such bleeding could be a sign of some serious disorder, it should be brought to the prompt attention of a doctor.

Melissa experienced a disconcerting situation for which no explanation was ever found. During the fourth month of her pregnancy with twins, her breasts started bleeding from the inside. Her doctor could not explain it and said under the circumstances she could not breastfeed. After the twins were delivered she had "dry-up shots." Melissa continued bleeding quite badly from both breasts, especially the right one. The doctor could not explain this, but eventually it stopped.

Melissa describes what happened when she became pregnant four years later:

> I was really interested in breastfeeding, and was excited when I passed my fourth month with no bleeding. At the end of my fifth month my right breast began to bleed. I immediately consulted a surgeon who thought that perhaps there were small tumors in my breasts which had become aggravated by my pregnancy. He said that an exploratory should probably be done, but not until after I had the baby. Breastfeeding was out as long as the breast continued to bleed.
>
> I was given dry-up shots after Brandy was delivered, but was still leaking colostrum when he was a week old. Since the bleeding had stopped, I decided to try and nurse him. I nursed him fifteen minutes on each side, no blood. At the next nursing, my right breast bled, so again I resigned myself to the fact that I would not be able to breastfeed.
>
> When Brandy was three weeks old, I noticed that I still had colostrum and no bleeding. I decided to try it again and the baby nursed like he'd been doing it all along.

Melissa experienced no more bleeding. She worked to build up her milk supply and treated the sore nipples. In less than three weeks, Brandy was completely nursed.

Cosmetic Breast Surgery

Silicone Implants and Injections

La Leche League International's Professional Advisory Board has been contacted by several mothers wondering whether they can nurse if they have silicone implants. The professional advisors have replied that the presence of silicone sacs implanted under the surface of the breasts will not affect nursing. Breast lobular and ductal tissue is not removed or cut across during implantation. The professional advisors feel, judging from their experience, that plugged ducts and breast infections are no more likely to occur in mothers who have had silicone implants than in those who have not. Nor do they feel that lactation would cause the sac to become detached and move within the breast.

Silicone injections into the breast are a different story. These probably interfere with lactation. A knowledgeable surgeon with whom I checked said that this procedure, which is now illegal throughout parts of the United States, incites an inflammatory response in the breast. The scarring secondary to the inflammation probably would cause such significant changes around the breast lobules and ducts that lactation and nursing would be difficult and possibly painful.

If you have had such injections and wish to nurse, you might try it. If the injections prevent you from attaining a *full* supply of milk, you might still be able to nurse your baby, as do some adoptive mothers who are not able to achieve a full milk supply. (See chapter 15, "Inducing or Reestablishing Your Milk Supply.")

If you are just in the stages of considering such surgery, and do plan to nurse a child in the future, perhaps a padded bra would do for now. It is certainly the safest course of action.

Reduction Mammoplasties

If you have had large breasts whose size was surgically reduced by removing the fat, you probably can nurse successfully. Unless significant amounts of secretory tissue were removed or several major mammary ducts transected, lactation will be normal. It's a good idea to tell your surgeon, before the operation, that you plan to nurse in the future.

Your Cheering Squad

Many mothers mentioned in this chapter nursed through unusual and difficult breast and nipple problems. Sometimes they did not even have the support of their own physicians, but they did have a great deal of determination and conviction that what they were doing was right for themselves and their babies. They kept the dialogue open with their doctors and, in the end, many of the doctors became "believers," too.

Many mothers have mentioned the importance of their husbands' encouragement during difficult times. Let your husband know that breastfeeding *is* important to you and gain his support. He can bolster your confidence a lot. He can help you in your dialogue with the doctor.

The support of breastfeeding friends can help your determination if it wavers. You can find the La Leche League group nearest you by checking local newspapers for announcements of meetings; by contacting a pediatrician; or by writing to La Leche League International (see address in Appendix: Organizations to Help the Nursing Mother). The leader may be able to check a Special Circumstances file to find a person you could visit or correspond with who has nursed under circumstances similar to yours.

Chapter 5

Nursing after
a Cesarean Childbirth

There have been many misconceptions and fears associated with cesarean birth and with breastfeeding after having a baby by cesarean. This type of birth *can* be the cause of certain discomforts and inconveniences for a mother. However, the surgery itself will not ultimately affect your milk supply, let-down reflex, the length of time it takes your milk to "come in," or the baby's desire to nurse. There are, in fact, certain benefits to be derived from breastfeeding after having a cesarean birth and these will be discussed later in the chapter.

Why a Cesarean?

There are many reasons why a cesarean may be performed. The baby may be too large to be born vaginally. The mother may be diabetic or have toxemia. She may have delivered a previous child by cesarean. Labor may be prolonged and ineffectual. The baby may be in distress or in such a position in the uterus that it is impossible for him to be born safely through the vagina. The umbilical cord or placenta may be situated so that the entrance of the fetus's head into the vagina would cause bleeding or an interruption in the flow of oxygen (placenta previa) or a premature separation of the placenta (abruptio placenta). Although a cesarean delivery may be anticipated before labor, this surgery is often an emergency procedure.

Types of Incisions

Cesarean is a surgical procedure in which a baby is delivered through an incision made in the walls of the abdomen and the uterus. In the past, a vertical or "classical" incision was made from the pubic bone to the navel. Now, a low horizontal "smile" or "bikini" incision is usually made. With this low cervical incision there is less postoperative involvement with "afterpains"—it's easier to have baby resting on your stomach —and the uterus is less vulnerable to future stress. Also, the scar is not noticeable when the pubic hair grows back, an important psychological plus for many women.

Once a Cesarean, Always a Cesarean?

If you deliver by cesarean, will you have to have all subsequent babies in this manner? Not necessarily. Some women have had vaginal deliveries following cesareans. It depends on several factors, including reasons for the previous cesarean, type of incision, and circumstances of the later pregnancy. You may want to speak to several doctors about the possibility of having a vaginal delivery after having had a cesarean since opinions and situations vary. It is certainly possible, but not in all cases.

Cesareans and the
Nursing Relationship

Having a baby by cesarean should not have any *long-term* effect on your nursing relationship. Nursing problems as such are likely to be secondary to baby-problems and mother-problems caused by the surgery.

Will Baby Have Problems?

Many cesarean babies are premature. This may mean pumping your milk, supplementary bottle feedings, trips down to the special care nursery, and lots of extra worry.

If you have a general anesthetic, the baby may be sleepy and may not suck well initially. He may nurse for a minute, just long enough to get a little warm milk down him, and then fall asleep. One hour later he may want to nurse again. You really have two options if the baby sucks sluggishly: you can try to keep him awake long enough to get a good-sized feeding, or you can nurse him frequently but for short periods for a day or so until the anesthetic has worn off and his suck is stronger.

Will Mother Have Problems?

What are problems other cesarean mothers have encountered? For one thing, there may be a delay in the start of nursing if the baby is in a special care nursery. Mother has had major surgery and will have some incisional pain and other discomforts. She may need a recovery time from anesthesia, so nursing may get off to a slower start.

Advantages

On the other hand, some mothers believe there is an even better chance to get a good start on nursing after a cesarean birth because of the long days in bed after the operation, with nothing else to do but nurse the baby. Karolyn, who had twins, says:

> I found that my recovery was much more rapid after having the twins by cesarean than when I'd had my first baby, vaginally. Of course, I was a more experienced mother by then, but I've always thought that the rest in the hospital made a big difference, too. You can talk about taking it easy at home all you want, but when you have newborn twins and a 19-month-old son, there isn't much taking it easy to be done.

Some mothers feel that their milk comes in sooner because they must rest so much more and must drink an abundant amount of fluids. Certainly your milk will come in at least as quickly as after a vaginal delivery *if* the baby is with you and has total access to the breast. The misinformation concerning the milk supply is incredible: I know of one professional who told a mother that cesarean mothers don't make milk!!

Many cesarean mothers have found that nursing fills a psychological need—a need which they often did not expect. Nancy Cohen, co-founder of C/SEC (Cesareans/Support, Education and Concern), has corresponded with thousands of mothers who, like herself, have had cesarean deliveries. Nancy says:

> Many times there are disappointments and angers and fears that accompany an operative delivery. Many women feel an intense *loss* of their babies. They feel that their infants have been taken from them, rather than having the feeling of giving birth. Breastfeeding often helps lessen the depression that follows many Cesarean births, bringing women closer to their babies and making mothers feel that although their bodies "failed them" (as they perceive it) in the capacity to deliver their babies, at least they function properly and can give the best that they have to their infants by successful nursing.

Multiple factors influence a woman's reaction to a cesarean delivery, including her (and her husband's) preconceived views about birth, and the reason for the cesarean. Anne, whose first baby was born by cesarean, shares her reaction:

> I never considered having a cesarean and it was very hard for me to accept. My husband and I had planned on as perfect and natural a birth as possible, with Richard helping to deliver the baby, no drugs, a Leboyer birth in a darkened room with a water bath, and my nursing on the delivery table. But everything turned out wrong—and it was all so uncomfortable, unnatural, and sterile. I felt cheated, gypped out of the best part of having a baby, and if I hadn't been able to nurse I think my world would have fallen apart. Nursing brought body contact, warmth, and reality to me and to my son, for he was the one experiencing the bright lights and having to be put in the inten-

sive care nursery right away. To be able to nurse him made me feel like a woman again.

Almost all the cesarean mothers who wrote to me remarked that in addition to the psychological benefits, breastfeeding helped them physically. Nursing helps you get back into shape faster by stimulating the uterus to contract and revert to its normal size. Nursing makes the recovery time easier, lets you feel your time in the hospital isn't wasted, and is a tremendous way to conserve energy. One mother, in looking beyond her hospital stay, said:

There were many people and nurses who thought I should coddle myself and let someone else feed the baby, but I knew that once the week was up and I was home—it was *my* business! Then *I* would be sterilizing bottles—and no thanks.

If Yours Is a Planned Cesarean

If you know that you will be delivering your baby by cesarean, there are some things you should do ahead of time. Talk with your doctor. Be sure you understand why you will need the surgery—it will help you psychologically. Discuss the various kinds of anesthesia and the advantages of each. Find out your doctor's attitudes concerning breastfeeding in this situation. You may want to talk about first going into labor. It may be psychologically (and physiologically) helpful. Contact your hospital; find out its policies regarding nursing on the operating table, nursing in recovery, nursing with a fever, etc. Can any of these policies be changed or bent if you are adamant and concerned? (See Hospital Policies and Doctors' Attitudes in this section.)

Get yourself ready physically. You'll want to prepare your nipples and maybe practice hand expression of colostrum. (See the discussion of nipple care in chapter 1, "What's Normal?," and Expressing Your Milk in chapter 2, "Nursing Techniques.") If you're in good health going into the delivery, it really helps.

Many mothers feel that the Lamaze physical conditioning seems to speed their bodies' return to normalcy. Certainly the total body relaxation will help ease the postpartum discomfort. See Bonnie Donovan's book, *The Cesarean Birth Experience* (1) for more exercises to ease postpartum discomfort.

You're going to be in the hospital for a while. Stock up on reading material, maybe a needlework kit. How about writing the birth announcements? Visit with other new mothers. And of course, rest and care for your baby.

What Do You Need to Know about Anesthetics?

Cesarean deliveries are generally performed under either general or spinal anesthetic. General anesthetic will almost certainly be used if your cesarean is a true emergency. It is much faster to administer and more easily controlled than a spinal. You will not be conscious during the delivery and will "wake up" in the recovery room or back in your own hospital room.

With a general anesthetic, it is not possible to nurse on the delivery table and your baby may nurse sluggishly the first time he's brought to you, because he will receive a certain amount of the anesthetic via the placenta. You may find that you have a sore throat for a day or so. (This is because there are tubes inserted down the throat to administer the anesthetic.) You may feel "dragged out" for several hours after leaving the recovery room, but should be out of bed and walking a bit a few hours after delivery.

It is possible to have your cesarean baby delivered with spinal or epidural anesthetic. You should discuss this possibility with your doctor ahead of time if you really feel strongly about being awake for delivery. Being conscious will increase your chances of nursing the baby soon after birth and may be especially important if you have prepared yourself for an "awake and aware" delivery. You should know though, that there is a chance of developing a spinal headache from this type of anesthetic. Although it is not serious,

115

the headache may prove to be uncomfortable for a while.

If you have a spinal, it's good to nurse before the anesthetic wears off so you can concentrate on a good, first-time meeting with your baby—before you're feeling the effects of the surgery.

One mother told me that she nursed 3½ hours after delivery, quite comfortably, lying on her side and assisted by a nurse.

Most hospitals routinely put babies born by cesarean into isolation for 24 to 48 hours. *This does not mean there is anything wrong with your baby.* Many hospitals are rethinking this in terms of new literature on bonding, imprinting, and the importance of early contact. Healthy, full-term cesarean infants are now going right to their parents' arms in many hospitals and can begin rooming-in as soon as requested.

Hospital Policies and Doctors' Attitudes

What about hospital policies? Are they ironclad? Do they truly fit the individual situation? Is there an administrator to whom you can present your case? Will he listen and come to a reasonable decision with you?

Policies do vary among hospitals and the rules are not necessarily inflexible. Anna, in comparing her first two deliveries, both by cesarean, says:

Fortunately for me, when our first baby was born I was in a hospital that treated birth as an exciting experience and the surgery as a minor part of it all. When our second child was born, it was at an old hospital where surgical deliveries were viewed as major problems. We were expected to remain in bed for several days, and nursing was out of the question. However, having already been through the experience, I had only a moment's hesitation before putting my daughter to my breast. She knew just what to do. The nursery nurse was so upset when the bottles went back full after every feeding and the baby slept for hours. The pediatrician didn't know what to advise as he had never had to handle a nursing mother after a cesarean. The obstetrician said okay since I had done fine with our first child. But the rule remained in effect for others.

Supportive doctors and hospitals can make the cesarean experience a better one. Your attitude is important in eliciting a positive response from them. "I want to be able to nurse my baby on the operating table or in the recovery room. I know mothers who have. What suggestions can you give to achieve this goal?" nets better results than, "Is it okay if I nurse my baby after he's born?" A C/SEC Newsletter (2) suggests that if any of the following are important to you, discuss them with your doctor and hospital. All of these *are* possible at many hospitals across the country.

I would like to . . .

have my husband with me for the birth and in recovery.

nurse the baby in the operating room.

have a "bikini" (low cervical) incision and dissolvable stitches.

have complete rooming-in.

have a close friend or relative with me (when father is not available) to help with the care of the baby those first days.

have the baby for night feedings, too.

have no extra pre-op medication.

be awake throughout the entire procedure.

have a cesarean roommate.

have an electrically operated bed.

see my other children while I am in the hospital.

have the baby "judged on its own merit" (eliminate or shorten the time a cesarean baby has to be in the special care nursery for observation).

come to the hospital the day of the cesarean so I can spend the night before at home with my family (have the preliminary tests done on an out-patient basis the day before or just prior to the birth).

go into labor before having the cesarean done.

have a trial delivery with the hope of delivering vaginally.

Some mothers, armed with a combination of knowledge, diplomacy and tenacity, have succeeded in persuading hospitals to rethink their policies. For example, at the Boston Hospital for Women, there are now several changes in what originally was "hospital policy" concerning cesarean deliveries. These include: husbands in the operating room and recovery room with the consent of the attending obstetrician; cesarean roommates; establishment of rooming-in as soon as possible (no mandatory observation period for cesarean baby in the special care nursery); and sibling visitation. This last point is very important to a cesarean mother and her children since they are separated for more than the usual number of days after delivery.

With an unplanned cesarean and no time to make any arrangements ahead of time, you still should be able to obtain some concessions from the hospital after the birth, if you request them. One mother says she began nursing 7 hours after surgery, but only after strong insistence and calls to the pediatrician. Another mother wrote that they weren't going to allow her the baby until 24 hours postpartum, but she said, "I kicked up a fuss with my obstetrician and he fussed too— to good effect, as I was allowed to have my baby at 12 hours and again at 15 hours."

Sometimes, doctors have not previously encountered a cesarean mother who wants to nurse her baby. They may try to protect you from "extra work," thinking that they're helping you to rest more and recover faster from your surgery. Your doctor needs to put medical considerations first, of course. However, he should be willing to take your feelings into consideration wherever possible. One mother delivered three babies by cesarean and nursed them all. She told me that "the obstetrician was not favorable toward breastfeeding, but I feel he responded to my evident need to breastfeed by at least not discouraging me."

After the Birth

You will find after surgery that you're physically weakened. You may have to force yourself to get moving, depending on the amount of pain. You're also probably tired and maybe a little nauseated. If you've had a general anesthetic, in order to prevent pneumonia and improve circulation, it's important that you move from side to side as much as possible, breathe deeply and cough deeply several times an hour postoperatively.

Coughing is easier said than done. We normally use our abdominal muscles to cough and those are going to be sore. You'll want to brace your abdomen so that you don't feel everything is falling out when you cough. You can do this by holding a pillow tightly against your abdomen when you cough. Or you can brace it with a towel. Fold it by taking hold of opposite corners. Pull tightly across your abdomen and hold it in place by pulling on the corners to ease the strain on those abdominal muscles.

Walk as much as you can, and gradually increase your time and distance each time. Walking helps you get back into shape quickly. Walk after nursing the baby, not before, so as not to get overtired while nursing.

As mentioned earlier, breastfeeding stimulates the uterus to contract and revert to its normal size. These uterine contractions, while important, may be painful for you. If they are, ask your doctor about safe analgesics he can prescribe. There is medication that will not adversely affect the baby and will help you move about and take care of your baby sooner. As Jane said:

> Without the medication, getting to my door was unbearable. With it I could walk down the hall without undue stress. Early walking means early return to strength. So don't try to do without medication to be brave. You'll do better for your baby, your milk and your strength by taking the medication when you need it in the first couple of days or so.

Nursing Tips

Because of post-op dehydration and because you're breast-feeding, you need to drink lots of fluids. You can drink liquids while still on I.V.

Hospital policy often dictates that nursing be stopped while mother has a fever. It's common (and normal) to run a low-grade fever after surgery. It's not necessarily cause for alarm and *not* necessarily *reason* to separate mother and baby. Also, engorged breasts can give you a low-grade fever. Ask to be allowed to feed your baby more frequently and see if this doesn't make the fever go down. If the staff is reluctant, ask that you and your baby be isolated *together*.

Until you are allowed to nurse, pump or hand express your milk every three to four hours. The hospital may have a breast pump you can use, or you may want to consider renting one. If you have abdominal clips, wait until they are taken out and then take cool showers when your breasts begin to feel tender. If they are very engorged, put warm compresses on them and then, gently, express enough milk to make yourself comfortable.

At first it will be hard for you to lift your baby and to move him from one breast to the other. Ask for help, not just in moving the baby, but for instruction in how to do it yourself by keeping your abdominal muscles limp and using your shoulder and back muscles to lift.

Keep the side rails on that bed up! Use them to help you move around in bed or switch sides during nursing. To change sides: Gently roll over onto your back. Change baby to the other side or put him on your chest and hold him with one hand. You'll get better momentum for turning if you swing your leg over your body (gently!) as you're starting to move, then use your arm and shoulder muscles to pull yourself over. Make a conscious effort to keep your abdominal muscles relaxed. If your baby came over to the other side on your chest, this gentle roll will often be enough to burp him!

You can also nurse without switching baby by nursing lying down and rolling your body slightly more towards the baby so that you can offer him the other (upper) breast. Leaning on the guard rail and using a pillow or two may be helpful. See also Comfortable Nursing Positions in chapter 2, "Nursing Techniques," for other positions to try.

But how do you nurse your baby when his bottom half wants to snuggle up against your sore tummy? Jane needed a little help:

> I very, very gingerly turned to my side and the nurses helped position my legs with a rolled blanket supporting the upper leg. My baby was positioned at my side. I also found my electric bed helpful. I pushed the button to make the head rise and sat tailor-fashion on the bed to nurse. The baby was partly supported by my knees and I'd lean forward slightly so she wouldn't rest on my incision.*

Paula found a couple of solutions:

> It helps to sometimes hold baby in the "football hold" position (see illustration in chapter 18, "Nursing Twins") to keep him off your sore stomach. Or sit in a chair. . . . I found a pillow at each side (to help support my arms) and a pillow across the stomach helped a lot.

Sharyn had several problems:

> I couldn't hold my baby in the upright nursing position because of the weight and couldn't nurse her in the reclining position because of very small breasts and inverted nipples. My husband came to my aid. He rolled up the bed to a folded position (sitting with bent knees) and laid two pillows across my lap which distributed the baby's weight. It worked perfectly!

---

* An electric bed is a very important plus for cesarean mothers. Request one!

Many breastfed babies do not need to burp. If yours does, and you're nursing lying down, you need not sit up to burp your baby. Instead, gently roll him over onto your chest or onto his tummy on the bed and rub his back. If you nursed sitting up, sit him up, supporting his chin with your cupped hand. Then gently rub the top of his head. Crazy, but it works!

Rooming-In

If you're uncomfortable because of your surgery and feel "all washed out," are you going to want to have rooming-in? Many mothers who had planned on rooming-in after a normal delivery, still want it after a cesarean, perhaps even more so.

The start of rooming-in may depend to a certain extent on how you feel. Some mothers seem to have no interest in anything but sleeping for a while. Other mothers, though, have said that the baby's nursing was the only thing that gave them a sense of time, and having the baby close by helped take the focus off the surgery.

You may want to ask someone to stay with you in your room so you can room-in—your husband, a friend, or another relative.

Time will pass more quickly and more pleasurably with your baby there, ready for a little snack or just some cuddling. It's a great opportunity to really get going—learning about each other and establishing good nursing patterns.

At Home

Because you have had major surgery and you have a baby, you're not going to have quite as much stamina as you'd like once you get home. It's going to take a while for you to work out a routine. Arrange for help if you possibly can, at least for the first couple of weeks. The money you save by breastfeeding could easily pay for someone to help you a few hours a day.

All the hints that are suggested for first-time mothers go double for cesarean moms. The dust will wait. Have friends bring casseroles, not baby clothes, or offer to do laundry for

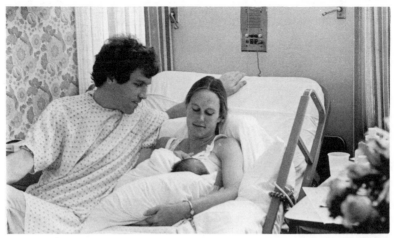

Sandra C. Wallace

Rooming-in is the perfect time for a father to become involved, if his schedule permits. He can be a real help with baby care, as he gets acquainted with his little one. Helping in this way can also lessen a father's disappointment at not being present for the birth.

you. Your doctor will most assuredly put a ban on lifting and housework; *listen to him!* La Leche League advises that you:

> Bear in mind that you have two very good reasons for lots of naps and bedrest. First, you are recovering from major surgery, and second, you're establishing a good milk supply. We emphasize that nursing in bed does much for both of these objectives. (3)

Some mothers put the baby beside their bed so they can easily nurse on demand. One mother told me she had a backrest next to the bed, which she used for night nursings.

Keeping the baby in bed with you eliminates lifting altogether. Even seven pounds can seem like a ton at first! Put a tall glass with ice cubes by your bed before you go to sleep. When you wake up at 2:00 or 3:00 A.M., it will have melted but still be cold and thirst-quenching. (Or, you can use a large Thermos.) Put diapers, and a snack, by the bed.

Your Cheering Squad

Where can you get physical and psychological help and support when you need it? Your husband can be your most valuable source. By helping you he is caring for both you and his baby. Dinner may not taste quite the same and the towels may not be folded so that they fit on the shelf exactly right, but all he needs is time. When you and the baby have "had it" at the same time, let Dad be the one to do the cuddling and cooing—to both of you!

If you're not feeling well, or have questions you think your doctor can answer, call him. Give him the chance to be compassionate and offer some support. He can also refer you to others who might be able to help.

A La Leche League leader is equipped with a lot of information. She can refer you to others who have had the same sorts of problems.

You may also want to get in touch with C/SEC. This organization was formed by two mothers, Nancy Cohen and Jini Fairley, both of whom had cesarean deliveries with their first babies and subsequently had vaginal deliveries with their second babies. These mothers felt there was a lack of information, education and understanding existing in the area of cesarean childbirth. See Appendix: Organizations to Help the Nursing Mother for information on contacting C/SEC.

Chapter 6

Nursing a Premature Baby

When your baby arrives weeks or even months before you expected him, you may feel the happiness of motherhood and at the same time experience shock, anxiety, and concern for his welfare.

There are many degrees of prematurity. Most premature babies are almost as developed as full-term babies, while some are so tiny and weak that their very survival is in doubt. Neva's baby weighed only 3 pounds, 5 ounces at birth. "I remember holding his head in my hand and being able to wrap my fingers and thumb around his head and face to shield his eyes. His cries turned into sighs of relief when I stroked his little face and talked softly to him."

A baby's size is not always related to his ability to nurse, and some three-pounders are able to breastfeed. Even though you may have to wait until your baby develops a strong sucking response, eventually he will be able to breastfeed.

Maintaining your milk supply until the baby can breastfeed may seem lonely and depressing. It does take determination and patience. However, following the weeks of uncertainty and inconvenience come months of happiness and satisfaction.

Special Benefits of Breastfeeding

Premature babies benefit from breastfeeding in many ways. Ideally, a baby is reunited with his mother immediately after birth. After some premature births, the baby is kept in an incubator and may be separated from his mother for weeks. The closeness and stimulation of breastfeeding are extremely important to these infants.

Premature infants are particularly vulnerable to infection and disease. Colostrum, the thick, yellowish milk present in the breasts when you give birth, is particularly rich in antibodies which protect your infant against infections. It contains almost six times as much protein as the later milk, and has scant amounts of the fats and carbohydrates which are not as easily digested by a newborn. Rich in vitamin E, colostrum helps the body maintain healthy red blood cells. This is especially important to premature babies who suffer from hemolysis (the separation of the oxygen-carrying component, hemoglobin, from the red cells).

Colostrum and breast milk are far more easily digested than any formula. In formula, there are larger curds which are more difficult for a baby's digestive system and kidneys to pass off as waste.

According to Dr. John D. Michael, a pediatrician who has worked with many premature babies at the Ross Valley Medical Clinic in Greenbrae, California:

> Breast milk has been shown to be the best nourishment for a premature infant. Studies done in England, the United States, and other countries convincingly show that in a premature infant with an immature digestive system including immature absorption, as well as immature enzyme systems, human milk is the most compatible and most efficiently utilized substance available. In other words, human milk is the nourishment of first choice for premature infants.

Human milk is especially important to premature babies because it contains high amounts of the amino acid cystine, an important component of protein. Premature babies lack the specific enzyme which is necessary to form cystine from another amino acid, methionine. Until their enzyme systems complete development, these babies must obtain their cystine directly from the food they consume. Among all sources of animal protein, human milk contains the most cystine. Cow's milk, meat, and other animal proteins have some, but they also contain large amounts of methionine which place extra metabolic stress on the nonbreastfed baby.

Human milk also contains many nucleotides, which are needed to form protein. Cow's milk contains some nucleotides, but they are mainly of one type, while human milk is rich in a wide variety.

Studies by B. D. Corner, author of "The Premature Infant" (1), show that the mortality rate from one month to six months is less for breastfed than for artificially fed premature infants. Other research indicates that the macrophages (cells which ingest foreign particles) contained in *raw* breast milk may prevent a very serious disease of high-risk premature babies, necrotizing enterocolitis, which affects a baby's intestines. Formulas do not contain these macrophages; they are present only in fresh human milk. (2)

Recognizing these advantages, some hospitals maintain a milk bank and routinely give all premature babies breast milk whether or not the mother plans to nurse.

Support of Doctor and Hospital Staff

How can you nurse a baby who is not yet able to suck? Can you maintain an adequate milk supply while you wait for him to develop a strong enough reflex to breastfeed?

First, try to surround yourself with people who will encourage you. One "doubting Thomas" can undermine your confidence. *Tell* (don't ask) your doctors and nurses that you are going to breastfeed. You must convey your determination to them. Make arrangements for the baby to receive your breast milk even if he cannot breastfeed right away. Discuss the advantages of colostrum and the studies mentioned in this chapter. Explain how much *you* can do to care for your baby even while he is in an incubator, such as touching, feeding, and diapering him.

Your doctor and the hospital staff may be surprised by your requests if they have never made such arrangements for premies before. This will be a good time for them to start. You can mention what happens at the St. Francis Premature and High Risk Nursery Center in Peoria, Illinois, one of the best centers in the nation for the care of premature babies. After routine admitting procedures are completed, parents may enter the nursery to see and touch their infant. The center has found these "touching" visits important for the baby and both parents. As the baby progresses, his parents are able to hold and feed him. A room is provided for breastfeeding mothers. Small, sterilized bottles are supplied for the mothers to bring their expressed breast milk to the hospital. The hospital suggests placing the bottles in an ice-packed, insulated container, such as a Thermos or picnic ice container. This milk is given to the baby through a tube or special nipple. As soon as the infant is strong enough to suck, regardless of his weight, the mother may begin breastfeeding. In the first attempts to breastfeed, a baby naturally tires easily. Breast and bottle feedings may be alternated temporarily. However, to avoid development of lazy sucking habits, total breastfeeding is encouraged as soon as possible.

Temporary Substitutes for Mother's Breast

If your baby is unable to breastfeed at first, he will receive his nourishment by dropper, spoon, or stomach tube. Bottles should be avoided if possible. While addressing a physicians' symposium in 1974 on the subject of breastfeeding and the premature infant, Dr. Richard Boette emphasized that it is most important that the baby not be given a rubber nipple. This confuses his sucking instinct and makes nursing at the breast much more difficult for him to learn.

Maintaining Your Milk Supply

If your baby is unable to nurse, start expressing your milk as soon as possible. Remember how valuable even a small

amount of colostrum is to him. Even if you have been expressing your milk regularly, you may have some engorgement when
the baby finally begins to nurse. This can be discouraging and
frustrating for both of you. He has to learn how to get hold of
the nipple. Since his sucking reflex may not be fully developed,
try expressing some milk before each feeding so that your
breasts are softer. Express some milk into your baby's mouth to
encourage him to suck, and guide your nipple into his mouth.

If you are told that nursing your baby is impossible because
he is not allowed out of the nursery, you may be able to compromise. Marilyn persuaded her pediatrician to let her nurse
her baby in the nursery as long as he was weighed at each
nursing to see if "he got enough."

A baby who is receiving a formula supplement in addition
to breastfeeding would be better off getting a breast milk
supplement in a bottle. By expressing milk between breastfeeding sessions your own milk can be given. Expressing your
milk regularly will maintain your supply for weeks or even
months. Pump or hand express each breast for five to ten
minutes every two or three hours during the day, and perhaps
once during the night. Or, you may find that if you sleep
through the night you'll have more milk because you are
rested. Often mothers discover their milk supply is greater
than baby needs. Try to keep it that way. Remember, his
needs will increase, and once your baby is home and nursing
frequently your milk supply will adjust.

Of course, pumping and expressing are *not* as satisfying
as nursing. "I remember thinking how easy it would be to sit
down every few hours and pump each breast," says Andrea.
"But during this waiting time I did get depressed, as my milk
supply seemed to diminish daily. Emotionally, pumping is a
long way from nursing a baby." These feelings are entirely
normal and eventually fade away. Even mothers of full-term
babies may experience periodic feelings of depression, the
"postpartum blues."

The waiting can be tough. It's hard to go home from the
hospital without your baby. It's a time of emptiness. By

expressing milk for your baby, you are really doing something important for him. "After all," says Grace:

> It seemed just about the only thing I could do for this tiny bit of life who had come into the world so prematurely and looked so small and helpless. It's a strange thing to gaze at your baby through a nursery window and know that it will be many more weeks before you are allowed to hold her in your arms; supplying the nourishment that nature intended for her seemed to make the waiting a bit more bearable.

Relactation

Even if you have been given "dry-up" medication, you can stimulate your milk production. Fern had twins, two months premature, one of whom survived and weighed just over 2 pounds. Fern had wanted to breastfeed but, thinking she couldn't, had taken "dry-up" pills at the hospital. A month later she became convinced that she could still breastfeed and that it would be the very best thing she could do. Fern explains how she built up her milk supply:

> I obtained an electric breast pump when Valerie was almost two months old. I did manage to get a few drops that first day, but I was very discouraged. I wondered what in the world I was trying to do, but kept pumping. I just couldn't stop yet; I had made some progress and the pump was far from easy to come by (we drove 125 miles to get it). In a few days I was increasing by an ounce a day.
>
> Five days after I started, my doctor said I should begin nursing in the hospital. This was really traumatic for me, because my supply wasn't up to where I thought it should be. Valerie did nurse, but not very well at first. Gradually, as the days passed, she caught on.
>
> Twelve days after I had started breastfeeding in the hospital, Valerie came home. I was so frightened. I had read that I should nurse her almost constantly for a couple

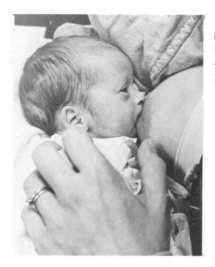

It may take some time for your premature baby to build his sucking response. Once he begins, the sucking will stimulate your milk production.

of days in order to increase my supply, but she was very sleepy. I had to waken her every three hours for nursing. I was afraid I didn't have enough milk. In fact, I had too much! The fact that she had colic also made me fear that I didn't have enough milk. As the weeks went by my confidence gradually increased. Valerie gained well and recovered from her colic by the time she was 4½ months old.

First Hospital Feeding

For many mothers who have been expressing breast milk for their premature babies, the long-awaited chance to breast-feed is met with a mixture of relief, happy anticipation, and apprehension. A mother can react this way to a first opportunity to bottlefeed, too.

One mother, Leona, who had been pumping to maintain her milk supply for 14 days, says:

When I was finally allowed to touch and bottlefeed my baby for the first time, I had to scrub my hands and put on a gown and mask. I was frustrated after 45 minutes, during which Laurel Ann drank just an ounce from the bottle.

I really had my doubts as to her ability to breastfeed if she couldn't even get the milk with a special premie nipple.

Two days later Laurel Ann went home and eventually learned to breastfeed very well.

Neva's first hospital feeding with her baby was breastfeeding. She says:

Three days before Jarret came home, I was allowed to come to the hospital for two nursings a day to see if he would nurse and gain weight on breast milk. I was extremely nervous at first. It felt too good to be true—just to hold him in my arms. The nurse watched to see if he would take hold. I coaxed, but it wasn't until he yawned that I was able to get the areola well into his mouth. He looked puzzled, then began to suck. The nurse couldn't believe it! Two more nurses came in to watch. One said as she left the room laughing, "That baby takes to that breast like he was born attached to it."

Let your doctor know how strongly you feel about breastfeeding your baby as soon as he can be out of the incubator for short periods. Even if your baby doesn't get one drop of milk, his contact with you is very important to his development.

Being calm and relaxed when you go into the hospital for your first breastfeeding may be more easily said than done. The nurses may hand you a surgical gown (which you'll have to wear backwards) and usher you and your sleepy baby into a closet-sized hallway saying, "You'll have 15 minutes." The rest is up to you. If a comfortable armchair is not provided, ask if one is available. If you want help, let the nurse know. If you'd be more at ease alone, say so.

Andrea says she was uptight and fearful before her first nursing experience. She worried that there wouldn't be enough milk, that her baby might dehydrate, and that the hospital would not allow him to come home unless she bottlefed. She experienced no let-down and thought her baby received very little milk. Andrea called her obstetrician, who ordered a prescription for synthetic oxytocin, Syntocinon, a nasal spray to help the milk ejection reflex. "Psychologically," says Andrea, "it was a real boost. Seeing the milk reassured me." Your baby may be getting plenty of milk without your feeling a let-down. Some mothers who never notice a let-down are very successful at breastfeeding.

Babies react individually to nursing. Dena had premature twins, both under 4 pounds. When they were able to breast-feed for the first time, she said, "Heath (the stronger of the two) took to nursing like a duck to water, but Sarah needed coaxing to make the switch from bottle to breast."

Discharge from the Hospital

Traditionally, professionals caring for infants believed it was hazardous to let them leave the hospital if they weighed less than 5 or 5½ pounds. This has been successfully challenged many times, and now the theory is obsolete. Dr. Robert Berg, reporting on " 'Early' Discharge of Low Birthweight Infants" (3), says that infants weighing as little as 3 pounds, 9 ounces were discharged from the hospital and were compared with infants discharged at an average weight of 5 pounds, 5½ ounces. He concluded that early discharge did not increase the risk of morbidity or mortality. All infants were followed up for at least three months, and some of the group were followed up for longer periods, and all showed normal or accelerated weight gain and satisfactory development.

Perhaps if doctors adopted the criteria set down by Dr. Berg at Beth Israel Hospital, Boston, they would feel better about changing their thinking on this. Dr. Berg's criteria, as reported in *La Leche League News* (4), are as follows:

- Vital signs are stable and normal in room air.

- Significant abnormalities have been corrected or treated to the point of stability.

- Intake by bottle or breast is adequate and the mother has been successful in feeding her infant in the nursery.

- Parents have been instructed in all aspects of care and are judged to understand their instructions.

- Parents have made plans for post-discharge care by a physician in private practice or at a clinic.

- The home is physically and hygienically adequate.

- The mother, or a substitute, is well and wants to undertake full care of the infant.

Homecoming

The day you finally take your baby home will probably be a hectic one. Homecomings bring with them an air of excitement which is more tiring than you may realize, and it sometimes makes the baby fussy.

You and your baby have a lot of catching up to do. Now you can really get acquainted. Though the idea of massive doses of loving contact, especially skin-to-skin contact, may be strange and new to you, other mothers have found such special attention helpful and rewarding. Take your baby to bed with you. Hold your baby close, stroking from head to toe. Babies love being in the bathtub with you; they feel secure there and may recall the time in utero.

Some mothers are afraid to take their premature babies home because they are so tiny. Anna says:

> Even though David was my third baby I shook so much that I could hardly dress him to come home from the hospital. We had been kept apart 33 days and suddenly he was all my responsibility. Finally, I just wrapped him and the booties together in the blanket. I simply couldn't get them on. A neighbor had to cut his fingernails for months; I was afraid of slipping.

It is quite normal to feel this way, and it is a good reason to request more contact with your baby during his hospital stay. If hospital personnel can handle your baby, you can, too.

If your baby is exclusively bottlefed during his hospital stay, you may have to help him learn to nurse. Try putting your milk in an eyedropper and squirting it into a corner of your baby's mouth while he is at the breast. This will encourage him. You can hand express your milk until it lets down before putting the baby to your breast. This way, the milk will be there as soon as he starts to suck and he won't become impatient waiting for it or be overwhelmed by that first let-down. Some mothers use a nursing supplementer like Lact-Aid. (See Supplemental Food section in chapter 15, "Inducing or Reestablishing Your Milk Supply.") Of course, once he is beginning to accept the breast these things won't be necessary at all. Some honey on the nipples is sticky but may help. Use very little, as it may discourage your baby's appetite, or, as at least one mother claims, may give him gas. If you try it, remember substitutes should always be as temporary and sparingly used as possible.

If your baby doesn't seem to have a rooting reflex and doesn't automatically turn towards you to nurse, try stroking, rocking, and singing to him. Take off blankets, clothes, and diapers—anything to arouse his interest. If he always falls asleep early in the feeding try rubbing the soles of his feet or changing his position.

If you feel it is necessary to supplement your baby's feedings when you're first home, offer him breast milk *after* he has nursed. If you spoon feed the milk, your baby will turn to you for his normal sucking needs. You may find spoon feedings quite successful, and feel reassured that baby is getting enough. Gradually decrease the supplemental amount until you are nursing completely.

The idea of doing little else but nursing your baby probably sounds exhausting. Forget the housework. Your baby is more important than a little dust and clutter. Tuck your baby in bed with you so you can rest, even nap, while he alternately nurses and dozes. Limit visitors to those who will really help with care of the house and the older children, and will let you care for the baby. You and your baby need each other right now. If your baby seems fussy, remember the extra attention he receives will *not* "spoil" him, but may even produce a happier, better-adjusted child.

Newborn Concerns

Jaundice

Even normal newborn jaundice might be considered severe in premature babies. Breastfeeding can be important in helping to reduce the seriousness of jaundice. It provides the fluids needed to help rid baby's system of the jaundice-causing factors and supplies the proteins and nutrients needed to help stabilize his condition. Dr. V. Smallpiece and Dr. P. Davies have done a convincing study that promotes the practice of providing breast milk to a newborn premature baby as a preventive measure as well as for nutrition. They found that there was less hyperbilirubinemia (high amounts of bilirubin causing jaundice), and symptomatic hypoglycemia was prevented when premature babies were given breast milk immediately after birth. (5)

Allergies

If you and/or your husband have allergies, you will want to be sure your baby receives your breast milk while he is in the hospital. According to pediatric allergist Dr. Vincent A. Marinkovich, the immune system of premature babies is less well developed than babies who come to full term. Since allergic reactions are more likely to occur under the circumstances of reduced immunity, the premature infant runs a greater risk of developing allergies than his full-term counterpart.

Even if your doctor has left orders for breast milk only, you should talk with nurses caring for your baby. They may not know that *any* formula given now could lead to a baby's developing an allergy to cow's milk when it is reintroduced into his diet.

Contact with Your Baby

Studies have shown that early and frequent handling of newborns is important for them to develop in a healthy manner.

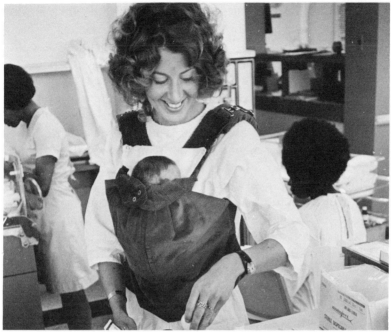

The Children's Hospital, Denver

Premature Baby Carrier

This premature baby is in a modified Snugli baby carrier. Hospitals using these are able to increase the amount of physical contact and stimulation for premature infants.

In his book, *Touching: The Human Significance of the Skin* (6), Ashley Montagu reports:

> There is good evidence that premature babies do much better when their mothers are allowed to handle them, after proper instruction in hand washing and gowning. Barnett and his co-workers at the Stanford University School of Medicine encouraged 41 mothers to handle their premature infants at any time of the day or night, with considerable benefit to everyone involved: infants, mothers, nurses and doctors. There was no increase in the much feared infections and no complications of any sort.

It may take some ingenuity on your part to communicate your love to your baby through touch if he is attached to life-measuring systems by wires and tubes. This was the case with Lane, born three months premature and weighing 3 pounds, ½ ounce. As reported in *La Leche League News* (7), Matir, Lane's mother, discovered she could roll Lane into a little ball with her right hand, put her left arm all the way into the Isolette, put Lane up onto that arm, and rock her. "The awkwardness was overcome by necessity," said Matir. "She *had* to know somehow that we loved her."

Breastfeeding was a necessity for Lane. She had not gained weight on formula, and when given a chance to nurse at three weeks she did indeed suck and gained 2½ ounces overnight. At four months she weighed a healthy 10 pounds.

When you first hold or stroke your baby, you may find very little response, or on the contrary, he may overrespond. There is a cycle of rest, activity, rest, activity that is typical for immature infants. In the rest period it is normal for him to be very sleepy, and seem unresponsive to you. During activity he may overrespond or tremble after just a mild touch. Don't worry, you aren't harming him. Continue your loving contact with your baby.

If the doctor wants your baby to be in the heated environment of the incubator, ask if an overhead lamp can be placed over your baby while you hold and nurse him. You'll feel more at ease with your baby when you bring him home if you've had opportunities for contact with him in the hospital. Otherwise a mother is apt to feel as if she is going through "adoption proceedings" with a strange, unfamiliar baby even though he is her own.

Baby carriers that hug the baby close to you (see Time and Energy Savers in chapter 2, "Nursing Techniques") can provide a premature baby with much additional sensory experience. Some hospitals use a modified Snugli carrier for their tiny patients, and the nurses find that restless, crying infants are lulled to sleep when nestled close. Hopefully mothers will soon be invited to comfort their own babies in hospitals.

Weight

It is normal for newborn babies to lose weight following birth. Whether breastfed or bottlefed, they usually regain their birth weight within one to three weeks. Naturally, there is special concern when a premie with a low birth weight loses weight. It may take him longer to regain his birth weight than a full-term baby because his digestive system is not fully developed.

If your doctor is doubtful about your breastfeeding successfully because your baby is so small, it may be helpful to share this story from *La Leche League News* (8) with him. Mari Kay's baby, Amanda, was born three months early, measuring just 13 inches and weighing 1 pound, 12 ounces. Mari Kay says:

> My heart really went out to our tiny baby whose will to live was so much greater than her size. So I asked if I could provide breast milk, thinking that this was one small thing that might help Amanda pull through.
>
> The nurses' and the obstetrician's first responses were quite negative. They felt that the whole process of providing milk before the baby could nurse was too complicated (or maybe they didn't expect the baby to survive and were thinking of me). However, Amanda's doctor was encouraging, and I decided to go ahead with my plans.
>
> I began expressing milk. At first I got only two ounces, but it was much more than Amanda could take. She had one cc. per hour by tube to her stomach (30 cc.'s equal one ounce). The hospital provided milk bottles which I filled, froze and returned to them. They would thaw and sterilize the milk just before use.*
>
> Amanda actually started nursing when she reached 3 pounds (she was two months old). This wasn't too suc-

---

* Research shows that fresh, raw breast milk is best because of the valuable nutrients and immunity factors. However, frozen or sterilized breast milk is always better than other substitutes.

cessful at first, and I was shaken by the thought that after all my efforts she would be unwilling to nurse.

When Amanda finally came home from the hospital, 2 months and 19 days after her birth, she nursed as though she had been doing it all along.

Death

Fear of losing a baby is understandable when you have a premature baby. Most premature babies live, but it takes some parents several months to feel secure enough to really relax and allow themselves the "luxury of loving."

However, some premature babies do not survive. Doctors, nurses, and parents react in different ways to breastfeeding an infant who may or may not live. Maria's premie was born with hyaline membrane disease. She was too exhausted to argue when the doctor said he was too small to nurse, so she agreed to an injection to dry up her milk.

Two days after delivery, Maria decided to try to breast-feed. With the help of a breast pump she expressed some colostrum the first day, and continued to produce a steady amount for her baby. Maria's son died when he was nine days old, and although she was never able to breastfeed Ricky, she at least had the satisfaction of knowing she had provided milk for her baby.

Maria writes about the loss of her son:

It is such agony to try to accept the death of your baby. There is no simple formula for dealing with it. You have such hopes for your child. You want a miracle so desperately.

The loss of a child cannot be equated with the death of a parent or spouse. A mother loves her child in a different way; when a baby dies, a part of the mother dies, too. Grieving is a process that cannot be set aside all at once. We go through stages gradually. At first denying the loss, I found myself thinking, "My baby's not dead. I can go to the hospital and see him." My denial stopped the day of Ricky's funeral. The finality of that tiny casket was overwhelming, and recovery from the initial stage of shock was gradual.

Day-by-day, normal routines became easier. Yet even now, 2½ years later, when I am alone with my memories, I cry for that part of me that I have lost. I will always be sad that Ricky died, but I can live with that.

Taking Care of Yourself

You will have a lot on your mind during the time your baby is in the hospital and may tend to pay little attention to your own needs. If you have had a cesarean birth or some complication, you may be physically weak. Your own recovery is important because your baby needs a strong, healthy mother. Remember that getting plenty of rest and an adequate diet is necessary for your good health and cheerful disposition. Consider hiring someone to watch your other children or to clean house. To avoid sore nipples remember proper care while baby is still in the hospital.

Later Concerns

Menstruation

With complete breastfeeding (no solids or supplements) for the first six months, the resumption of ovulation and the menstrual cycle is usually delayed for 7 to 15 months. However, Andrea says, "The six weeks of pumping before my baby came home did not provide enough stimulation to prevent menstruation. This increased my depression at the time. However, once we were nursing full-time, menstruation ceased until many months later."

Catching Up

Premature babies tend to catch up with their full-term counterparts in growth and development by age two. Most premature babies are not abnormal, just born early. All the vital organs and systems are present, and fairly well formed by the sixth month of pregnancy. It may encourage you to know that Isaac Newton, Voltaire, Charles Darwin, and Winston Churchill were all premature babies.

Solids

You might think that a premature baby will need solids sooner than a full-term baby. Actually, solids aggravate an immature digestive system. At her doctor's suggestion, Fern tried to feed her 10-week-old baby solids. No success. "So we forgot about the solids and I just nursed until Valerie was 5½ months old. Even at that age, we introduced solid foods very slowly."

Another mother who started her premature baby on solids at eight months says:

> My baby did all right with fruits and vegetables. When meats were introduced during his tenth month, he developed constipation. Luckily, my pediatrician was a supporter of breastfeeding and recommended taking him off solid foods and just nursing. At 11 months I gradually reintroduced solids with no further problem.

Our premature twins received only breast milk for 4½ months. When Karen started on solids, Sharon was content with only breast milk for another month.

Iron Supplement

Most breastfed premature babies never need an iron supplement. Breast milk prevents the anemia often associated with cow's milk formulas. Anemia may be associated with a lack of vitamin A, vitamin E, and/or iron. Vitamin E in mother's milk helps baby assimilate the trace amounts of iron in breast milk, plus any natural iron in solid foods started later.

Grace's doctor was about to prescribe iron for her 6-month-old baby (born 2½ months premature), when he realized that the baby was now eating banana and strained liver. Based on that, he decided the iron supplement wasn't necessary.

If you are concerned about iron count and delaying solids until your baby seems ready, a hemoglobin test may be the answer. On a doctor's request a lab technician takes one drop of blood from the baby's heel to be tested. The results are usually obtained in five minutes.

Weaning

After all you have overcome to breastfeed your premature baby, you may wonder how long he will continue nursing. There is a wide variation in ages of weaning for all babies. Our twins still nursed occasionally when they were two years old.

Andrea says:

> By 13 months Daniel was eating table food and had weaned himself. Since he had been in an incubator for so long with little of the physical contact of nursing, cuddling, and stroking, I thought he would nurse for at least 2 years to compensate. Probably, as a result of all we had been through, *I* didn't want to give it up. But he didn't feel that way, and was happy and content without nursing. Once a baby has decided to stop, there is no way to keep him nursing. Today Daniel is a happy, well-adjusted 4½-year-old. If I ever have another premature baby, I will definitely breastfeed again.

Your Cheering Squad

To be successful in nursing a premie, a mother needs to convey her determination to her husband as well as to her doctor and hospital staff. A husband will take his cue from his wife on the importance of breastfeeding. It is important to share your feelings with him. There is a tendency for fathers not to become as involved. Encourage him to share with you the pleasure of loving his child, and experiencing something which can give joy and special meaning to his life.

Friends can help your morale a great deal. Contact your nearest La Leche League group to get in touch with mothers who have successfully breastfed a premature baby. It will be a help if you can turn to them for encouragement and suggestions. There also may be an organization near you that offers to help parents of premature babies through difficult times, such as the Premature and High Risk Infant Association, Inc. To contact these groups, see Appendix: Organizations to Help the Nursing Mother.

Chapter 7

Newborn and Infant Problems

When our twins were born, Karen didn't seem to know how to nurse at first. I had to help her by putting my nipple directly into her mouth. She would suck a couple of times, then turn away, and cry. It took several starts before she would suck without pulling away. This lasted for about two weeks, when Karen finally seemed to realize what nursing was all about. In the meantime, our other twin, Sharon, had no problems at all with nursing. Sharon was a vigorous nurser from the start. If I hadn't had twins, I might have thought that Karen's problem was due to something *I* was doing wrong. Many newborn problems are like ours with Karen—annoying, frustrating, but overcome within a few days, or a few weeks. Some babies are, of course, born with serious problems. Some remain in the hospital, or return periodically to the hospital or require a great deal of care at home. Some babies have handicaps, such as a cleft palate or brain injury, that almost prevent them from sucking.

In the past many mothers who have had a sincere desire to breastfeed have given up in a few days or weeks from a lack of information or support. "Wean the baby" has been a common solution proposed for any problem, even for opposite concerns such as "the baby is too fat," or "the baby is too thin." However, the answer to a problem does not usually lie in bottles. Bottles can bring with them problems of their own, including severe allergic complications. After encountering such complications, some mothers have returned to breastfeeding.

It's not easy to be patient while a problem resolves itself, but it's worth the wait. If you have a problem, don't give up. Find out about the problem and what you can do about it, rather than switch to bottlefeeding.

This chapter will explore some of the problems that can affect newborns. Other, more serious long-range situations that affect newborns and can complicate breastfeeding are discussed in later chapters.

Nursing after Birth

Many studies have indicated the desirability of nursing your baby as soon after birth as possible. For example, I. A. Archavsky, in "Immediate Breast-Feeding of Newborn Infant in the Prophylaxis of the So-Called Physiological Loss of Weight," (1) observed that the sucking reflex is at its height 20 to 30 minutes after birth. If a baby is not permitted to suck the reflex diminishes rapidly and only reappears 40 hours later.

Early and frequent nursing has advantages which contribute to the best possible beginning for breastfeeding. The nipple stimulation causes your pituitary gland to release pitocin into your bloodstream, causing your uterus to contract, reducing bleeding and hastening the return of your uterus to its nonpregnant state. The result of early, frequent nursing is almost always an uninhibited let-down and a contented baby.

Marshall H. Klaus and John H. Kennell, in their book, *Maternal-Infant Bonding* (2), also describe a maternal sensitive period soon after birth. They cite several studies showing the effects on breastfeeding of early contact between mother and baby. In one study, for example, a group of 19 mothers was given their babies on the delivery table during the episiotomy repair and then allowed to stay with them in privacy for 45 minutes. An equal group of mothers was separated from their babies shortly after birth, before nursing. Except for this difference in initial contact, the care of the two groups was identical. All babies were brought to their mothers to start breastfeeding at 24 hours. Six months after birth, the group which had been allowed to breastfeed their babies immediately after birth had significantly more mothers who were still breastfeeding. They reported fewer episodes of infection, and the weight gain was greater.

The sooner after delivery that breastfeeding is begun, the more colostrum your baby will receive. Dr. Robert Jackson, a member of the Professional Advisory Board for La Leche League International, has also pointed out these interesting facts about colostrum: The proportions of the constituents in human milk gradually change; the colostrum of the first day is not the same as the colostrum of the second; with the transitional milk there is a gradual consistent change intimately related to the needs of the baby. Dr. Jackson says that no matter how much artificial formulas are improved, it's never going to be possible to manufacture formulas for the first day, the second day, the third day, and so on, that are as suited to baby's developing needs as is his mother's own milk. (3)

So, the sooner you nurse your baby, the better. The American College of Obstetrics and Gynecology recommends "provision of adequate sucking stimulation by permitting the baby to nurse at least six times daily, beginning as soon as practicable after delivery, when mother and baby are in good condition." (4)

Many mothers nurse their babies on the delivery table, and with rooming-in, or a home delivery, feed them on demand, which may be every two or three hours, or sometimes more often.

Doctors who have delivered thousands of babies and allowed them to nurse right after delivery attest to the safety of this practice. Dr. James Good, a La Leche League International Professional Advisory Board member, comments when asked about a problem of a tracheo-esophageal fistula (an abnormal connection between the windpipe and the esophagus), "This is a very rare instance (about 1 in 4,000) and there is a simple test the doctor can do in the delivery room, by slipping a tube down the baby's throat, if a major symptom makes him suspect a T-E fistula." Dr. Lewis A. Coffin, pediatrician and author of *The Grandmother Conspiracy Exposed* (5), also states that if a baby is fed colostrum, and, because of a T-E fistula, it is aspirated into his lungs, it will *not* produce any severe lung problem. This is in contrast with damage from cow's milk or even sugar water, which is usually given a newborn who might have this problem. The colostrum apparently is reabsorbed in the lung, whereas the others act as "foreign bodies" and can cause problems in the lung, such as aspiration pneumonia.

How will your doctor react to your desire to nurse on the delivery table? Hopefully this is something that you have discussed and agreed upon during your pregnancy. He may hesitate giving approval in advance, preferring to wait until delivery to make sure you and the baby are both feeling well enough.

How will your baby react to your offering to nurse immediately? Some babies suck vigorously. My own babies were not interested on the delivery table, but did nurse contentedly when brought to me a few hours later. Even if your newborn is disinterested in nursing, you can spend the time holding and stroking your baby. This is not just a time for physical feeding but also for emotional nourishment.

There are two situations which might make your doctor apprehensive about early nursing. If you have been completely anesthetized (as for a cesarean delivery), you may have an anesthetized baby, and it may take several hours before both of you are in shape for nursing.

The other situation that a doctor might be concerned about is a *very small* premie. If your baby is not big and strong enough to nurse, your doctor may want him in an incubator, getting extra heat and oxygen.

If, however, your doctor routinely insists upon artificial warmth, there is no reason why the heat lamp can't be placed over a strong, healthy baby while he is nursing.

Sleepy Baby

If you have drugs during labor, the longer you wait before having them, the less effect any necessary medication will have on your baby. If your baby remains sleepy from drugs used during labor, the effects may last a week or more, according to

Dr. T. Berry Brazelton, professor of pediatrics at Harvard Medical School. (6) Dr. Reuben E. Kron, psychiatrist at the University of Pennsylvania Medical Center, found that babies of mothers who had received barbiturates during labor did not suck as well and that the effect lasted at least throughout the first week of life, and in some cases for several weeks. (7)

During this time breastfeeding needs careful management. Your baby needs nourishment and fluids to help rid his system of the drugs. You need regular emptying of the breasts to help establish an adequate milk supply. If your baby is still weak and tired after your milk comes in, you can empty your breasts after nursing with a breast pump or hand expression. The milk can be frozen for later use or fed to your baby by spoon, dropper or nursing supplementer until this drowsy period has passed. The extra nourishment, plus extra handling, extra body contact, may be just what your baby needs to perk up.

Checking the number of wet or soiled diapers daily will help to measure your baby's progress. Disposable diapers are convenient but are hard to assess in terms of wetness. Cloth diapers will give a better picture of your baby's output. Six to eight wet diapers daily are sufficient for a totally breastfed baby who receives no fluid other than breast milk.

The use of bottle supplements, nipple shields and pacifiers should be avoided with a sleepy baby. They only serve to confuse an infant's sucking reflex as each requires a different technique and a lazy baby may soon learn that bottle milk flows most easily. It can be a battle to keep your baby at the breast during the first few days at home until he is convinced that breastfed is best fed. Many mothers have given up needlessly under pressure from those around them who do not understand why the baby fusses at the breast and seems to prefer the bottle.

Placid Newborn

A placid newborn may regularly sleep four to five hours between feedings. Often everyone remarks on how good the baby is. Then comes the first weigh-in at the doctor's. The baby may have gained little or no weight; some even show a loss! Now everyone is concerned.

Supplements and solids may be recommended. A better plan is to stimulate your milk production with more frequent feedings. Waking your baby for feeding every two hours during the day and at least once at night will add several feedings to the day. (You can even try nursing him while he sleeps.) The extra milk and extra stimulation should begin to produce a weight gain in a few days.

Slow Weight Gain

Weight gains which are less than average are often given as a reason for discontinuing breastfeeding. However, according to Los Angeles pediatrician Dr. Paul Fleiss, who has cared for many babies with low weight gains, it is rarely necessary to stop breastfeeding because of a "nonthriving" infant. (8)

Sleepy babies and placid newborns are not the only candidates for low weight gain. There can be many other reasons.

Normal Slow Growth Pattern

It may be normal in your family to have slow growth patterns. One mother who had been told to wean each of her first four babies because of their slow weight gain was determined she would breastfeed her fifth. When the suggestion again came to wean, she was prepared with growth charts from the first four babies showing that even on formula her babies were just slow gainers. She continued breastfeeding her fifth baby, and the child did indeed gain at approximately the same rate as the first four.

According to Dr. Fleiss, there are some infants who are very active physically and develop according to normal milestones but do not gain weight in the first six months of life as other infants do. By a year they have usually caught up with other babies their age, in height and weight.

There can be, however, definite reasons why a baby is

gaining weight slowly. If your baby's slow weight gain does not seem to be due to his own particular pattern of growth, it is worth considering the following.

Should You Alter Your Breastfeeding Habits?

Are you feeding your baby often enough? Sometimes mothers expect that their babies need to be fed on a four-hour schedule. Although a few breastfed babies do thrive when nursed this infrequently, *most* breastfed babies do best when fed on demand, which is usually every two or three hours for a newborn. If you've been feeding your baby on a four-hour schedule he simply might not be getting enough milk to gain weight. Frequent nursings are best for optimal milk production.

Are you supplementing your nursings with bottles of water or any other fluid? If your baby does not nurse well because he is full of another fluid, your breasts will not be stimulated to produce the proper amount of milk. Also, drinking from a bottle is easier than nursing from a breast (though not as good for jaw development) and some babies who learn the easier bottle technique do not nurse well. Gradually decrease the supplements and/or give them with a spoon.

Are you holding your baby so that he can properly grasp the areola? This is necessary so that he empties the milk ducts well, thus stimulating the production of an adequate milk supply. Cradle him in your arms and draw him close to your breast. If your breasts are large or engorged, press your breast away from his nose so that he can breathe. If you have small breasts, you may find that a pillow in your lap helps you hold your baby comfortably close. Change positions—lie down, sit up, use the "football hold."

Most mothers nurse from both breasts at each feeding. Your baby may not be getting enough milk and adequate calories for weight gain if he falls asleep before nursing from both breasts. Try nursing him a shorter time on one breast (about 10 minutes), then switching to the other breast. Some activity part way through a feeding, such as changing his diaper, may rouse the baby enough to keep him nursing.

Baby's Problems Affecting Milk Supply

A sick baby, as well as one with an immature sucking reflex, may not suck well enough to adequately stimulate your breasts.

Weak Nurser.   If your baby was born with a malformation of the nose, mouth, lips, or tongue, improper sucking could make breastfeeding difficult but not impossible. Other babies who, because of improper sucking, simply may not be capable of taking enough milk from the breast for adequate nourishment include premature babies, brain-damaged babies, and those with heart defects or lung problems.

Often, time along with a large dose of patience will solve the problem. Your baby may need help to receive enough milk for adequate growth. Small, frequent feedings will help him learn to suck better as he practices what should be instinctive. You can express any milk left after about a 20-minute feeding (total time) and feed it to your baby, or add the expressed milk to the next feeding, using a dropper, spoon, or nursing supplementer.

Infection.   Infections of a newborn's urinary tract, respiratory system, or central nervous system will interfere with the strength of the baby's sucking. He will be weak and will not be able to suck well. Once the infection is treated his strength will return and the former sucking response should be restored.

Nasal Congestion.   Nasal congestion due to allergy or upper respiratory infection can interfere with proper nursing since a congested baby cannot breathe and nurse at the same time. Some doctors recommend saline (very mild salt water) nose drops followed by gentle aspiration of mucus with a nasal syringe.

Jaundice.   Whatever the cause, jaundiced babies are often passive and placid and some do not nurse well. Jaundice can be treated while breastfeeding continues. (See Jaundice later in this chapter.)

Mother's Problems Affecting Milk Supply

Breast or Nipple Problems. If you have engorgement, sore nipples, a breast infection or abscess, are you nursing less often because of the pain or fear of the pain? Actually, along with producing more milk for your baby, you will be *more* comfortable if you nurse frequently.

Nutrition. Be sure to eat nutritious foods and avoid fad diets. A malnourished mother may produce less milk and possibly even milk of lower nutrient value. Drink plenty of liquids.

Drugs. Some drugs will affect both the amount and the composition of the milk you produce. Usually, substitutes can be prescribed. Drugs such as barbiturates, sleeping pills, and alcohol should be eliminated if your baby is not gaining weight.

Hormones. Lactation is influenced by several hormones. Hypothyroidism or another hormone deficiency problem could hamper milk production, which could result in inadequate weight increases in your baby. Check with your doctor. If you are taking birth control pills, they probably will reduce your milk production.

Emotions. Any anxiety-producing situation may interfere with the let-down reflex and therefore inhibit lactation. If you are constantly upset, for example, by your neighbor's barking dog, or a worrisome family situation, your let-down reflex may be affected. The more peaceful and happy your surroundings, the more apt you are to produce enough milk for your baby.

To relax at feeding time, it may help to set up a routine for feedings. (See *Taking Care of Yourself* in the section on Treating Illnesses at Home, chapter 12, "When Baby Is Sick or

Hospitalized," and How to Insure a Good Milk Supply in chapter 2, "Nursing Techniques.") With your let-down functioning well, your baby will get not only the fore milk but also the richer hind milk which will add needed fat and calories and help him gain weight.

The sleepy baby, the placid newborn, the weak nurser and the "nonthriver" or slow-weight-gain baby all have common needs. While finding the cause is important, careful attention to nursing techniques will help you maintain an adequate milk supply so that your baby can gain at least a few ounces weekly. Demand feedings may have to be given in reverse; instead of waiting for your baby to wake and nurse on demand, you may have to do the waking and "demand" that your baby nurse.

An example of a situation involving a combination of poor sucking and inadequate milk supply can be found in chapter 21, "Nursing during Stressful Times," in the section Some Stressful Situations, *Baby Who Doesn't Gain.*

Rapid Weight Gain

Mothers are sometimes told that a fast-gaining baby should nurse less and be put on a diet because of the concern that infant obesity leads to weight and health problems in adults. However, a totally breastfed baby who becomes "roly-poly" is developing healthy muscle tissue, not blowing up with fluid retention and excess fat cells. Breast milk alone is still the best nourishment for the first half year or so. (9)

One mother I know, Jody, had *both* fast-gaining and slow-gaining babies. She is slender, while her husband has a large frame. Of their four sons, two gained weight at average rates. Their first son, David, gained more slowly, and Bennett, their third son, gained much faster than average. With both David and Bennett, the doctor was not satisfied with their weight gains. Jody says:

It's really hard to have the perfect weight gain. If Bennett had been my first child and David born later, I might have been really worried about David being a slow gainer. David was started on solids at 3½ months, but he continued to gain slowly. He was perfectly healthy even though he hadn't doubled his birth weight by 6 months.

By contrast, Bennett had *tripled* his birth weight by five months and was a picture of health. At one year he wore size 3 clothes. People expected him to answer when they asked him his name, but he hadn't learned to talk yet! My doctor and I had several discussions about Bennett's weight. Around three months he said, "Hmm, well, we're not *really* concerned about babies gaining this fast" (but his tone implied he *was* concerned). He suggested vitamins. I asked, "Why? Isn't he doing well already?" "That's true," the doctor admitted. Another time he suggested I change Bennett's diet. "What diet?" I asked. (Bennett was still totally on breast milk.) Later the doctor suggested I start solids and I asked, "Why? He's doing so well on breast milk." The doctor replied, "Well, I guess you're right." Then he brought up the possible need for iron. I asked, "Oh, does he look like he needs to have his hemoglobin checked?" and the doctor looked again at Bennett and said, "No. He looks perfectly okay."

Around seven months Jody and the doctor talked about how Bennett's father is 6 feet, 2 inches tall and has a large skeletal structure. The doctor agreed that considering this, Bennett's weight gain seemed perfectly normal for Bennett. Jody says:

I was concerned about one thing—that Bennett wasn't as mobile as other babies his age. However, I have known other big babies who have been active and I realize now that so much activity just wasn't Bennett's "style" as a baby.

With each child I have learned it is good to keep his individuality in mind with size and weight as well as other growth patterns such as walking and talking.

Colic and Other Discomforts

Many babies have a "fussy period" during the day. It often begins before the family's dinnertime and lasts several hours. If you find that as dinnertimes approach, you are tired and anxious to finish preparing the meals, try to plan your days so that dinner preparations are done ahead of time and you can take a nap or at least relax for a while in the late afternoon. This may help you to cope with your baby's fussiness.

When babies have long periods of hard crying and seem to be in some sort of physical discomfort for no apparent reason that you or your doctor can discover, they are often said to be colicky. Colic seems to be a catchall explanation for babies who fuss, cry, or scream a lot.

It is often thought that colic is related to some difficulty in digestion. Perhaps the best guess is that some babies have more sensitive nervous systems and have difficulty relaxing enough to nurse contentedly. They start to nurse, then pull away from the breast. Some rocking and gentle handling before nursing may help to calm your baby. Pick him up as soon as he stirs, feed him, then change his diaper when he is finished nursing from the first side. (See also Crying and "Spoiling?" in chapter 1, "What's Normal?")

Some babies are upset by a full breast obstructing their breathing and may pull away, screaming in protest. The instinct to breathe is so strong, they may become afraid to nurse. You can express some milk before feeding so your breast is not so full, and also depress your breast away from baby's nose as he nurses.

With much crying during a feeding, your baby may be uncomfortable partly because of swallowed air. Again, careful management can help relieve the problem. Burp him gently several times.

Some colicky babies latch on hungrily when nursing, nurse well and, if allowed, will also down a bottle of formula or water, too. It's easy to wonder if you have enough milk since your baby never seems satisfied. However, like a goldfish, the colicky baby can easily be overfed. Try feeding every two hours and offering only one breast for any nursing needed during a two-hour period. Offer the other breast during the next two hours. This way your baby won't get too hungry, and he'll still have ample opportunity to suck without getting overfed.

A mother of a premature baby explains how she handled her situation:

> Every night after nursing, about 8:00 P.M., my baby would get the colic. It would last for three hours until his next nursing. After weeks of experimenting with drugs, heating pads and walking the floor, I discovered a method of dealing with it. After I nursed, I would rock my baby to sleep. Instead of putting him in the bassinet, my husband would recline the chair back for us, and I would lie there with him asleep on my chest until the next nursing. During that three-hour period my husband would take care of our older son and do anything else that needed immediate attention.

Other forms of colic may result from a food intolerance. Your baby's immature digestive system may react to something in his diet (if he has started solid foods) or to something in your diet. However, if a breastfed baby is colic-prone, he will usually have greater difficulty on formula.

Delaying the introduction of solid foods gives a baby the time he needs to develop the ability to easily tolerate foods other than human milk. For the allergic baby, this time is even more important. The average baby needs about six months. Very allergic babies may need several more months. Most mothers' diets need not be changed for breastfeeding. Very sensitive babies can react to items in mothers' diets. By adjusting the diet and waiting for the baby's system to mature a bit the problem can be controlled. If your newborn is upset after you have eaten a piece of chocolate cake, for example, you may be able to eat a chocolate chip cookie (which contains a smaller amount of chocolate) instead. In a few months a piece of chocolate cake may cause no problems at all for your nursing baby.

Families with a history of severe allergy must be extra careful. Dr. E. Robbins Kimball, a pediatrician who has had many years of experience with severely allergic babies, says that even if an infant reacts when fed breast milk, breastfeeding should be continued. The properties of mother's milk far outweigh those of any commercial formula. (For more about allergy see chapter 11, "Dealing with Allergies.")

Overabundant Milk Supply

Many times mothers seem to have too much milk for their babies in the first few days and even for a few weeks afterwards, until the milk supply adjusts to the baby's needs. Your baby may cough, or cry, and not be comfortable with a forceful flow of milk coming at him. Of course, you're probably glad you don't have to worry about having enough for your baby, but still you'd like more relaxed, calmer feeding times. What can you do about it?

First of all, you can express some of your milk before starting to nurse, so that the milk is not under as much pressure (see chapter 2, "Nursing Techniques"). Catch this initial surge of milk in a diaper, and start feeding your baby after the flow subsides. Also, choose nursing positions in which the baby has to nurse uphill so that gravity does not make the milk flow faster. Mother lying on her back with baby on top is a good position for this.

Sometimes, one stream of milk may shoot up at an angle and hit a different part of the palate and the baby needs to get used to this. Different positions may be helpful, such as the "football hold" (see illustrations in chapter 18, "Nursing Twins").

It is best not to try to decrease your milk supply in the first six weeks. According to the ups and downs of growth spurts, your baby may sometimes need more milk, sometimes less. Allow your body to respond to signals from your hormones and baby's stimulation, and to find its own pace without interference. However, after about six weeks, if you still feel you have a problem with an overabundant milk supply, you might try nursing from only one breast at a feeding. This will mean each breast will be stimulated less frequently, and will probably produce less milk.

Whenever there is an overabundant milk supply, a mother needs to be aware of the problems of engorgement and plugged ducts. (See The First Days of Nursing in chapter 1, "What's Normal?" and Plugged Ducts in chapter 4, "Breast and Nipple Problems.")

Newborns in Distress

Some infants are born with or develop hyaline membrane disease, infections, or pneumonia from having aspirated amniotic fluid during labor or delivery. Your baby may be so sick that he must be fed intravenously and/or be in an incubator and receive oxygen for a while. During this time you can hand express your milk or use a breast pump.

You may arrange to stay with your hospitalized baby or else visit a few times a day to nurse, taking in expressed breast milk for the times when you are not there. If your baby cannot nurse at first, ask that nursing be allowed as soon as possible, and that you at least be allowed to provide your milk for his feedings in the meantime. What do you do when you want to nurse and the doctor hesitates? Discuss your feelings with him, and tell him how you want to help. You want the best possible care for your child, and that includes the best possible nourishment. Your baby already has enough problems without adding possible complications from formula. It may help to discuss with your doctor some of the advantages of breastfeeding.

When your baby comes home from the hospital, arrange to do nothing else but rest and nurse him for a few days, as he builds up your supply.

The following examples show how some mothers have handled hospitalization of their newborns, and present ideas which you can adapt to help you manage through your own time of stress.

Laurel Ann was born six weeks prematurely, with pneumonia and hyaline membrane disease. Later she was found to have jaundice and still later a hole in the heart (ventricular septal defect). She was placed on the critical list and given antibiotics and oxygen in an incubator. Her mother, Leona, says:

The next morning I had a conference with my doctor about breastfeeding. He checked with the nurses and said that it was impossible for me to pump my milk and give it to my baby. It was against hospital policy because of the danger of contamination.

I suppose I could have fought harder to provide milk, but at the time I was glad she was alive by any means. I took no dry-up medication and began to pump with a hand pump. It was frustrating to have to discard the milk in the hospital. At home, I saved the milk, which only averaged about two ounces daily.

Meanwhile, my daughter was still battling pneumonia. In addition to intravenous fluids, she was fed two times a day with a special premie nipple and formula, and two times she was tube fed. I didn't get to touch her for 14 days. We brought her home when she was 16 days old.

Home at last, all was fine until Laurel Ann got hungry. I tried to breastfeed; she still cried. Two formula feedings later, I had to remind myself that breastfeeding was best. So I picked her up when she was not so hungry and put her to my breast. She began to suck, and sucked more vigorously than she had with the premie nipple. I was encouraged. From then until her next doctor's visit one week later, I breastfed her on demand with no bottle feedings.

The night after I began to breastfeed Laurel Ann, she became constipated. Later I learned that it is not unusual for a baby to become constipated after a transition from breast to bottle or vice-versa.

At first Laurel Ann seemed to sleep all day and want to be fed every hour during the night. She was gaining *very slowly*. Her not eating during the day for six to eight hours at a time worried me. So I expressed some breast milk and sterilized a spoon and spoon fed her during the day to help her gain more. That was very successful. At the next doctor's visit her weight was fine. The hole in her heart gradually closed.

Laurel Ann's recovery was fantastic. But more than that is my feeling of closeness to her through breast-feeding. I feel now that she is mine in every respect, but I didn't when she first came home. She was like a stranger.

Laurie's son was born with a rare skin disease called urticaria pigmentosa. She explains:

This caused him to have welted skin which was reddish pink and lumpy. Although congenital, a person can exhibit it at any time and it varies in severity. Jake was born with a very severe case. It was three days before it was diagnosed, but I was not allowed to nurse him for seven days due to the danger of infecting his open skin. We couldn't even touch him except with the plastic gloves in his Isolette. I used a breast pump so he got my milk, even though he was in the hospital and I was at home.

We brought Jake home when he was ten days old. Two days later he had a huge swelling in his chest, which turned out to be a staph infection. He had to go back to the hospital and was there another week. When he was rehospitalized, the doctors took him off breastfeeding entirely. I kept insisting that Jake and I were already exposed to the same germs, and finally, after 48 hours, I was allowed to breastfeed him in the hospital and supply milk for nighttime bottles. Since Jake later proved to be extremely allergic to cow's milk I am most happy that I persisted in breastfeeding.

Jaundice

A newborn problem that can have a number of causes comes under the catchall heading of jaundice, a yellowing of the skin and eyeballs. It can be quite harmless, or it can be dangerous, resulting in brain damage or death. In rare instances it may be due to a substance in a mother's milk. Jaundice often clears up without its cause being identified.

The time of onset of the jaundice gives a clue to its cause or causes. Dangerous jaundice, caused by blood incompatibility, infection, or drugs used by a mother, will appear on the first day. Breast milk jaundice, which is a reaction to a hormone present in some mothers' milk, does not appear for several days; it takes that long for a baby to have had enough of his mother's milk to show an effect. Several conditions may exist simultaneously which can cause the baby to appear jaundiced.

While tests are being done to determine the cause and severity of the jaundice, breastfeeding should continue in frequent sessions. No water or formula should be given. If the cause is a hormone in the breast milk and the blood bilirubin level becomes high, your doctor may recommend temporary weaning (for a day or two) until the level drops. Then you will be able to resume nursing. If your doctor feels the jaundice should recede quickly, he may want to use one of the treatments to lower serum bilirubin levels. For example, exposure to ordinary sunlight or to fluorescent light (of a specific wavelength) may help lower the level of jaundice. Either is preferable to even temporary weaning.

In our family, two of our four children had jaundice. With our son, it was very mild and disappeared in a few days. With Sharon we needed to take her to the hospital once a week for a blood test to determine the bilirubin level. This continued until she was ten weeks old. Sharon seemed to have no ill effects from the jaundice. Her fraternal twin, Karen, never had any trace of jaundice.

Before giving further examples of jaundice, here is some information that will help you understand this complex condition.

Physiologic or "Normal" Jaundice

This is a common short-lived form of jaundice which carries with it no harmful effects. Estimates on the number of newborns who develop this range from 30 to 75 percent. It usually appears between the second and fourth day of life and slowly disappears in a week or so with no treatment.

What causes it? In the later weeks of pregnancy your baby builds up extra red blood cells to insure an adequate supply of oxygen. After birth, he doesn't need these extra red blood cells, since he can breathe freely. The cells are broken down and the iron is stored in the liver. If this breakdown occurs rapidly, or if your baby's liver is not mature enough to clear the blood of the broken down cells, your baby will appear jaundiced. Theoretically, the later the cord is cut, the more extra red blood cells your baby will receive, and the more likely he is to appear jaundiced, but also a greater amount of iron is available for later use. So the cause of this type of jaundice can even be considered beneficial since it reduces the chance of iron-deficiency anemia later on.

Any stress during delivery can increase the risk of jaundice. Moreover, if you are diabetic or are seriously ill at the time of birth, your baby is more likely to be jaundiced. Probably this will not be a dangerous type of jaundice.

Pathologic or "Abnormal" Jaundice

This type of jaundice may be caused by infections, or drugs such as sulfa drugs used by a mother or given to the newborn. It can also be caused by blood incompatibilities (erythroblastosis), which occur if your blood is type O and the baby's is type A or B or if one of you is Rh negative while the other is Rh positive.

Your baby's bilirubin level should be checked frequently. Blood transfusion or exchange may be necessary. However, it has been demonstrated in several studies that breastfeeding remains the preferred method of infant feeding in these cases and will not harm your baby in any way. (10) This type of jaundice usually appears within 24 hours of delivery.

Breast Milk Jaundice

This is a rare type of jaundice that begins after the fourth day and may be prolonged. In the 1960s Drs. Irwin Arias and

Lawrence Gartner studied nursing mothers whose babies had prolonged jaundice which could not be explained by any known causes. Two-thirds of the babies nursed by these mothers developed jaundice while none of their bottlefed babies became jaundiced. The doctors discovered a steroid hormone called pregnane-3 (alpha), 20 (beta)-diol, previously found in cattle but considered not to occur in humans, in the milk of these mothers, and this seemed to cause the jaundice. In all cases, the mothers were healthy and the development of the babies was entirely normal. In some cases the jaundice was severe enough to cause concern, and breastfeeding was interrupted for three or four days.* This resulted in a rapid reduction of jaundice. After that, breastfeeding could be resumed without the jaundice becoming severe again.

In a statement printed in *La Leche League News,* January/February 1966, Dr. Arias declared: "Because of the rarity of breast milk jaundice and its thoroughly benign nature, we do not feel the existence of this syndrome should be used in any way to discourage the breastfeeding of infants."

In answering a question in the *Journal of the American Medical Association* (11) about jaundice in breastfed babies, Drs. Arias and Gartner said, "Among the many reports in the literature of late-onset, prolonged jaundice related to breastfeeding, there are none suggesting that this syndrome has resulted in brain damage or any other type of residue." The doctors recommend continuing nursing if the baby is mature and the serum bilirubin level is "15 mg per 100 ml or less during the first week of life, 18 mg per 100 ml or less during the second week of life, and 20 mg per 100 ml or less thereafter. If these conservative limits are exceeded then a four- to six-day period of artificial feeding should be undertaken, followed by resumption of nursing."

---

* During this time of interrupted breastfeeding, if possible, arrange for your baby to have donated or purchased breast milk. A formula which is least likely to cause allergy problems would be the next best choice. Be sure to express your milk or use a breast pump to maintain your milk supply and prevent engorgement.

Bilirubin

This is a waste product in the blood resulting from the breakdown of red blood cells. It is the liver's job to get rid of this waste matter. Bilirubin testing is done from a sample of a baby's blood, usually obtained from his foot.

With premature babies, the bilirubin count will rise more rapidly than with mature babies. Up to 20 mg% is considered safe if a baby is otherwise normal, but sick, premature babies can develop brain damage at a much lower level. Above 20 mg%, brain damage becomes a danger, but most babies can tolerate higher levels. The danger drops sharply after the sixth day of life.

Transfusions

Exchange transfusion is a procedure in which a severely jaundiced baby's blood is removed through the umbilical cord to rid the body of excess bilirubin so that kernicterus (permanent brain damage caused by very high bilirubin levels) can be prevented. The doctor removes small amounts of blood and replaces it with fresh blood free of damaging antibodies until a thorough exchange has taken place. The process is slow and risky but many infants have survived to grow strong and well.

Exchange transfusions are not always necessary. Sometimes the baby does well with small transfusions (additions) of blood.

Phototherapy

This is light treatment for jaundiced infants which helps the breakdown and removal of bilirubin. It is a treatment that has greatly reduced the need for exchange transfusions. Breastfeeding can continue during phototherapy. It has been shown that intermittent phototherapy is just as effective as continuous phototherapy.

Babies with Jaundice

Two mothers explain how they successfully nursed their babies. Judy's daughter, Carolyn, both nursed and had formula:

> Carolyn started developing jaundice on the second day. My husband is Rh positive and I am Rh negative, and there was the question as to whether or not this jaundice was stemming from Rh incompatibility. As a precautionary measure, Carolyn was moved to the nursery for premature babies where she was placed under special lights. Our pediatrician said I could go downstairs at every feeding time during the day and nurse her. An aide or one of the nurses went with me each time. At night they gave Carolyn formula.* Her blood test was okay by the fifth day and we were allowed to go home as planned.

Kathleen nursed her son, and expressed milk to be used when she wasn't with him:

> When our second baby, Sean, was born he appeared somewhat jaundiced. They tested his blood right away. It was not at a dangerous level. Just before we checked out a few hours later, they took another blood test. We went back for two more tests the next day. At 10:30 P.M. of the second day, our doctor called and said the last blood test showed a bilirubin level of 17.5 mg%. Since there was a possible ABO blood incompatibility, she was worried because the level went up so high so fast. She said that I should stop nursing, give Sean water, and bring him back to the hospital immediately.
>
> I wanted to keep nursing Sean, even if he had to stay in the hospital. The admitting room doctor mustn't have read the studies on jaundice because he said as he observed me nursing, "If you're going to nurse, you're going to kill your baby." I knew that wasn't so, but still it shook me up to hear that from a doctor. Then we went to the

---

* Expressed breast milk would have been better.

newborn floor with Sean. The doctors there said I would be allowed to nurse whenever I wanted. I felt greatly relieved.

Sean stayed in the hospital. For three full days he was under the lights. Researchers say that sunlight causes the best artificial breakdown of the bilirubin. The fluorescent lights were used as a substitute.

My husband and I drove twice a day to the hospital and I nursed Sean there. In between times I expressed my milk, and took it to the hospital on the next trip. They gave him water if they ran out of my milk. I found that having a nursing toddler at home really helped my let-down reflex.

On the ninth day the bilirubin level had gone down to 9 mg%, and the doctor thought Sean was probably going to be okay. The level was at 5.7 the next morning, and the doctor told me "You have nothing more to worry about. The count will never go up again." *

Based on their studies of breast milk jaundice, Drs. Gartner and Arias found that there was a wide variation in the intensity and the duration of the jaundice. In most cases, the babies were weaned for a few days, the bilirubin level went down, and then breastfeeding was resumed. In one case, breastfeeding continued without any weaning and the bilirubin level went down rapidly. The level became normal on the twenty-sixth day of life. (13)

Coping with a Handicap

When a newborn has a problem, parents may feel guilty, helpless and angry all at the same time. Some blame each other, and vent their frustration on each other or on the hospital staff. This is a time for patience, prayer and persever-

---

* If the bilirubin level goes down consistently from 15 mg% for a couple of days in a healthy full-term baby, many doctors feel he can safely be taken home. (12)

ance. Parents can come through an ordeal stronger and more loving toward each other as they concentrate on the needs of their helpless newborn, coping with each day and stress as it comes.

Sometimes mothers are urged *not* to nurse handicapped children, not to become too attached . . . just the opposite of what is needed.

Many parents find that they can happily raise their little ones who are born with less than perfect health or physical stature. These children can bring much pleasure to their families as they grow at their own special pace. Provided with stimulation, nourishment, love and opportunity, your child will develop his potential to his fullest. Parent groups, such as those listed in Appendix: Organizations to Help the Nursing Mother, offer support intended to help each of us do our best for our children.

Chapter 8

Malformations of Baby's Nose, Mouth, and Digestive Tract

If your child has been born with a malformation of his nose, mouth, or digestive tract, you may find breastfeeding difficult. Improper sucking can cause you to develop sore nipples, and minimal sucking stimulation may make it difficult for you to maintain an adequate milk supply. If your baby does not have a normal digestive passage, he may need to be fed your milk directly into a tube leading to his stomach from the outside.

Breastfeeding is not always possible for a baby with one of these conditions. You and your family will be under a tremendous strain and a lot of pressure. You may become upset and frustrated if things do not go the way you expected. If you feel resentful of the effort involved in breastfeeding, if breastfeeding is causing friction in your family life, and *if bottlefeeding would be less traumatic,* then bottlefeeding might be your best procedure.

Some mothers have found that a compromise solution works well for them. They express their milk and feed it to their babies with a bottle, tube, eyedropper, spoon, nursing supplementer, or a special feeder. This can mean feeding exclusively by an artificial means or nursing first at a feeding and then finishing off with a bottle or other feeder.

However, many mothers *have* successfully breastfed babies who had malformations of the nose, mouth or digestive tract. It depends on the malformation, the baby, you and your family. Many parents feel that nursing gives a baby an extra measure of security as he faces the stressful experiences involved in correcting his problem.

Choanal Atresia

Margaret's son was born with choanal atresia, a nostril blockage that made it impossible for him to breathe through his nose. Surgery was required to open up the cartilage in one nostril so a tube could be inserted in the opening to allow him to breathe.

Margaret says:

Joe was in the hospital three weeks. After the tube was inserted, I went once a day to nurse him. The rest of the time I pumped my milk, froze it, and took it to the hospital for him. I would have felt so lost without providing my milk during that time. The doctors and nurses could do *almost* everything for Joe. But this was something *I* could do—give my baby my breast milk. At first I tried a hand pump. Then my La Leche League leader suggested hand expression. She said it would be much faster,

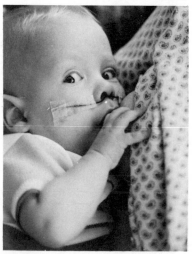

Sandra C. Wallace

A blockage made it impossible for Joe to breathe through his nose.

and it was. Still, it's not any fun to get up at 2:00 A.M. and pump for a baby in the hospital.

While Joe was in the hospital, my milk supply dwindled and he had to have formula once a day. But as soon as he came home, I had enough for him. He loved nursing, even though we had to stop five or six times to use a suction machine that removed milk and mucus from his tube. Bottles would have created more problems, because the milk comes out much more quickly and causes the buildup of more mucus.

I'm really glad I nursed Joe, because of the special feeling of closeness that has grown between us.

Cleft Lip and Cleft Palate

Fortunately, science has made great strides in repairing clefts. If your baby has a cleft lip, repair will probably be done within six months after birth or as soon as the surgeon feels it is advisable. A cleft palate repair usually is not done until after the baby is a year old. Your surgeon will determine the best time. Following surgery to repair either cleft lip or cleft palate, a child should be kept from crying as much as possible and should receive a great deal of attention, affection, and diversion—two excellent reasons for talking a reluctant hospital staff into letting you stay with your baby.

You may be wondering if you can breastfeed your baby. Many mothers have—both in the weeks or months before repair surgery and then again after surgery. The severity of the cleft will affect the ease with which you are able to accomplish breastfeeding. A simple cleft lip or cleft lip and alveolus (an opening of the lip and gum that does not extend into the palate) does *not* interfere with breastfeeding. A cleft palate may cause inefficient sucking which results in slow weight gain. With help in improving their feeding methods, infants with these conditions are able to breastfeed successfully. Babies with clefts of both the lip and the palate are the most difficult to nurse.

If your baby has a cleft palate, you will probably notice that some of the milk comes out of his nose as he nurses. For this reason you may find it necessary to stop the feeding fairly often to let your baby have a breathing spell. Actually most babies seem to handle this problem quite well.

Most mothers who have breastfed cleft lip or cleft palate babies have found that it is usually easier for the baby to nurse if he is held in a sitting position, as opposed to lying completely flat. This doesn't mean you cannot nurse your baby in bed, only that you might raise his head slightly with a hard pillow. This elevation helps to minimize the problem of milk in the baby's nose and prevents fluid from getting into his ear.

Depending upon the type of cleft, your baby may find it easier to nurse on one side. Try offering him the other breast while holding him in the "football hold" (see chapter 18, "Nursing Twins").

Sometimes things do not go smoothly in the first few weeks. Many mothers say that it took time for their babies to nurse really well at the breast. However, as the baby grows, his ability to nurse improves.

When your baby is ready for repair surgery, discuss with your doctor his plans for feeding the baby after the operation and his reasons for those plans. He may ask you to refrain from nursing for a period of time following surgery. You can request making this time of temporary weaning as short as possible by stressing how important breastfeeding is to you and how beneficial it is to both you and your baby. But remember that when you first offer nursing, your baby may refuse. He may not breastfeed until he is feeling much better.

If your baby is not able to suck well enough to get sufficient milk you can still give him your milk from a bottle or nursing supplementer. Human milk is especially beneficial because babies with clefts are particularly prone to upper respiratory and middle ear infections. (1) Babies fed breast milk have far fewer infections.

It may be hard for you to accept bottlefeeding your baby if you had your heart set on breastfeeding. But after all, that's how artificial feeding started—to feed problem babies. Sometimes bottles are necessary, at least temporarily. If you bottle-feed as though you were nursing, you and your baby can still enjoy much of the warmth and closeness of the breastfeeding relationship.

One mother says, "Our baby never held the bottle herself, although she was almost 20 months old before she weaned. She had a lot of touching and rocking during feedings and bathings to make up for the closeness she was missing by not being fed at the breast. She is still a cuddler and loves to be loved."

If your baby was born with a cleft lip, you undoubtedly were aware of it immediately. However, if your baby has a cleft palate, you may *not* notice this right away, depending on its severity. Some symptoms of cleft palate are inability to suck, regurgitation of fluids through the nose, and difficulty in swallowing and breathing.

Edith Grady (2) says she started nursing her twins without realizing that one of them, Andrea, had a cleft of her soft palate. She noticed that Andrea had trouble holding onto the nipple unless Edith held it in Andrea's mouth. After a few frustrating days, Andrea was crying hard at feeding time and Edith noticed a gap in the back part of the roof of her mouth. The doctor confirmed that there was a cleft in the soft palate but did not indicate that it would cause a feeding problem.

Two weeks later the baby was still having trouble and the doctor suggested letting her nurse a bit and then giving her a bottle of expressed breast milk to fill her up. They stumbled along this way until Edith noticed that Andrea had learned to milk the breast with her gums and tongue. Edith found that by placing her index finger on the top or upper edge of the areola and her middle finger on the lower outer edge of the areola and pressing down or back towards the chest wall, she could cause her nipple to protrude as it normally would during nursing.

Edith says, "It made sense that if I could hand express using my fingers without any suction available, then Andrea could milk my breast using her gums and tongue as I used my fingers." Edith would also hold Andrea's head close to her breast throughout the entire feeding. Having another nursing baby (the twin) was more work, but helped to keep up the milk supply.

When Andrea was 4 months old and weighed ten pounds, she was strong enough to obtain all of her milk supply from direct nursing. For the next 2½ months, she was a totally breastfed baby in every sense of the word, with no other type of food or liquid supplement. At 6 months, she no longer had to have the nipple held in her mouth or to be held especially close to the breast. Instead she would grab the breast with both hands, pull it into her mouth, and hold it there until she finished nursing or fell asleep. Between the sixth and seventh months, solid foods were introduced. Andrea continued to nurse happily until she weaned herself a couple of years later.

Edith says:

> In the beginning I had many personal doubts about whether I would succeed in breastfeeding Andrea. I have to admit now that I used the bottled milk as a mental crutch to prove to myself and to my critics that Andrea was getting the nourishment she required. But, feeding Andrea from a bottle only served to confuse her as she tried to learn how to nurse directly. With bottle feedings, she got used to having the milk run into her mouth as soon as the rubber nipple entered her mouth. With breastfeeding, she had to "milk" my nipple a little before the milk flowed freely. If I had to do it over again, *and* given my present knowledge, I would have nursed her exclusively from my breast.
>
> I have also come to realize that although Andrea was a very fussy baby, she would have been so even if she had no problems. But when your baby has a problem such as mine did, it's easy to blame every difficulty you have with the baby on the problem, instead of attributing it to personality, immaturity of body systems, or upsetting outside situations.
>
> Andrea's milking action was rather weak, especially at first. This could cause a mother to worry if she wasn't expecting it. But, though she was gentle, she was a very

effective nurser. When a baby is nursing from your breast without suction, you should not expect to feel much sensation. This does not mean that the baby is not obtaining sufficient milk.

Dr. Robert Mendelsohn, Associate Professor of Preventative Medicine and Community Health at the University of Illinois College of Medicine, and a La Leche League professional advisor, believes that many physicians who specialize in cleft palate have almost no experience with babies who are *totally breastfed*. Therefore, he says, any mother with a baby with a cleft palate would do well to consult Edith Grady, who not only is familiar with the available scientific literature, but also has had firsthand experience with her own baby and with many doctors.*

Susan's baby had the most complicated of the cleft problems: a complete bilateral cleft of the lip and palates, both hard and soft. She says:

> Both my husband and I were acquainted with a variety of birth defects because of our experience in special education. Having seen so many serious disorders, we did not feel overwhelmed by a cleft. Meghan was a gorgeous healthy baby; she just had no apparent upper lip.
>
> Meghan's defect meant that the central portion of the upper lip was not connected to either side and that the roof of the mouth was open to the nasal cavity. This made it impossible for her to form a suction. Even though Meghan willingly latched onto my breast, she could not suck the milk out. But, after trying several different

---

* Edith Grady is a La Leche League leader in Indiana. She sends out an information packet, including her own experiences, which you may obtain by writing to her at 8742 East 100 N. Lafayette, IN 47905. Send your name and address and two first class stamps.

Sheri Hansen is another La Leche League leader who is experienced with cleft-related problems, whose own baby had a cleft lip and palate, and who is willing to help other mothers. Sheri is past president of the Cleft Parent Guild of Los Angeles, and may be contacted through that group. (See Appendix: Organizations to Help the Nursing Mother)

La Leche League International is also planning to issue a Cleft Palate, Cleft Lip Information Sheet.

methods of nursing, I learned to hold her tightly so that my breast covered one hole in her lip. With my thumb or index finger, I covered the other hole. The suction was not strong, but milk came out.

For the next two weeks, I spent most of every day feeding Meghan. She would exhaust herself nursing and fall asleep. Finally, she began to gain back a tiny bit of the weight she had lost, but she continued to dehydrate on occasion. I knew we had to get more breast milk into her, so we tried an eyedropper. First she would nurse, then we would feed her an ounce or two with the dropper.

My milk supply was low due to her poor sucking so I obtained an electric breast pump. After several days, I was getting three ounces at a pumping every four hours, day and night. Then, our consulting orthodontist introduced us to a special feeder to replace the eyedropper, the Beniflex Feeder by Mead Johnson. (See section on Special Feeders and Feeding Techniques in chapter 2, "Nursing Techniques.") From then until she had her lip surgery at six weeks, I spent about ten hours a day on Meghan's feedings. She would nurse, then take my milk from the feeder, then I would pump. It was well worth the effort, for with the addition of the breast pump and the special feeder, Meghan's weight climbed rapidly.

During the week Meghan was in the hospital for repair surgery, I continued pumping and took the milk to the hospital for her. With running to the hospital and caring for our other daughter, my supply dropped, but other nursing mothers donated their milk and she did not have to take formula supplements. Meg was in peak condition for her operation and recovered from the anesthesia and surgery so rapidly the doctors were delighted. Some felt it could be attributed, in part, to the benefits of the breast milk.

After surgery, Meghan was not allowed to nurse until the lip healed. After a month of special syringe feeding, we were allowed to try nursing again. But although her suction was a little better, she was unable to get enough to give up the supplemental feeding and pumping. When she was three months old, Meghan caught a cold and completely refused to nurse. She took the breast milk fine from a regular bottle with the special nipple, but would not nurse. After her cold was gone, she would not resume feeding at the breast, so she weaned.

I felt badly but was determined to continue pumping for awhile longer. Meg was obviously thriving and healthy. She consumed six to eight ounces of milk, four times a day. I pumped every three hours from 6:00 A.M. to 10:00 or 11:00 P.M. As she grew older, her capacity increased and I began pumping every 2½ hours. I finally weaned myself from the electric breast pump and this gave me tremendous freedom, for I could hand express anywhere there was privacy, rather than being limited by having to use the electric pump at home.

By the time Meghan was five months old, her daily demand exceeded my supply by four to six ounces and at the pediatrician's suggestion I began to supplement breast milk with skim milk. In order to prevent the ear infections so prevalent in cleft palate children, we did not feed her solids until she was seven months old. At that time, yogurt, cottage cheese, and cream of wheat were added to her diet and she continued to consume a quart of breast milk a day.

Surgery to close the soft palate and place drainage tubes in the eardrums took place when Meghan was just over nine months old. At this time she could drink from a cup and eat many solid foods that were prepared in a baby food grinder. After much soul-searching I cut down my milk expression about a month before the operation and slowly weaned myself.

Birth Defect Involving
Small Nose and Mouth

Phyllis wanted very much to nurse her baby, Janeen, but had great difficulty for many months. Although she was a full-term baby, Janeen was small, weighing slightly less than 5 pounds. Sometimes when Phyllis tried to nurse her, Janeen would root and root for the nipple but would scream rather than suck.

The baby's father eventually discovered the problem. While nursing, Janeen flipped up the tip of her tongue so that the nipple was underneath. When she sucked, she got nothing. Although nipple shields improved Janeen's sucking for a few feedings they caused great nipple soreness. The best technique seemed to be to place the breast nipple directly under Janeen's nose and straight down over her lip. Then when she opened her mouth, the tongue fell down more naturally.

During nursings, Phyllis manually worked milk from high in her breast into the nipple. Many times she squeezed the milk into Janeen's mouth. But the baby's tongue would flip up so that she couldn't swallow and the milk ran out of her mouth. Janeen was unable to empty the breast during nursing, and she was losing weight. Phyllis hand expressed or used an electric breast pump after, and sometimes between, feedings.

Besides the problem of Janeen flipping up her tongue and nursing with the nipple underneath her tongue, several other problems became evident. Janeen had such a tiny nose she could barely breathe, and her mouth was so small she could not get enough of the areola into her mouth to compress the milk ducts. An extremely high palate made it difficult for her to get the nipple firmly between tongue and palate, so after the initial let-down she couldn't get any more milk from the breast.

Because of her low weight, Janeen was not allowed to go home from the hospital until she was 13 days old. During this time one of Phyllis's friends offered to help keep up Phyllis's milk supply by visiting regularly with her two-month-old nursing baby, Mike, and letting Mike nurse from Phyllis.* The visits continued after Janeen came home, with the friend now nursing Janeen some of the time. (Since Phyllis had flat nipples this foster nursing hopefully would help Janeen learn to nurse correctly.)

---

* Great care must be taken when considering having another mother nurse your baby. See Foster Nursing, chapter 13, "When Mother Is Sick or Hospitalized."

After a few days, Phyllis tried breastfeeding Janeen without assistance from Mike and his mother. At each feeding she would nurse Janeen, then offer breast milk she'd expressed after the previous feeding, then formula. Finally she would express what was left in her breasts.

In the weeks that followed, Janeen gained very little weight, and slept six hours at a stretch unless awakened. Even then, she usually wasn't hungry. Perhaps the supplemental formula was causing Janeen to feel full for too long. In order to avoid formula, several other mothers donated breast milk until Phyllis could build up her own supply. Janeen did begin to gain a little more weight, but she did not improve in her ability to nurse from the breast. After a few weeks, Phyllis felt it was unfair to impose any longer on the donors since Janeen had not shown any adverse reactions to formula. Phyllis continued to nurse Janeen, offer her own breast milk in a bottle, and then feed formula.

A slow growth pattern is to be expected with Janeen's birth defect. The pediatrician approved the mothers' sharing procedure, to try to increase Janeen's weight gain. After the first few months he said that the struggle had been worth it since Janeen's survival had been in doubt. He said that perhaps she is a baby who is alive because she got the best—breast milk.

Since Phyllis's breasts were never completely emptied, her milk supply gradually decreased. Eventually Janeen became a bottle baby. She subsequently had repeated bouts with diarrhea which was finally traced to a cow's milk allergy. However, for the first four months of her life, about 85 percent of her intake was breast milk—and she didn't have a trace of even a cold.

Esophageal Atresia

Atresia means absence or closure of a normal body opening. In esophageal or tracheo-esophageal atresia, milk is prevented from reaching the stomach because of a blockage somewhere between the throat and the stomach. Many times there is also a fistula, which is an abnormal hole or connection between the windpipe and esophagus.

In order to receive nourishment normally, your baby will need surgery to open a passage to his stomach. Until he has a normal passage for his food, he will have a tube from the outside to his stomach through which food can be provided. Your baby may suck on a pacifier while being fed through the tube in order to maintain his sucking and swallowing reflexes. Even if the surgery to complete the esophagus is done within the first week of life, it *may* still take a long time for your baby to swallow normally.

If the surgical area tightens, the opening may be so small that your baby will have difficulty getting food down into his stomach. Some may "spill over" into the windpipe, causing him to cough during breastfeeding. It takes more effort for a baby in this condition to nurse, and for you it means more than normal frequency of breastfeeding. You and your doctor may have to decide whether your baby can thrive with breastfeeding or whether he must be fed entirely through a tube. But, as one mother whose baby had esophageal atresia told me, "Just because breastfeeding will be hard or a lot of work for a mother and baby, that should not be the major factor in the *doctor's* decision as to whether or not it should be done! A lot of loving closeness through breastfeeding can result in a very special bond with a baby who has been through many medical difficulties."

Another mother, Zelphia, often nurses her baby at the same time as she administers his meal through the tube so that he can benefit from the breastfeeding experience. He was premature, born with esophageal atresia, but without the fistula. Zelphia says:

> From his second day of life our son has been fed by a gastrostomy tube. When Danny was five weeks old a cervical esophagostomy was performed to drain saliva through an opening made in his neck. Once that was healed I was allowed to nurse him while I also fed him through the tube. At first he did not nurse at every feeding but now he

does so enthusiastically for at least 10 of the 20 minutes I take to feed him by syringe.

At mealtimes I undress Danny down to the diaper, pin one diaper around his neck and place another over my arm. During nursing, the milk drains out of the neck opening into the diaper. As often as possible, I hand express milk so that his feedings are about half breast milk and half formula. By hand expressing and nursing I feel I am helping my baby. My husband is especially impressed that when he has fed our baby and I am out, the baby is unhappy until I get home and nurse him, even though his stomach is already full.

Conditions That Cause Vomiting

Vomiting, ranging from simple regurgitation or spitting up to the projectile type associated with pyloric stenosis, can result from a number of causes. Overfeeding, a strong let-down, a gag reflex, immature muscle control, allergies, diseases, and infections all can cause vomiting. Infants who spit up or vomit frequently need gentle handling. Babies prone to vomiting should be fed upon waking, before they have cried for very long because swallowed air can force up a feeding. Propping the baby in an infant seat or carrier after feeding will help keep the milk in his stomach. Many of these problems are outgrown during the second half of the first year, as the digestive system matures.

With all the vomiting, don't be discouraged about breastfeeding. It's easy to think that once your baby has vomited up "all" the milk there is no more milk until the next feeding. But your breasts are constantly producing milk. If your baby seems happy, avoid feeding him until he acts hungry. Give his stomach a chance to quiet down. Some babies seem to vomit every feeding, but still go on gaining satisfactorily. One distinct advantage to breastfeeding is that there is no sour milk odor when your baby spits up!

See also *Vomiting* in section on Treating Illnesses at Home, chapter 12, "When Baby Is Sick or Hospitalized."

Pyloric Stenosis

This condition, caused by a thickening of the pyloric muscle at the entrance to the stomach, prevents the normal passage of food through the stomach to the intestines. The milk is forcibly ejected from the mouth. The problem usually doesn't show up for several weeks, but it occurs later when a baby is breastfed, and is less severe, because breast milk digests more easily. The lipase that breast milk contains partly digests the milk even before it gets to the stomach. Therefore it passes much more easily through a partially obstructed intestine.

If your baby develops this condition, there will be waves across his stomach and milk will be vomited out with great force, either during or shortly after the feeding. Occasional projectile vomiting does not mean your baby has pyloric stenosis, but if it occurs once a day or more, see your doctor.

Babies suffering from pyloric stenosis lose weight and often become dehydrated and malnourished. The condition is cured by simple surgery involving splitting fibers or is treated by careful feeding and an antispasmodic drug.

The usual technique for breastfeeding a baby with pyloric stenosis is to feed from one breast at a time with short intervals between. Keeping your baby upright during and just after feeding helps the milk stay down. Plastic infant seats were originally designed for babies with this problem.

Some researchers feel that pyloric stenosis may be caused by a baby's reaction to an irritating element in the milk. Whole milk and eggs in the mother's diet may be the cause. Changing to cheese, yogurt, and other sources of calcium and limiting eggs during pregnancy and lactation can help the problem.

Intussusception

Vomiting that comes on suddenly later in infancy, especially if there is pain or if there is green bile in the vomitus, may mean obstruction of the intestines, as in intussusception or strangulated hernia. (3)

Intussusception is an unusual condition in which one part

of the intestine telescopes into another part, resulting in an obstruction. It causes a baby to have sudden, severe cramps, several minutes apart. Repeated vomiting is likely. After a number of hours a movement is passed containing mucus and blood, a "currant jelly" stool.

This condition requires immediate attention. If it is not attended to, gangrene can occur, then bowel rupture, followed by peritonitis, and eventually even death. With adequate early treatment, however, the chances of recovery are high and recurrences are uncommon. (4) Intussusception occurs most commonly between the ages of three months and one year, though it can occur at other ages.

Surgery is frequently used in the United States, but medical treatment is more common in other countries, especially England. Intussusceptions can sometimes be eliminated or reduced by hydrostatic pressure of a barium enema, which pushes the obstructing intestine back into place.

Mary describes her son's experience with this condition:

Tommy was nine months old when he had intussusception. The day before, he had been perfectly happy and healthy. But the next day, he got cramps. He would draw his legs up and his stomach was very hard. He wanted to nurse, for comfort. After a while his stomach would relax and he would fall asleep, exhausted. This pattern repeated itself several times that afternoon. Finally, the cramps would not go away. He cried inconsolably.

We took Tommy to the hospital, but hours passed before they discovered the cause of his pain. When it was finally determined that Tommy had intussusception, he was scheduled for surgery immediately.

After surgery, Tommy was put on I.V.'s to give his stomach a rest. They gave me lemon swabs for his thirst, but he wouldn't take them. Everyone was concerned about dehydration. He begged me to nurse and hold him. But all I could do was stroke his arms, head and legs and talk to him. On the third day his tears turned to despair. He just gave up.

Early the fourth morning they removed the I.V.'s and

tried to feed Tommy. He refused bottle, cup, and baby food. They called *me* to come in. When I walked into the room, Tommy was quiet and staring out the window. I called to him. He turned, looked at me for a minute, then started shaking all over. I picked him up and offered to nurse. He just lay in my arms and sobbed for about 15 minutes. Finally he was calm enough to nurse. For the next three days we just sat in a rocking chair and Tommy nursed constantly, no longer screaming or crying.

Tommy was different after his hospital stay. For the next ten days he nursed like a newborn. He refused to be placed on his back so I carried him in a baby carrier. He had separation anxiety for a long time after the hospitalization. Nursing was a great comfort to him, to both of us.

Breastfeeding meant even more than comfort to Sharon's son. For Michael it was literally lifesaving. Michael had intestinal problems, including *repeated* intussusceptions, until the age of four months, when he outgrew them. These caused him severe pain and projectile vomiting. Sharon explains her son's situation:

When Michael was vomiting so much on breast milk, we tried thick cereal to see if it would stay down better. It didn't. He vomited even more violently, had colic and rashes. Then when he started to lose weight we tried to supplement nursing with an ounce or two of many different types of specially made high calorie formulas. The results were the same as with the cereal. He could tolerate *nothing* but breast milk. He was a good nurser, which helped, so we nursed every one to two hours for four months (around the clock). Many times the breast milk came up. We would wait 20 to 30 minutes and nurse again. The breast milk apparently came up only because Michael had a very immature digestive system and a great intolerance of any strange protein of any kind. With frequent feedings of breast milk only, Michael slowly started gaining weight.

Even after the intestinal problems were overcome we waited until six months before even trying *very* gradually to introduce any type of food. Finally by one year he could eat anything except milk and milk products (still nursing of course).

Today Michael is 8½ years old, a healthy, all-American boy with no problems. We only have one food problem and that is "Give me more, Mom."

I might add that never once did any of our doctors say to quit nursing. They all said, "You keep nursing and your baby will live."

Imperforate Anus

One of the most common malformations at the lower end of the digestive tract is a defect known as imperforate anus (no anal opening). A temporary surgical measure (a colostomy) is taken, without which babies with this condition would probably die. This involves making an opening and bringing the intestine to the outside of the body. Your doctor will probably want to defer the corrective surgery until your baby is bigger and stronger. In the meantime your baby can be breast-fed as before any other type of surgery.

Linda's son was born with imperforate anus, lacking about an inch of intestines and the anal opening. She says:

I was allowed to nurse him on the delivery table. That blissful moment of nursing made the next few days, with filling breasts and no suckling baby, easier to bear. Adam was just 12 hours old when he underwent his first operation, making a colostomy for him. (The doctors planned to wait until he was bigger to do the corrective surgery which would hopefully allow him to function like any other child.) I didn't get to nurse him for three days because he was on I.V.'s. We stayed together on the maternity floor for another nine days, nursing on demand. Adam became badly jaundiced due, no doubt, to the abdominal surgery, and nursed rather lazily. The improvement the first week home was astounding. He became much more eager to nurse.

Adam's corrective surgery was to be done when he

was a year old. It was a two-stage operation—3 weeks apart. Part one was to construct an anus; part two was to close the colostomy. For part one, I didn't nurse Adam for 3 or 4 days out of a week's stay. For part two, I didn't nurse for 7 days out of a 14-day stay. I did remain in the hospital with my baby for the entire time, using their electric breast pump and visiting my baby. During the last operation my milk supply reached a very low level. I was pumping a total of only half an ounce every six hours. Luckily, Adam wasn't especially hungry at first so he slowly built up my supply.

Adam is almost four years old now. There have been other hospitalizations, unrelated to the imperforate anus, and I have always stayed with him. Nursing in the hospital has meant security and love during much pain; it was often the only way I could help Adam. I wouldn't have been able to function as well as I did without that bond. It was sanity in the midst of insanity.

Handling Your Situation

Everyone wants a perfect baby. When there is a birth defect, doubts, fears, and worries are understandable. Parents are often under a tremendous emotional strain, sometimes without fully realizing it. Guilt feelings are nearly inevitable and can be overwhelming. They may not be "rational" at all. One mother of a cleft palate baby told me, "I used to lie awake nights wondering what I could possibly have done, though I knew it wasn't my fault. Eventually I did get over it."

You may be quite upset over the appearance of your child and have feelings of rejection. This may increase your feelings of guilt, for naturally you feel you should accept your child wholeheartedly. A mother of a baby born with imperforate anus told me:

> I was repulsed by my baby's stomas (the ends of the intestine that were brought to the outside since there was no anus). My baby was (as I only realized later) unhappy and in pain and hated to be held. If I didn't *have* to pick

him up to nurse him every two hours, if I could have given his care to someone else, I would have. Thank goodness I had no one but myself to depend on during the day. I loved him too much to see him like this and I constantly dreamt of "accidents" in which he would be killed. I felt terribly guilty for having these thoughts. But, through the touching and closeness that only nursing *demands*, I slowly was able to look at his colostomy and, later, to tend to it as I would have an anus. We touched more and more and my love for him grew.

It's easier to accept your own baby's defect if you have already known other babies with defects. One mother wrote that both she and her husband and her brother were acquainted with birth defects. She says:

As long as Mike didn't have any other more serious problems, we were happy. A cleft lip and a cleft palate can be fixed. Most people don't think in those terms. When my brother first saw Mike he said, "Hey, if it wasn't for his cleft—he'd beat the hell out of the Gerber baby!"

You'll find it helpful to get in touch with other breastfeeding mothers and people who have experienced a situation similar to yours. For parents of cleft palate babies, there are many parent groups across the country. Although you may not find many mothers in the group who have breastfed, they will be very concerned and happy to help you in any way they can. See Appendix: Organizations to Help the Nursing Mother for the address of the Cleft Parent Guild.

For breastfeeding help and encouragement with *any* problem, be sure to get in touch with a La Leche League group. The leader might even be able to put you in touch with another mother who has nursed a baby having the same problems as yours.

Remember, you have a perfectly normal child who happens to have special needs in a very limited area. He will be a more normal baby and a more normal child if you treat him that way and this will ultimately be more important than anything the doctors can do for him medically.

Chapter 9

Problems Related to Baby's Altered Body Chemistry

The nutritional benefits of breast milk are valuable for any baby, and this is especially true for babies who have serious metabolic problems. For various reasons, these babies have difficulty processing nutritional substances to supply their energy and growth needs. They are far better off with mother's milk than with any formula.

With certain problems, breast milk can also help a child who has been weaned months, or even years, earlier. If a mother is nursing a younger baby at the time, she can often supply all or part of her older child's needs for recovery. Breast milk also can be purchased from a milk bank. Sometimes it is donated by other nursing mothers.

There are also metabolic problems which may interfere with a baby's being able to take full advantage of his mother's milk. The amount of breast milk allowed may be minimal, or none at all may be allowed, as with galactosemia.

Hypoglycemia

Hypoglycemia is the body's impaired ability to sustain normal amounts of glucose, a body sugar which serves as a principal source of energy. This is an uncommon metabolic problem of infancy and childhood, affecting 3 of every 1,000 live-born full-term infants, and 43 of every 1,000 premature infants. A baby may be prone to hypoglycemia if he is full term but of low birth weight, or if his mother is hypoglycemic or has Rh negative blood. Among babies of diabetic mothers the frequency of hypoglycemia may be as high as 50 percent. (1) (2) It is important to realize that there are many different causes of hypoglycemia, and treatment varies according to the cause.

Your newborn may be hypoglycemic, but show no symptoms. Or, he may have difficulty in feeding; appear listless or irritable; experience episodes of cyanosis (blueness of the skin, caused by lack of oxygen in the blood); exhibit pale skin and low body temperature; cry in a weak, high-pitched tone or go through tremors, eye-rolling or convulsions. These symptoms may indicate any one of several serious conditions in newborns and should be investigated promptly by your pediatrician.

Brain damage can accompany severe or prolonged hypoglycemia. The likelihood that there will be brain damage is greater the sooner hypoglycemia begins, and increases with the length and severity of the disorder. *Brief, mild,* low blood sugar doesn't seem to affect children if treated early.

Premature babies are especially susceptible to hypoglycemia. Studies have shown that immediate feeding of undiluted breast milk to premature babies is one means of prevention. (3) Hypoglycemia can also be prevented by early feeding of formula, but breast milk provides the baby with many other advantages.

Frequent feeding is vital to hypoglycemic children, and these frequent small feedings may continue even beyond the early months. One mother reported that her son at ten months was still nursing every two hours around the clock, even with solid food.

Diabetic Infant

Diabetes results from a deficiency of insulin in the blood. With too little insulin, the digestive system is unable to absorb normal amounts of sugar and starch.

At birth, diabetic babies are usually small, with a very low insulin level and a very high blood sugar level. Medical supervision is absolutely essential. Breastfeeding is the ideal nourishment, but you may have difficulty finding a cooperative pediatric endocrinologist. A general pediatrician with a good background in diabetes who supports nursing is fine if you can't find a supportive pediatric endocrinologist.

It is possible that your baby may not require insulin, and the diabetes may disappear after a few weeks or months. Meanwhile, you will probably need to keep an eye on the clock to make sure you feed your baby on a regular schedule.

If your infant's diabetes is still present when he starts on table foods, careful attention in making the whole family's diet as well balanced as possible will set good eating patterns and help your diabetic child feel more comfortable with any food restrictions.

(For diabetic mothers, see Diabetes, in chapter 22, "Mothers with Special Physical Problems.")

Malabsorption Problems

Diseases which cause malabsorption involve the functioning of the small intestine. The common feature is the absence of one or more digestive enzymes, which may be lacking in the intestinal wall or the pancreas.

Cystic Fibrosis

Cystic fibrosis is a serious disease affecting children's lungs and digestion, which occurs once in approximately 1,600 births. (4)

In babies born with cystic fibrosis the glands of external secretion do not function properly. The mucous glands secrete an abnormal, thick, gluey mucus and the sweat glands produce an unusually salty sweat. It is the thick mucus which creates two principal problems: difficulty in breathing and in digestion.

Normal mucus is thin and slippery and helps keep the lungs and air passages clean, carrying off germs and dust particles. The sticky mucus of cystic fibrosis clogs the small bronchial tubes in the lungs and makes it hard for a child to breathe. The bacteria which collect in the clogged tubes can then multiply and lead to infection.

The mucus also plugs the tiny ducts of the pancreas, an organ lying along the intestine just below the stomach. The pancreas supplies enzymes to the small intestine, to help digest foods. When the openings from the pancreas are blocked by mucus, the digestive enzymes cannot reach the small intestine to do their work. Food passes through the bowels only partially digested.

The salty sweat produced by the sweat glands usually does not create any major problems; however, it is helpful in diagnosis. By using the sweat chloride test, finding more salt in the sweat than is considered normal indicates cystic fibrosis. Mothers and grandmothers often have been the first to give the doctor a hint by reporting that the baby tastes salty when kissed.

There are striking variations in the severity of cystic fibrosis, ranging all the way from conditions that are undetectable (except by laboratory tests), to those which are serious in the extreme. Many cystic fibrosis babies have a constant cough and have had two or three respiratory infections by the time they are three years old, depending on the severity of their condition. They often look thin, pale, malnourished. If they don't have enzymes added to their diet, they need to eat twice as much as normal children to get all the necessary nutrients. They may also need extra salt in hot weather.

Although cystic fibrosis usually affects both the lungs and intestines, it may affect only one organ. This is the case with Gladys's daughter; only her digestive system is affected. Gladys says:

> After Amy was born, I realized she was gaining very slowly, and by her 6-week checkup, she had only gained a pound. My pediatrician thought it was mainly because I didn't have enough milk, but I was quite sure I did, because she had enough wet diapers and extra large bowel movements. He suggested more frequent nursings. I had been demand nursing about every four hours, but now I

woke her up every two hours. This was extremely frustrating, because she didn't want to nurse that often. She was normally a very contented and happy baby, but became very fussy. At her 3½-month checkup, it was apparent that besides gaining no weight, Amy was not developing properly and was anemic. A series of tests were run, and finally the cystic fibrosis was discovered. I continued nursing, and by giving her the prescribed enzymes, she began gaining weight immediately. It was such a relief to know what her problem was because then we were able to do something about it.

Another mother with a baby whose digestive system was affected by cystic fibrosis describes her method of feeding the additional enzymes:

Our first specialist had me feeding Renée formula, with enzymes added. It was awful. The enzymes kept clogging the nipple and I had to constantly stop Renée from sucking, to shake the bottle. My baby was very frustrated. She also developed an allergy to the formula.

I wanted very much to nurse and the doctor finally agreed I could try. Renée was three weeks old. I'd been keeping up my milk supply with a breast pump and in two days Renée was nursing beautifully and starting to gain weight.

Many cystic fibrosis babies suffer from malnutrition. Without the additional enzymes they can't even digest breast milk properly. I'd had to figure out a way to give her the enzymes (which come in a powder, like sugar) and my solution was to add them to a spoonful of applesauce *
and feed this to Renée immediately before nursing. Later, Renée had tablets, instead of the powder, before meals.

Supplements or solids are often prescribed for babies with cystic fibrosis, but Renée didn't start solids until seven months and did fine on breast milk alone until then.

---

* The enzymes could be put in breast milk instead.

Celiac Disease

After cystic fibrosis, the most frequent cause of malabsorption in infants is celiac disease. This condition makes it impossible to digest gluten, a protein found in all cereal products except corn and rice (soy and potato flours are also gluten free). When a celiac patient eats gluten, the tiny fingerlike protuberances on the walls of the small intestine clump together and become sore and inflamed, eventually making the digestion of all food impossible. (5)

A baby born with celiac disease will show no signs of it for several months, and growth does not usually slow down until 6 to 12 months of age. As foods containing gluten—wheat, rye, oats, barley—are introduced, the baby cannot utilize them, which causes excess mucus to be produced in his digestive tract and his stool to become voluminous, pale and frothy, with a very offensive odor. Often children with celiac disease have inadequate caloric intake in addition to malabsorption.

Where there is a family history of celiac disease, a gluten-free diet for at least the first half year will help postpone the problem. Breast milk alone can supply all the needed nutrients during that time. Patsy says that her two bottlefed sons had such severe celiac symptoms that her doctor had even suggested an abortion when she was expecting her third child. She breastfed her newborn and carefully followed a special diet when solids were introduced. Jeff's first year was problem free, and it wasn't until his second year that celiac symptoms appeared as he weaned. Some donated breast milk during the most serious times helped him recover much more quickly than his brothers had.

In describing the difference between formula-fed and breastfed infants in *The Medical Value of Breastfeeding* (6), there is this statement:

> The celiac infant appears normal at birth and if he is formula-fed he usually becomes a feeding problem with vomiting and poor appetite—or perhaps he eats well and has episodes of diarrhea. . . . The breastfed infants who

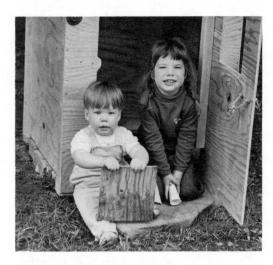

Bryan (16 months) and Rebecca (4 years).

Both children developed celiac disease. Rebecca outgrew it, while her brother still suffers from the gluten intolerance.

develop celiac disease remain well while they are on mother's milk and for many months thereafter and usually don't become ill until the second year.

There is a varying threshold for gluten tolerance among children with celiac disease. Some require dietary management throughout life; others outgrow it after a few months.*

Kathie's baby, Rebecca, was 15 months old when she started having diarrhea problems—four to seven movements a day. (In a completely breastfed baby this would be normal, but not in a baby on other foods.) Kathie says:

> Thank heavens we were still nursing! At least I didn't have to worry about dehydration on top of everything else. We were frustrated for 2½ months until finally we found a doctor who suggested gluten intolerance. We tried avoiding gluten-containing flours and foods that may contain the flours as fillers (such as frankfurters), and it worked.

---

* Mrs. E. Hartsook, Clinical Research Center Dietician at the University of Washington Hospital, Seattle, Washington, will provide upon request a packet of materials which includes Gluten-free Diet Instructions, a Gluten Content of Products List and the latest newsletter from their Gluten Intolerance Group.

Rebecca was affected by the gluten intolerance until she was 2 years old, when she finally outgrew it. Our second baby, Bryan, began having problems at age 16 months, and he too was diagnosed as celiac. Bryan still has the gluten intolerance at 26 months.

I nursed Rebecca until she was over two years old and Bryan is continuing to nurse at this age, too. I especially enjoy nursing because with celiac disease there are so many restrictions. At least I feel sure of the nutrition Bryan is getting from my milk.

Acrodermatitis Enteropathica

The malabsorption associated with this extremely rare disease is the result of poor availability of zinc. For a nursing infant, the condition usually begins at weaning, and for non-breastfed babies it appears at several weeks of age. The symptoms include a very severe skin condition, loss of hair and nails, and diarrhea.

Treatment involves the use of zinc supplement for a child who is not being breastfed. Breastfeeding is important and preferable for babies with this disease. The zinc in breast milk is absorbed better than the zinc in cow's milk or zinc supplement. Soybean formulas cause more problems than cow's milk formulas since soybean protein impairs zinc absorption.

PKU

Phenylketonuria, called PKU, is an inherited disorder which is relatively rare. Children with PKU are unable to properly metabolize an essential nutrient, phenylalanine, which is necessary for normal growth. It is one of 20 amino acids which are the building blocks for proteins. Proteins in turn form an important part of muscles, bones, and the brain—in fact, of all tissues.

High-protein foods such as meat, fish, eggs, and milk contain the most phenylalanine. The proteins in these foods are ordinarily broken down during digestion into amino acids which the body uses with the help of enzymes. In PKU, a particular liver enzyme is lacking. As a result, the amino acid, phenylalanine, is not broken down and it collects in large amounts in the blood, interfering with normal brain development. In addition to mental retardation, a child with untreated PKU may also have convulsions, abnormal behavior, skin rashes, a musty odor to the sweat and urine, and light hair and skin color.

It is impossible for a child with PKU to obtain enough protein from ordinary foods without obtaining an excess of phenylalanine. He must therefore be fed a special chemical formula called Lofenalac. Because *some* phenylalanine is necessary for normal growth, a certain amount of additional protein, usually in the form of cow's milk or breast milk, is allowed.

If your child has PKU, periodic testing to determine the amount of phenylalanine in the body is necessary, and his diet will be adjusted accordingly. Probably when he is six to eight years old his diet may be liberalized, but the phenylalanine still must be kept within reasonable limits. Some clinics are now taking a number of children off the diet completely when they enter school.

Since a low-phenylalanine diet assures normal mental growth and development, it is important to establish the diagnosis of PKU early in life. Many states require by law that a PKU test be run on all babies.

This diagnosis can be established only if a child is already taking some phenylalanine in his diet. Cow's milk contains more protein than breast milk, and leads to a more rapid rise in the blood phenylalanine level. The test therefore usually becomes positive earlier for babies being fed cow's milk.

Medical authorities say, however, that it is not necessary to give a baby cow's milk formula for the PKU test, since the testing can be done on breastfed babies almost as easily. On the contrary, there is good reason to avoid the formula since it is known that early introduction can trigger allergic reactions later on.

A lot of babies have had positive screening tests for PKU and later were found not to have it. Many clinics allow a baby to continue a normal diet (formula or breastfeeding) during a testing period as long as the blood level of phenylalanine remains within a safe range. One mother describes her situation:

> My daughter was tested and the initial results indicated that she was a PKU baby. I kept nursing and she was periodically retested. It took five or six tests, but finally her level came down to the normal range. At five weeks it was determined she needed no further testing, and since then she has shown no signs of the disease. (7)

A child with PKU cannot be raised on breast milk alone because it contains too much phenylalanine. If tests show a considerable worsening of the PKU level, breastfeeding will probably be stopped and Lofenalac formula substituted.

Dr. John W. Gerrard, recipient of the 1962 John Scott Award for work done in the development of a special diet for phenylketonurics, feels that additional breast milk may be allowed as long as the level of phenylalanine in the blood remains reasonably low. The amount of breast milk will need to be specifically determined, and a baby may be allowed more of this than cow's milk, since it is lower in phenylalanine.

If breast milk is to be fed by bottle, you may wish to mix it with the Lofenalac formula since the milk and formula have different tastes. A baby who is offered each separately *may* start to refuse the Lofenalac, even though it must remain the major part of his diet.

Though the breast milk your baby receives may be fed from a bottle, you and your baby may find it more satisfying if the baby can be partially breastfed. This was the case with Marti and her son Andy:

> Two positive screening tests alerted us that Andy had PKU. By the time he was four weeks old he was hospitalized to bring his blood level down to the safe range and he began the restricted diet.*

---

* Children who are started on the PKU diet by the age of four weeks show no discernible brain damage.

Two weeks later, when Andy came home, he was on a strict schedule, alternating nursing with a bottle of Lofenalac every three hours. I weighed him before and after nursing to determine his intake. During the first three months I used a breast pump every time I gave Andy a bottle of Lofenalac to insure that my supply of milk would meet his demands. Then at four months I stopped using the pump and relied on fairly regular nursings to regulate the supply.

Andy's blood level of phenylalanine was tested weekly, and it stayed within the therapeutic range of five to ten times normal on the breast milk and Lofenalac diet. The only deviation came when he had a cold and fever, which caused the level to shoot up.

I began offering solids at 6 months, and took him into bed with me for more comfortable night nursing. Now at 10 months, he usually takes his Lofenalac in two bottles, and nurses several times during the day on demand. He also enjoys foods allowed on his diet plan, such as fruits, vegetables and saltine crackers.

Two other mothers I met have also partially nursed their PKU children. One baby had a diagnostic level of 50 at 3 weeks. She is now 8 months old and has 18 ounces of breast milk a day, plus solids and 65 grams of Lofenalac. The other child had a diagnostic level of 45 at 3 weeks. He partially nursed until he weaned himself from both breast and bottle at 11 months. Both started solids around 6 months, and are active and healthy children.

Galactosemia

This is an inherited disease, which occurs rarely. The disorder results from an enzyme deficiency which inhibits the body's use of galactose. Mental retardation, cataracts, vomiting, diarrhea, jaundice, poor weight gain and malnutrition can result from the continued use of foods containing galactose. As much as 40 percent of the blood sugar in normal infants on a milk diet may be galactose, which is obtained by enzyme action on lactose, or milk sugar. The problem may be worse for breastfed babies than those on cow's milk formulas because there is more lactose in breast milk.

Instead of breastfeeding, you will need to feed your baby a lactose-free milk substitute such as Nutramigen, Isomil or Prosobee. With your baby on a galactose-free diet he will resume normal growth. After a few years your child may be able to tolerate a normal diet because growth is slower and the galactose content of the diet is smaller in relation to body weight. Meanwhile, give your baby lots of holding and cuddling during feedings, even though he cannot be breastfed.

Your Special Concerns

It is natural for all parents to have worries when raising a child. Parents of children born with metabolic problems sometimes have even more concern because of the special diet. Some of the worry may come from well-meaning relatives and neighbors who do not understand your child's condition and think it is cruel to deprive the child of foods *they* happen to like. Simply explain to them that as long as dietary control is maintained, your child can gain weight and grow normally.

If you are discouraged about the diet and feel sorry for yourself, you are not alone. Many parents share these feelings at times. Jenny says:

> For about two years Renée was allergic to eggs or anything containing eggs. Maintaining a constant watch on her diet was a chore at first, but with time it became very routine. One day toward the end of the second year, Renée's older brother gave her a hard-boiled egg. I panicked; I pulled all the egg I could from her mouth, but she was swallowing as fast as I was pulling. I calmed myself, sat and read her a book and kept an eye on her. At naptime she went to sleep as usual, and nothing happened.
>
> I feel like a "Monster Mom" when people offer Renée "forbidden foods" and I have to say "No." Any new food is a temptation, especially when other kids are enjoying

it. I've had to be especially careful with teenage baby-sitters and warn them of the consequences of giving Renée foods she shouldn't have.

Now that Renée is older, it's easier, because she declines on her own by saying, "No, thank you, I'm allergic."

When a child is on a special diet, your facial expressions can have a lot to do with his acceptance or rejection of a particular food. A mother who was feeding her PKU baby the Lofenalac formula said that while it may look like milk, it doesn't taste or smell like it. She disliked the smell so much that without thinking of the effect on her child, she would make a face when she gave it to him. Because of this, he refused it for several days, until she and her husband realized what was wrong. They changed their attitude to thinking only that "this wonderful diet will make it possible for our child to have a happy life." (8)

Marti describes how her son with PKU responded to her loving method of feeding the Lofenalac formula:

It is absolutely essential for parents to accept the bottles of Lofenalac, to teach themselves to enjoy giving their baby his bottle. I hold Andy close to me while he takes his bottle and now that he is eight months old and able to hold the bottle himself this leaves my hands free to stroke him as I would if I were nursing. It is me he looks at, not his bottle. It is me he looks to for his nourishment, not his bottle, despite the fact that he has had 10 to 14 ounces of Lofenalac daily since he was four weeks old.

The mother of a child with cystic fibrosis said that looking back to her daughter's babyhood, the one thing that she regrets is the neglect her 2½-year-old son went through. When his sister was born, he was hurt, jealous and bewildered by the sudden shift in his parents' attention, and wanted the baby to go away. Mother and father let the baby, at first, control their every move, and they couldn't see how their son was suffering from neglect. Two months later, they finally realized what he had been going through and changed their attitudes. Their daughter was accepted as a baby who needed help with a special problem, while at the same time their son deserved his fair share of love and attention.

If you are concerned about your child and his diet management plan, it may help to talk with your doctor, a nutritionist or social worker. Professional counseling can also help if your child's condition is affecting family relationships. Find out if there is a local organization of parents whose children have the same problem as your child. Discussing common problems can benefit parents as well as children. See Appendix: Organizations to Help the Nursing Mother, for a list of addresses.

Chapter 10

Nursing a Baby with Special Developmental Conditions

Acceptance of a Child with a Handicap

Acceptance is important to the welfare of both you and your child. With a handicapped infant, acceptance requires a conscious effort. This means overcoming feelings of guilt, anger, despair, and shame and coming to grips with your expectations. It also involves understanding what will be necessary to take care of your child and preparing yourself to do it.

Nursing can play a major role in developing a loving, warm, accepting relationship. From the moment a handicapped child is born, he needs tremendous quantities of love and acceptance, which breastfeeding can provide. This doesn't mean that a bottlefed baby cannot receive these same things. But breastfeeding is so much more intimate, so much more meaningful for a baby who's handicapped. The relationship is established early and continues for many months— months when a handicapped child is most vulnerable both physically and emotionally.

The care and acceptance of a child with a handicap place great demands on parents. You may have been planning to breastfeed, but now have doubts about it. Medical personnel and family may discourage you, while you yourself are torn between doing something to help your baby and protecting yourself from more sorrow if he does not survive.

Conditions discussed in this chapter include mental retardation, cerebral palsy, epilepsy and varying degrees of responsiveness. While it is the general belief that no treatment can restore a damaged brain to normal functioning levels, the tender loving care associated with breastfeeding is the best aid to health any baby could receive. This nurturing, combined with medical treatment, can help a handicapped child attain his highest potential.

The Importance of Touching

Touching is important to all babies, but especially to those who are not responding to their environment in a normal way. Vera, in telling about her autistic son, says:

A child learns more through his sense of touch than through his visual sense. Breastfeeding is more likely to be a tactile experience than bottlefeeding. We live in a society that tends towards alienation. The crib, playpen, and other restrictive baby equipment accentuate this, which is especially harmful for a child who may already be inclined towards alienation. Autism is an extreme condition. But other children, perhaps having just mild brain damage, may also not be as receptive. You never know how much touching and caressing a child needs. You don't know at first how the child is responding, so it's important to keep giving him lots of loving and touching. Babies are "touch-hungry." You can give them too little, but never too much.

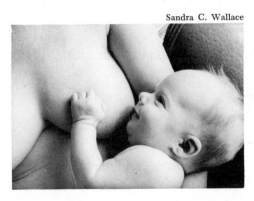

Sandra C. Wallace

The importance of touching to baby's development can't be stressed enough. Breastfeeding allows for the greatest amount of contact between mother and baby.

Stimulation of the skin causes stimulation of all the organs of the body. This is a very important factor in maximum development of the brain, especially one that has been injured. This stimulation occurs best during breastfeeding.

Benefits of Breastfeeding

Some of the advantages of breastfeeding are especially important to babies with developmental problems.

According to Dr. Clemens Benda, author of *Down's Syndrome: Mongolism and Its Management* (1), "The very best thing you can do for these children is nurse them. Breast milk is a perfect food for their often immature digestive systems. Breastfeeding helps to develop good tongue thrust and jaw development."

Human milk is aptly called the superior food for infants. According to *The Uniqueness of Human Milk* (2), it contains over a hundred constituents perfectly suited for babies. Of particular interest is the fact that it supplies specific fatty acids and high levels of cystine (an amino acid) and lactose (milk sugar) for growth during early infancy and particularly for brain development. Because breast milk is such a complete food source, solids can be started at a later age, an important consideration when there is a developmental problem involving the digestive system.

Breastfeeding also improves breathing and therefore gets more oxygen into the bloodstream and subsequently to the brain. Ashley Montagu states:

> The cutaneous stimulation the baby receives from the mother's caressing, from the contact with her body, its warmth, and especially the stimulations received during suckling about the face, lips, nose, tongue, mouth, are important in improving the respiratory functions and through this means the oxygenation of blood. (3)

He also cites a study of 383 Chicago children which found that breastfed children were physically and mentally superior to those who were artificially fed, and that those breastfed from four to nine months were in these respects more advanced than those breastfed for three months or less.

Breastfeeding plays an important role in communication. Many mothers feel that the communication and understanding between mother and child is unparalleled during this time. Kristin's 2½-year-old son is severely retarded, hydrocephalic, and suffers from cerebral palsy. He can't chew or sit up, has no speech (except a few sounds), but is slowly improving. She describes how nursing brought them closer:

> Nursing—how can I measure what it has meant to us? Matt nursed until he weaned himself at two years. The greatest thing for him, emotionally, was the comfort, love and security of Mom. Nursing was the only response I got from Matt for months; there was no eye contact; no smiles, no recognition except that he knew how to nurse.

Amy, mother of a child with a spinal defect, describes the value of breastfeeding in helping parents accept such special children. She says:

> Psychologists have determined that, when all else has failed, "mothering" of these babies has done more than "doctoring." Survival obviously is crucial, but survival alone is not enough. To secure a child's life and neglect the emotional bond is not fulfilling the circle of healing. . . . As a mother, I needed this breastfeeding experience to become more at ease with my baby, whom I simultaneously loved and feared. I loved the beautiful pink face, so full of trust, but feared the defect. The initial rejection of the baby, which is felt to varying degrees, is greatly reduced through breastfeeding. The bond of mother-infant love is made great enough to overcome negative reactions and fear.

As you read through this chapter you will find other benefits that nursing mothers have found, as well as ideas on how they have handled their situations.

There is a wide range of severity in the problems discussed. No two babies are alike (even though their problems may have the same name), and no two mothers are alike, either.

With extremely severe problems, breastfeeding in the usual sense may not be possible. But even though the normal route may be impossible, tubes or other special apparatus can enable your baby to receive breast milk.

Sucking Reflex

One of the most frequent problems for babies with muscular and developmental conditions is a poor or absent sucking reflex. A great deal of patience is needed to help a baby learn to suck.

A further complication occurs when a baby is born seriously ill and his mother is not even allowed to offer to nurse him. She must keep up her supply until she can nurse and not become discouraged.

Once your baby can suck, even poorly, the practice of breastfeeding will improve his sucking ability. Bottles are to be avoided *if possible*. Scientific research shows that babies who are given bottles do not develop such a strong sucking motion. If your baby is being given bottles of water or milk, he will be less interested in breastfeeding. (4)

If your baby's suck is so weak at first that he cannot get enough milk for adequate nourishment by breastfeeding, there are other ways of giving him your milk: by tube, spoon, eyedropper, or nursing supplementer. See chapter 6, "Nursing a Premature Baby," for alternate ways to feed and to maintain your milk supply.

Difficulty of Diagnosis

Diagnosis of developmental problems may be difficult with a young baby. Some infants seem perfect at birth and their problems are not obvious for several days, weeks or months. Some parents feel that their babies have a problem but are unable to pinpoint it or if they can, perhaps they cannot convince anyone else, including their doctors, that something is wrong.

Even if the diagnosis of a problem is made a few weeks, months or even years after birth, it can still come as a shock. Yet, knowing for certain that your baby does have a problem helps you know what to do about it.

Hydrocephalus

Hydrocephalus is an enlargement of the head caused by an abnormal accumulation of cerebrospinal fluid. Normal drainage of this fluid is blocked by an obstruction. Depending upon the amount of pressure on the brain caused by this poor drainage, there may or may not be brain damage. (5) The increased pressure on the brain can cause severe headaches.

There are several causes of hydrocephalus: prenatal developmental defects of the openings of the cavities in the brain; tumors; a scar or adhesion on the absorbing surfaces occurring after meningitis; or hemorrhage from a brain injury. (6)

Once your baby is diagnosed as hydrocephalic, treatment will probably be started at once to minimize or prevent brain damage. The surgical treatment consists of inserting a synthetic tube to form an artificial passage which bypasses the point of obstruction and diverts the cerebrospinal fluid to another area of the body, where it can be absorbed and excreted. (7)

After surgery, your baby will be observed carefully and fed intravenously. He will probably be kept flat for two to four days to avoid complications, and will be given fluids by mouth when he can tolerate them. Ask your doctor to request that your expressed breast milk be given to your baby rather than formula. When your baby's condition becomes stable and he is strong enough, you can get permission from your doctor to start or resume breastfeeding. If your baby's head is markedly enlarged so that you have difficulty holding him, you may find it easiest to nurse lying down.

Lesley, a mother who gave birth to a son with hydro-cephalus, said:

> David was born two months premature, and was put on intravenous feeding. My doctor would not allow me to breastfeed, so when he was about 14 days old, I began feeding him with a bottle. The entire time, I really felt something was missing. David improved and finally we were allowed to bring him home. At my postnatal checkup my doctor suggested that I might try to breastfeed.
>
> When I put David to my breast I only had a trickle of milk, and felt I had to help him out with formula. After a trying week, I almost gave up. But then a girl-friend's enthusiasm gave me the boost I needed to try and reestablish my milk supply. The baby was seven weeks old when I really decided to feed him, and soon he no longer required any supplement. (8)

Spina Bifida

More than 12,000 babies with spina bifida are born every year in the United States. While developing in utero, every infant's backbone remains open until about the twelfth week. In spina bifida, one or more of the individual bones of the back (vertebrae) fail to close completely, leaving a cleft or defect in the spinal column. (9) Part of the spinal cord and the membranes covering it may bulge through the defective closure like a hernia, forming a visible external sac. Body functions below the defect are usually affected.

If your baby is born with spina bifida, you will probably be unable to hold him for several days. However, most inten-sive care units recognize the importance of bonding and will allow parents to visit and touch their infant.

Your baby is likely to undergo surgery soon after birth, and will be placed in a prone position to protect his incision. He will be fed intravenously at first, but in a short time may be ready to be put to breast. You will be shown how to hold your baby properly so that the surgical site is protected and under no strain.

Maurie's son, Erik, underwent surgery 12 hours after he was born, and she was unable to begin nursing him until he was three days old. She describes the positioning:

Erik couldn't be on his back at all, or cradled in my arms. The nurses suggested I use a rocker-recliner chair placed back at a 45-degree angle. I then put my feet up for comfort and arranged two bed pillows under my arm on the side Erik would nurse. The nurse placed Erik across my stomach so that we were tummy to tummy and he could easily reach the nipple. He was comfortable and began to nurse immediately. Eleven days after the back was closed, the stitches were removed and I was finally able to nurse him in a normal sitting position.

Diane's son was placed in an Isolette and fed intravenously immediately after birth due to complications from spina bifida. Diane says:

After some persistence, I was allowed to nurse him for the first time, while the tubes were still attached. It was awkward and more than a little frightening but Matt latched on right away. I stayed with him as much as possible and nursed him on demand. When I couldn't stay, I expressed my milk every two or three hours and sent it in bottles for him. At three weeks, Matthew was doing well and gaining nicely, so we could take him home.

Children with multiple problems such as those with spina bifida are often involved in lengthy outpatient visits. One mother stressed that "nursing was the safety valve for us after long waits in reception rooms and the emotional encounters one has in obtaining medical advice and treatment."

Cerebral Palsy

Cerebral palsy, the major cause of crippling disease in children in the United States, is a defect of motor power and coordination related to damage of the brain. Children are affected in varying degrees: some are mentally retarded; others are capable of considerable improvement; others may be so mildly affected that treatment is not necessary. A very small number of cases are so severe that the child must be bed-ridden. (10)

Some infants with cerebral palsy can be diagnosed soon after birth. They may have a feeding problem related to a poor suck and difficulty in swallowing, excessive drooling, or asymmetry in body movements. Diagnosis may not occur until two or three years of age if delay of motor development is the only symptom. Other symptoms which may be associated with cerebral palsy include visual defects, hearing defects and emotional disturbances. (11)

Dr. Alfred Scherzer, director of the Division of Pediatric Rehabilitation, New York Hospital, and Clinical Professor of Pediatrics at Cornell University Medical College, states: "Feeding a child with cerebral palsy presents many challenges, both in management and in learning. . . . Early stimulation of the lips is essential. . . . The older child may not be able to close his lips and retain food because of inadequate oral development." (12)

With severe cerebral palsy, instead of the normal wave-like motion by which food placed on the front of the tongue is moved back in the mouth and then down the throat, the movement may be reversed. As a result, each mouthful of food the child tries to swallow may be pushed out of his mouth. (13) Breastfeeding, of course, is an excellent stimulant for the lips and entire mouth area and promotes good oral development. It is therefore most desirable for a baby with cerebral palsy.

Breastfeeding your newborn may be difficult at first because of his weak suck or difficulties with tongue thrusting and swallowing. Your baby may be slow in learning how to latch onto your nipple or may lose it easily. He may tire quickly because of his efforts and perhaps not be able to nurse fully at each feeding. (This is also true of many normal, premature babies.) Try more frequent nursing sessions and offer one breast at a time, perhaps every hour or two, until he is more successful. This can help conserve your baby's energy, but it does mean nearly constant nursing for a while. Your baby will gradually develop a better sucking reflex, which not only will help him nurse well but also help avoid tongue thrust and drooling.

While his suck is still poor, you may find that you are not producing as much milk as the baby needs. Try expressing from your breasts either by hand or by breast pump to build up your supply.

Problems with swallowing, such as coughing, sputtering or a hyperactive gag reflex, may occur, especially during your milk let-down. To help avoid this problem, encourage your let-down by expressing before you start to nurse or by temporarily taking the nipple out of your baby's mouth when you start to let down. You can just let the milk flow onto a diaper or allow it to flow into a sterile container and freeze it for future use. After the let-down your flow of milk will be gentler and easier for your baby to handle.

If biting is a problem, it will probably occur at the beginning and end of a nursing, as with normal babies. It may be helpful to run a finger along the inner cheek and outer gum on both sides and along the front of your baby's mouth before nursing. This "desensitizes," or diminishes, the biting reflex.

Hypotonia

Hypotonia is diminished tone, strength or tension of the muscles. Often distinguished by apathy and disinterest in nursing, it is a symptom of a more general problem stemming from brain or nerve damage. It is associated with cerebral palsy, spina bifida, hydrocephalus and Down's syndrome.

Margaret's baby was hypotonic and had delayed motor development. Several years passed before a very mild case of cerebral palsy was diagnosed. Margaret describes how her baby's condition affected nursing:

Michelle had no problem in learning to nurse although she did tend to lose her grip on the nipple. She would latch on again quickly with each suck, making a clicking sound. Fortunately, I was loaded with milk and would let down three or four times per nursing, so she got plenty.

She slept for hours at a time, then would wake up and nurse for an hour or an hour and a half before dozing off again. I found I had to be a clock-watcher and wake her for nursings, so she would get the nourishment she needed. This continued for about five or six months. She was not very active, and seemed even "floppy," but there was no need for alarm because she was progressing gradually and gaining well.

Michelle is now six years old and vastly improved, obviously bright with excellent speech and understanding although she is not physically as strong or coordinated as her peers. She nursed right through my next pregnancy and then after it right along with her baby sister. She still nurses (one suck) occasionally at bedtime. Our doctor has been very supportive and thinks it is great that we still nurse.

Overresponsive Infants

An overresponsive baby is one who overreacts to stimulation by being hypersensitive, highly irritable and highly active. He is not easily comforted, doesn't like to be touched, is extremely fretful and cries in a high-pitched voice much of the time. All these things may prevent him from relaxing enough to feed at the breast very successfully. Other labels for this type of child are hyperactive, hypertonic, and hyperkinetic.

Some babies seem to be irritable or fussy because their mothers are taking medications and the babies cannot tolerate the small amount present in breast milk. Medications are rarely the cause of a problem, but it is well to have a knowledgeable discussion with your doctor before taking anything. If a medication you are using does seem to be upsetting your baby, ask your doctor for a different prescription.

If you find that your baby is highly sensitive or irritable in some way, you may need to modify your environment to help him feel secure. Avoid loud sounds that can be startling, and talk to him in gentle tones. Have father pay special attention to this; the lower tones of a man's voice can frighten a baby. Avoid strange or new environments until he settles down and can cope with them better. Pad any surface where you might lay him down for a diaper change or bath, always hold him securely, and use a baby carrier often. Do not feel awkward about refusing to allow others to hold your baby if it upsets him. Think of your baby's emotions first and offer an explanation.

Mable describes her experience:

Patrick was an extremely active baby right from the start. He was easily startled and was awake for longer periods than he was asleep. He was fed on demand, and I did notice there were certain predictable times when he'd want to nurse. For example, he wanted to nurse at lunchtime when everyone else was eating, but if lunch were delayed for others, he'd be likely to wait longer before asking for that nursing. He always wanted to nurse at bedtime when the house was very quiet. Patrick wanted to nurse more frequently than my other babies, and I got upset until I accepted this as part of Patrick's personality. Patrick weaned later than my other children, because nursing was such a source of comfort for him.

Jeri said her son, diagnosed years later as having minimal brain dysfunction with some hyperactivity, was very unhappy as a baby and cried constantly except when nursing. Jeri explains their breastfeeding relationship:

David had a "strictly business" attitude when he nursed: he'd spend ten minutes on each side and then want me to put him down. I wanted to caress him more, but due to a tactile sensory problem, handling was painful to him. Bringing David into bed to nurse didn't work because he would usually stop nursing before falling back to sleep.

He just would not nurse any longer than he had to for nourishment. David continued to nurse through my third pregnancy and weaned himself just barely past two years of age. It's unusual he nursed this long, because children with this problem usually remain emotionally detached and will not nurse, except for food. Obviously David must have enjoyed it to some extent, because he nursed to that age.

Down's Syndrome

Down's syndrome, formerly called mongolism, occurs in about 1 of every 1,000 live births. (14) These children have 47 chromosomes in each cell instead of 46. The risk of having a child born with Down's syndrome increases as the mother's age increases. It rises to 1 in 50 births for mothers aged 45 years and over. (15)

Indications of Down's syndrome may be recognized at birth. Typical characteristics include eyes that slant slightly upward and give an Oriental appearance, a protruding tongue and muscle weakness. The relatively large tongue and generalized muscular hypotonicity often cause weak sucking and slow nursing.

Growth and development are slow. Generally, the ability to sit, to walk, and to talk develops later than in other babies, sometimes requiring many extra months or years.

There are varying degrees of physical problems associated with Down's syndrome. Some newborns may simply be sleepy with a poor or nonexistent suck. Others may be in more serious condition due to a heart defect or an intestinal obstruction. Some infants may have breathing difficulties at first even though there are no heart problems. But, if your baby's condition is good after birth, you should be able to nurse him soon after delivery, perhaps even on the delivery table.

How successful you are at nursing depends on the extent to which your baby is affected by the condition. One mother was never able to get her baby to breastfeed because of the baby's muscular inability to suck effectively at the breast. The baby was fed intravenously at first, then at 3 weeks she was given formula in a bottle through a large-holed nipple. At 2 months, this infant had gained only a pound; she weighed less than 6½ pounds. By 3½ months solids were introduced, but because of eating problems she would scream every time she saw her food, and vomit afterwards. A neighbor, experienced with her own premature baby, suggested that breast milk be put into the bottle. She expressed a few ounces to be given to this baby, now 6 months old and only 9 pounds. The baby accepted the breast milk willingly and retained it. Other nursing mothers also contributed milk which was given to the baby in addition to her other food. Within three weeks, this baby had gained a full pound and has continued to thrive and gain satisfactorily.

A baby with Down's syndrome who doesn't nurse well needs to be treated like a premature baby. His sucking reflex may be underdeveloped at first, but he will eventually mature to typical newborn level. One mother said that for the first few weeks it was difficult to get her son to "latch on" as his tongue was always pressed against the roof of his mouth. She had to push his tongue down with her finger and push the nipple into position so that he could start sucking.

Another mother pointed out that because these children are often not demanding, you may have to be a clock-watcher for a while. Her baby needed to be on a two-hour schedule for four to six weeks, then every three hours until three months, then four hours until six months.

Susie's daughter was born with Down's syndrome, and additional complications meant immediate surgery. Susie describes how she began breastfeeding Emily:

> Her operation involved the intestine so she was allowed nothing by mouth for some time. In the meantime, I had obtained an electric breast pump to keep my milk supply in. After being fed intravenously for 10 days, she was finally allowed to nurse, but she had no normal sucking reflex. It took two weeks for the nurses and me to stimulate

any sucking instinct, and then it was only with the easier-to-suck rubber nipple. She gained slowly, but finally, 28 days after admittance, Emily came home. I was still determined to nurse, but even when we got home, we made little progress. On the advice of a friend in La Leche League, I tried a rubber breast shield and it worked.*

Then one day several months later as Emily lay on my lap, ready to nurse, I dropped a towel. As I leaned over her to retrieve it, she began to suck on my real nipple. We threw away the breast shields and Emily nursed until the age of two, then weaned herself.

Other Types of Retardation

Retardation is often associated with many of the conditions discussed in this chapter. It can range from mild to severe and is not always easy to detect in the early weeks of an infant's life unless there are other related problems.

Mothers have described their retarded infants as having some of the following symptoms:

Unusual posturing, with either limpness or rigidity

Apathy, disinterest, lack of eye contact

Excessive drooling

Difficulty in swallowing

Lack of enthusiasm about nursing at any time

Weak sucking

Retardation varies in its effects on breastfeeding. These mothers suggest that smaller, frequent feedings may be necessary if the baby vomits when too full. When he begins

---

* Susie used the breast shield discussed in Shields Used during Nursings, chapter 2, "Nursing Techniques." Cleanliness is very important with these to prevent infection and soreness. La Leche League does not recommend breast shields in most cases, since babies can become dependent on them. Fortunately, it worked well for Susie and Emily.

solids he may need to be nursed first if he tends to gag with solids plus breast milk in his stomach.

One mother who had a difficult time getting her retarded baby to nurse after he'd been bottlefed for three weeks in the hospital, offers these hints that worked for her:

- At first, place the breast nipple in his mouth, then place your finger under his chin to coax him to close his mouth and begin to suck.

- Hold the breast, otherwise the weight will pull the nipple out of his mouth.

- At the beginning of each feeding, put him to the breast to encourage nursing. When he tires or becomes frustrated, then give the bottle.

These babies are often prone to be slow gainers. Don't panic. Remember a fairly steady gain is all you need, and the amount is not important.

Maybe your baby's tongue is relatively thicker or his mouth smaller than normal and this can cause difficulty in sucking. Also, if he is not holding the nipple properly he may be swallowing air. Burping is important for any baby who tends to gulp and swallow air.

Don't force solids; you can wait until six months or even later.

Autism

Autism is a rare condition which is characterized by severe problems in communication and behavior, and an inability to relate to people in a normal manner. It may be suspected as early as a few weeks or months after birth, or not until two years of age or later. (16)

No two autistic children are exactly alike, but they all have language difficulties in common. They may appear withdrawn, apathetic or unresponsive or resistant to change. An extreme disinterest in people and surroundings may be countered by an unusual interest in inanimate objects. They may exhibit repetitive movements, such as hand shaking, prolonged rocking and spinning, and head banging. Autistic children often have sleeping difficulties and feeding problems (such as a poor suck) and may show no desire to be held. (17) Some cry constantly, some not at all.

An autistic baby who sucks very poorly may become more vigorous as he matures. (18) It is well worth the effort to attempt to breastfeed even if you must use special aids until your baby learns to nurse. He may not be able to suck enough from your breast for his nutritional needs but you can express your milk and feed it to him by other means, until he can nurse reasonably well on his own. It is important to put your baby to your breast as frequently as possible to help stimulate his sucking reflex and to provide the closeness, security, and warmth so necessary to him. A baby who persistently objects to close cuddling could still be nursed by resting him on a pillow if you are sitting. Or you might lie down with him, with his body angled away from yours (as you might nurse a baby in very hot weather) until he accepts closer skin contact. Some infants may have a hyperactive gag reflex; remedies for this problem are discussed in the section on Cerebral Palsy in this chapter.

Vera's son seemed to have problems right from birth, even though he was not diagnosed as autistic until he was two years old. Mark spent his first nine days in an Isolette, being fed by bottle. When he came home he adjusted to his mother's breast with little difficulty. Up to about six months, Mark took a long time with nursings, often several hours, and when he wasn't feeding he was either asleep or crying. Vera explains how breastfeeding affected their contact and communication:

> The long nursings left me no time to do anything else. But that was what Mark seemed to need. With breastfeeding you *can* let your baby suck for hours. With bottlefeeding you can't.
>
> Mark found inanimate objects very appealing, and with bottlefeeding he could have run off to a corner, alone

with his bottle. With breastfeeding we were constantly touching, something that is very important when dealing with autism. Mark could see me better and identify with me better than with bottlefeeding. He did not cry while he was nursing and didn't object to the body contact. As an older baby, if he was ever touched (except when nursing) he would stiffen and cry.

Around eight or nine months of age, Mark started long periods of rocking by himself, on his hands and knees. He was becoming increasingly resistant to being held, but was still breastfeeding.

One day, when he was 11 months old, he bit me while nursing. I knew that to stop a baby from biting, a firm "No" usually does the trick. Unfortunately, Mark would never nurse again. He acted as if he had never seen the breast before. He went on the bottle then and he refused to be held any more. If I had a chance to do it over again, I would try some other method of stopping the biting, such as closing his nostrils.

Though Mark wasn't diagnosed autistic until he was two years old, by being aware that something was not right, I feel we were able to make the problem less severe.

Your Cheering Squad

A supportive husband, doctor and friends can help carry you through the times of questioning, disappointment and discouragement. Louise put it this way: "I mustn't underestimate my husband's help with Erika. He bolstered my ego in times of depression, and encouraged and consoled me. With his help I have been able to think of Erika first as a child and secondarily as a child who has a handicap."

Husbands need moral support too. Who can give this better than their wives? Louise's husband wrote, "It is easy to accept a normal, healthy infant, but it is much more difficult to accept a handicapped youngster during those first minutes and hours. A nursing mother somehow puts her husband at ease as she cuddles his child to her breast."

It is not unusual for one parent to feel differently from

the other. As parents adapt, they often go through stages of wanting to be alone, then wanting to share their feelings with someone close, and finally reaching out to others. (19)

One mother said that at first she had not been able to face meeting with other mothers whose children had no problems. She wanted, though, to talk with other mothers of handicapped children. Such families need each other for moral support and information. For a list of groups to contact for help and advice consult Appendix: Organizations to Help the Nursing Mother.

Other people, besides you and your husband, may be involved in your child's development. Susie, in writing about her daughter who has Down's syndrome, said, "Emily has many teachers to help her with all phases of development. A home trainer comes every week, she sees a physical therapist every few months and we are working with the people from a clinic for the developmentally disabled. One of Emily's favorite helpers is not among these professionals, though; it is her four-year-old brother, Alan."

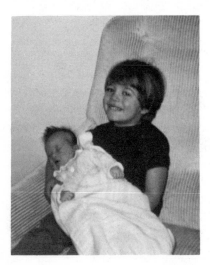

Alan (4 years old) holding Emily (1 month old) on her first day home from the hospital.

Chapter 11

Dealing with Allergies

Breastfeeding to Avoid
Potential Allergies

According to a report from the National Institute of Allergy and Infectious Disease, it is estimated that 35 million Americans suffer from allergies (about 17 percent of the population). (1) Nearly a third of the days lost from school are due to asthma alone. (2)

Avoidance, or lessening, of allergic symptoms is one of the main reasons why many mothers choose to breastfeed their babies. According to Dr. Jerome Glaser, pediatric allergist and author, breastfeeding is the most important single measure in the prevention of allergic disease. (3)

As long ago as 1936, Grulee and Sanford, in a study involving more than 20,000 infants observed over a five-year period, found that eczema (a skin rash characterized by dry scaly areas, itching, and progressing in more severe cases to the formation of patches of oozing, tiny blisters) developed in seven times as many infants fed cow's milk as in infants fed breast milk. (4)

In a more recent study, at the University of California Medical Center, San Francisco, Herbert S. Kaufman, M.D., and Oscar L. Frick, M.D., observed 94 infants from birth to age two. All of the mothers and 36 of the fathers suffered allergies. But the 38 children who were breastfed "inherited" significantly fewer allergies from their parents than did bottlefed youngsters. While almost 18 percent of the bottle-fed infants developed asthma, only 5 percent of the breastfed infants did. And fewer of the breastfed infants developed allergic skin rashes. (5)

Further corroboration of the value of nursing in preventing allergy is given by John W. Gerrard in an article in *Pediatric Annals* (6) where he states:

> The evidence that breastfeeding prevents allergic disease is based on five factors. First, pediatric allergists such as Glaser, who practiced when breastfeeding was common, noted a greater prevalence of allergies in infants brought up on formula than in those brought up on the breast. Second, breast-fed babies, after developing allergies when given supplemental foods, recover from their allergies when these foods are avoided. Third, babies on the breast alone may develop allergies that subside as soon as the food to which the baby is sensitive is eliminated from the mother's diet. Fourth, some babies—approximately 20 percent in our experience—grow out of their cow's milk allergy by the age of 12 months. (Such babies, if brought up on breast milk and not given cow's milk until the age of 12 months, would not be expected to develop cow's milk

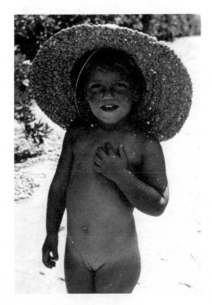

Lada's daughter,
Eleanor, 2 years old.

"Due to her allergic condition, Eleanor was unable to tolerate any foods besides breast milk, white rice, and honey. Her childhood has not been normal, but except for the night she was born, she has never spent a night in a hospital. Breastfeeding has given Eleanor beautiful skin, free from eczema, and perfect teeth. She has an ebullient personality which I attribute to all the cuddling she has had and the fact that most of the time she has been free from allergic episodes."

Lada

allergy.) Finally, it has been our experience . . . that babies with gastroenteritis due to cow's milk allergy often develop normal gastrointestinal function when given breast milk alone.

Breastfeeding can also have far-reaching effects beyond the beneficial quality of mother's milk. "In avoiding allergies, it's not just the breastfeeding that's important," said one allergic mother, "it's the mothering that goes along with it. Your allergic child is liable to be unhappy. He doesn't feel well. His stomach may hurt, he may itch or he may have headaches or all sorts of little problems, and you can't do any better in the mothering department than you can as a nursing mother."

What Are Allergies?

An allergy is an oversensitive reaction to a normally harmless substance that enters or comes in contact with the body. By reacting to the substance as if it were an enemy, and trying to protect itself against the "foreign agent," the body produces an allergic reaction. This involves an overproduction of certain antibodies which combine with the invading substance; chemical mediators such as histamine are released which can adversely affect body organs and tissues. The symptoms may cover a wide range of complaints. Almost any substance ingested, inhaled or contacted can cause an allergic reaction in someone at some time. No age is exempt.

Allergies in infancy are apparently the outcome of a relatively immature immune system. Some children do lose their sensitivity to certain allergens after a while. However, many children never do so. By breastfeeding, you help your child avoid allergic symptoms at a very critical time. Allergies, once established, may persist with varying manifestations and degrees of severity throughout life.

Other factors besides food which are involved in the production of allergy symptoms include: infections, fatigue and emotional stress; the presence of other allergens such as house dust, pollen, mold, wool, synthetic materials, dyes; and even weather changes with extremes of cold or heat. If you have a potentially allergic baby (a baby who has one or more allergic parents or siblings) you will want to be aware of these other factors as well as your baby's diet. Environmental allergens are not usually considered a problem for infants. It is generally thought to take several pollen seasons for these to materialize.

An allergic reaction can manifest itself in various ways. Many babies with allergies have colic and spit up considerably. Some have rashes, diarrhea, frequent night waking, dark circles under the eyes ("allergic shiners"), and stomach cramps. They generally do not feel well. Asthma, hay fever, eczema and hives are familiar symptoms, but there are many other symptoms that are often unrecognized.

The following is a list of symptoms which you may not have associated with allergies:

Noisy breathing
Sneezing, wheezing
Runny or stuffy nose after eating
Seasonal colds
Frequent respiratory infections
Ear infections, itchy ears, dizzy spells (middle ear irritation)
"Clogged up" ears (edema—watery swelling—of eustacian tube)
Voice changes or hoarseness (from swelling)
Itchy skin
Clicking noises with tongue (itchy palate)
Facial grimaces (itchy nose)
Conjunctivitis—reddened eyes, itching, excess watering, child rubs eyes
Colic
Poor appetite
Anemia (usually milk allergy)
Excessive burping, gas
Constipation
Vomiting, nausea
Constant crying, fretfulness

Lethargy
Hyperactivity, irritability

Don't jump to conclusions; many of these may appear as symptoms of conditions other than allergies.

The Role of Inheritance

The tendency to be allergic is inherited, but any or all of the four major allergic disorders—asthma, hay fever, hives, atopic (allergic) dermatitis—may occur in various family members. For example, if you develop hives when you eat wheat, your child might have a tendency to have asthma when he is around cats or dogs. Parents who have skin allergies or respiratory allergies—with no specific food allergies—can have a baby with food allergies.

It is estimated that a child has a 50 percent chance of developing an allergy if there is a history of allergy on one side of the family, and a 75 percent chance if both family lines are affected. (7) Occasionally children are allergic in the absence of any family history of allergies. Genetic possibilities are not the only factor. The amount and frequency of the food consumed and its own nature also play a role.

When Do Allergies Occur?

Allergies may appear dramatically soon after birth. One mother's child was given a bottle of sugar water in the nursery, and soon afterwards he began jumping and twitching all over his bassinet. It was discovered later that he was extremely allergic to corn in any form, and the sugar water he was given contained corn sugar. However, delayed reactions are more common.

Some babies become allergic to a substance when exposed to a minute amount. Others require a massive exposure before they have an allergic reaction. Usually, an allergy does not appear on first exposure to the substance, but only after two or more exposures. However, it can be difficult to trace previous exposures when a reaction occurs. For example, the offending substance may have been given in the hospital or given by an older child who let the baby have a "taste" of his food without the mother realizing it. Or the substance may have been encountered during pregnancy or lactation.

During pregnancy, an excess of one food can sensitize a susceptible baby. Dr. Glaser tells of one mother who ate large quantities of peanuts during pregnancy. A short time after birth, before any feedings, the infant showed a marked local skin reaction when touched with a peanut.

In another case a woman drank considerable amounts of orange juice during pregnancy. Shortly after delivery and before breast or other feeding (at the suggestion of the father, a distinguished allergist), a few drops of orange juice were given to the baby; this resulted in the development of eczema. Later the child was shown to have an intolerance for orange juice and it had to be omitted from her diet for many years. (8)

Some babies react to one substance only when they encounter it in connection with another substance. For example, they may not be able to eat certain foods during the hay fever season although at other times they can enjoy them with no apparent reaction.

If the effect of the *combination* of factors involved in the production of allergy symptoms in your baby (such as his diet, health, surroundings) remains below his allergy tolerance threshold, his allergies will not be apparent. If the flood of allergens exceeds the tolerance threshold, the allergic symptoms appear. Sometimes an allergic child may safely eat one of several foods to which he is mildly sensitive, but if he eats two at the same time, he is likely to suffer a reaction. It is possible that everyone has a tolerance threshold which can be overwhelmed if the allergic load is heavy enough. Those with an inherited predisposition to allergy seem to have a lower threshold than those with no family history of allergy.

No matter what form your baby's allergic reaction takes, it has the potential of developing into a very serious problem.

Some Allergic Manifestations

Tension-Fatigue Syndrome

The tension-fatigue syndrome is an allergic manifestation that is often overlooked by parents and doctors. It is character-ized by fatigue, lethargy, irritability, alternating periods of excitement and listlessness, pale complexion with dark circles under the eyes, and nasal congestion. An allergic child may exhibit all or some of these symptoms and life can be difficult for a child with an undiagnosed syndrome. Dr. Vincent A. Marinkovich, a pediatric allergist, sees breastfeeding as nature's protection:

> The classical form of tension-fatigue syndrome is caused by cow's milk. Removing all sources of the offending allergen from the diet is sufficient in uncomplicated cases.

Digestive Disturbances

Digestive disturbances caused by allergy can involve the gastrointestinal tract anywhere from the mouth to the anus. Common conditions in infancy include colic, diarrhea, and constipation.

Pearl, an allergic mother who has nursed all six of her children, said:

> In my own experience and from talking with other mothers, two weeks after birth is often when problems begin. One of my daughters began to have mild colic and diarrhea at two weeks, and by six weeks was in severe pain, con-stantly passing blood in her frequent, slimy, greenish stools. Cow's milk turned out to be the culprit. I found that breast milk was perfect for Becky as long as I eliminated from my diet *anything* containing cow's milk products. After a year I gradually began to eat foods containing cooked cow's milk, and there were no longer any obvious allergic symptoms shown by my daughter.

If your baby has colic you should not automatically assume it is because of what you are eating. Check what else might be the cause. Try burping the baby several times during a feeding. Is the baby's mouth positioned properly around the nipple while nursing? Is the baby ill? He may be fussy because he has an ear infection, or is teething earlier than expected.

Allergic diarrhea is usually caused by foods. It is caused by swelling of the mucous membranes or by smooth muscle spasms, and results in many loose, smelly stools a day.

It is important to make a distinction between diarrhea and the normal bowel movement of a totally breastfed infant. An article in *La Leche League News* (9) on diarrhea states:

> Breastfed babies can have very small, runny, soupy, frequent stools, sometimes only a stain on the diaper, which may vary considerably in color and consistency even from day to day or week to week.
>
> Even the appearance of mucus need not necessarily be a cause for alarm in an otherwise healthy and thriving baby. This particular kind of stool is sometimes thought to be the result of a sensitivity to a foreign protein or substance which has been passed on to the baby through the mother's milk. This may occur in babies whose families have a history of allergies, and the "treatment" for it is not to take the baby off the breast, but rather, to ignore it and eventually it will go away. If it seems to contribute to a sore bottom, one could treat the bottom and at the same time try eliminating from the mother's diet for a couple of weeks certain of the more allergenic foods—milk, cheese, eggs, or chocolate. Even the mother's vitamins (especially those with fluorides) can cause a problem for the baby. But remember, the last thing you do is stop nursing, because such babies almost always react even more strongly to any substitute for mother's milk and do not do well at all.

When a baby has diarrhea it is very important that he receive enough fluids. Many babies who are not feeling well increase their nursings, while others are lethargic and may need to be encouraged to nurse well. Breast milk may be the only nourishment the baby will be able to accept and to digest.

Some doctors will recommend solid foods in order to make the stools firm. This does not usually work too well and may cause added problems.

When Dana's baby developed diarrhea, her doctor put the baby on cereals at 3½ months in order to "tighten" his stools. She explains how she found an alternative to solids:

> James became very constipated so I took him off the cereal. I went to see another doctor whom I'd heard was pro-breastfeeding. He suggested that I stop eating or drinking anything that contained cow's milk. He also said that if James did have a cow's milk allergy it would take a mini-mum of two weeks to get it out of both our systems. He recommended I continue breastfeeding and not give any solids until at least six months. This regimen worked, and James's condition improved.

Unless intravenous feeding is necessary, breast milk is the best possible food for a baby or a young child with diarrhea. There are also cases of dramatic improvement in older children who are given human milk as a treatment for diarrhea.

Constipation due to allergies has also been alleviated by breast milk.

Marge's son was four years old when he was given breast milk. He had been found to be very allergic to milk and several other foods, and as a result was losing hair, was underweight, glassy-eyed and had big brown blotches on his face. He also suffered from constipation and bronchitis. Marge describes how breast milk proved to be the answer:

> I had tried soybean formula and goat's milk but Ron couldn't tolerate them. One day I told my doctor that I remembered reading that one thing a child is never al-lergic to is his own mother's milk, and I wanted to give Ron some of mine (I was nursing Ron's four-month-old sister at the time). He agreed, so I expressed some milk and gave it to Ron. The first week he drank about eight

ounces a day. His hair stopped falling out. His eyes lost the glassy look, and he quit coughing. I pumped up to a quart and a half a day for him for three months. Gradually, I tapered off. The doctor agreed that the change in Ron was due to my milk. Certain foods to which he was found to be allergic had been eliminated from his diet before I added the breast milk, but Ron's condition had not improved. It was when I gave him the breast milk that the dramatic improvement came about.

NOTE: It is wise to enlist the cooperation of a pediatrician in finding the solution to such serious medical problems as those experienced by Ron, even if it means changing doctors or getting a consulting opinion.

Skin Problems—Eczema

Authorities state that mother's milk itself never causes eczema in a baby. If your baby is getting nothing but breast milk (no juices, vitamins, or other supplements) and develops an eczemalike rash, the cause may be an external irritant such as wool, laundry products, jewelry, or diaper pins. An exception may arise if you are taking medication for a prolonged period. Your doctor should be consulted if the trouble persists.

Eczema may be the warning flag of allergy in the older baby eating his first solid food. The most important among the triggering allergens are foods such as cow's milk, eggs, fish, nuts, chocolate, citrus fruit, and wheat. It is important to introduce solids in such a way as to minimize sensitization. (See section, Starting Solids, later in this chapter.)

Respiratory Problems—Asthma, Bronchitis

Asthma, with its accompanying cough and wheeze, is the result of an increased resistance to the flow of air out of the lungs. This occurs as a product of three simultaneous changes in the lungs. There is a spasm in the muscle lining of the major air passages, causing a narrowing of the channels. The lining of the passages becomes swollen, and there is an increased secretion of thick mucus. Bronchitis may coexist with and even trigger an asthma attack, especially in infants. Infection, allergy, and irritation from noxious fumes can bring on an asthma attack.

When a baby has an attack it is sometimes difficult for him to nurse because he is using all his energy to breathe. The younger the baby, the more difficult it is for him to coordinate the two efforts. The rapid breathing creates downward pressure on the stomach, which makes it difficult to retain the milk. One mother found that small, frequent feedings helped; she nursed every hour for just a few minutes.

It is difficult for baby to sleep during an asthma attack. Several mothers have found that their nursing sessions are the only times during the day that the baby can relax enough to fall asleep. For a baby who has trouble breathing when lying down, nursing is easier because he *can* feed in a vertical position.

Preventive Measures

The best protection against allergy is prevention. The formation of an allergic response can be minimized or prevented by not exposing an infant to proteins which are foreign to humans (such as cow's milk proteins) until his intestines have matured sufficiently to keep undigested proteins from passing through the intestinal mucous membrane into the bloodstream. Cow's milk in any form is the principal cause of allergic disease in early infancy, so breastfeeding is a definite advantage for your baby. Eggs and wheat are the next two commonly involved foods. But allergies can develop to *any* food.

Your Diet during Pregnancy

As previously mentioned, a baby can become sensitized to a food his mother eats during pregnancy. If you have a family history of allergies there are some precautions you can take while pregnant. Here are a few guidelines gathered from people who have studied the relationship between allergy prevention and diet restrictions:

- Cow's milk (and foods containing cow's milk), if taken at all, should be limited. Powdered skim milk or boiled milk are preferable since they are less allergenic. However, milk can be avoided entirely and calcium supplements can be taken in addition to calcium-rich vegetables such as beet greens, chard, collards, kale, mustard greens, spinach, turnip greens, and broccoli.

- Limit or avoid eggs.

- Limit wheat, gluten and corn. Rice and oatmeal are less allergenic grains. You can use soya bread instead of wheat bread.

- Limit or avoid chocolate, nuts, citrus fruits, and peanuts.

- Limit fish. Shellfish are the most allergenic.

- Do not "binge" on any one food, as an excess of a food creates a greater likelihood of undigested foreign protein passing through your digestive tract and across the placental barrier into the baby's bloodstream.

- Eat a wide variety of foods.

According to Dr. Glaser, the severity of allergic conditions in the immediate family should be an important factor in how strict you will be about your diet. An absolute indication for a strict dietary regimen is the presence in the immediate family of significant asthma or eczema. Dr. Glaser also advocates that such a diet be started at least by the eleventh week of pregnancy. (10)

Kathy and her husband are both allergic, so the chance of their having allergic children is very high. With this in mind, when Kathy began nursing her first child, she avoided

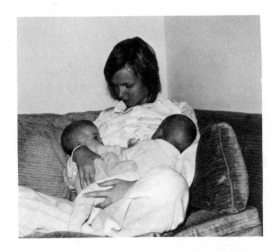

Kathy, nursing her potentially allergic twins Nels and Jared, who never developed any allergic symptoms.

highly allergenic foods until her baby was in the second half of his first year. Today, at six years of age, her child has no allergic problems.

During her second pregnancy, she followed a diet recommended by a doctor: milk and eggs were limited after the sixth month of pregnancy, and only small portions of wheat, orange juice, and fish were allowed. She supplemented this with vitamins and calcium.

Kathy gave birth to six-week-premature twin boys. Both she and her pediatrician were concerned that they receive only breast milk during the first few months. She began pumping milk but it was slow in coming in, so other mothers donated milk which was fed to the twins by a gavage tube through the nose (their sucking reflex had not yet developed). Kathy describes her efforts to nourish the twins:

> I "borrowed" a two-month-old baby for two nursings which helped build confidence that my milk would come in, and I used an electric breast pump. After 11 days one twin came home while the other remained in the hospital. They both were able to receive breast milk, because two friends agreed to nurse the baby who was in the hospital, when I was at home with the other. The mothers who donated

milk observed strict health rules: no colds, illnesses or medications. They scrubbed their hands, washed their breasts, put on surgical gowns backwards to nurse and wore a cap and mask. Admittedly there is much more risk of transmitting germs when other mothers are involved, but we felt it was worth the risk to have our son nursed, when I was unable to do it myself.*

Around eight months, we started the twins on poi, a Hawaiian food of high nutritional value. Until that time, they were totally breastfed; no solids or juices and no formula. Poi is a starchy paste made by pounding the root of the taro plant, and is one of the most allergy-free foods that is known. It is highly digestible with a good vitamin and mineral content, and is a good first food for potentially seriously allergic infants. We obtained the poi from a local Japanese market, and when I also called several "ordinary" markets, they nearly all said they could order it and have it within a week.†

The boys are now almost 3 years old and have no allergies at all. After 15 months we allowed them to eat any type of food. I believe that with the twins we did everything we could to eliminate the possibility of allergies. Because of nursing we feel our children have the greatest chance of being allergy free.

NOTE: Such thorough preventive measures as these taken by Kathy are usually not necessary, but may be seriously considered if there is much allergy in the immediate family.

Your Diet during Lactation

Many mothers do not need to restrict their diets at all when nursing potentially allergic babies. The babies are fine as long as they are on breast milk alone. Dr. Gregory White, a

---

* If possible, with allergic or potentially allergic infants, the donor mothers should be on the same diet as the mother.

† A stable freeze-dried poi preparation may be ordered direct from Honolulu Poi Company, Ltd., 1603 Republican St., Honolulu, HI 96819.

La Leche League Professional Advisory Board member, says that allergy to breast milk itself probably does not exist. Infants may be allergic to foreign proteins, such as cow's milk proteins which the mother has consumed. However, any baby who has trouble with the cow's milk proteins passed in breast milk is going to have *more* trouble with any substitutes. It is better to be aware of this and try excluding suspected foods from your diet to keep your baby healthy and content. Sometimes, this may also be accomplished by *limiting* the intake rather than totally excluding a food. For example, your having one glass of cow's milk or one serving of a dairy product a day, and one egg a week may be easily tolerated by your baby. Each mother and each baby is different and food allergies change as infants grow.

A mother who found her baby's tolerance increased as he got older said that during the first two months of lactation, any dairy product that she ate caused abdominal cramping in her infant. These cramps appeared a few hours after the feeding that followed her intake of the dairy product. Between three and six months, mother's one serving a week was tolerated well by the baby. After six months, three or four servings a week were tolerated.

"Binging" should be avoided during lactation as well as during pregnancy. Overeating any one food seems to increase the possibility of a baby's being sensitive to that food. An intolerance level for your baby might also be reached if you have reasonably small amounts of *several* different foods which are all in the same food family, all in one day. Servings of milk, cheese, cottage cheese, yogurt and ice cream (all from the dairy group) in the same day could be enough to trigger a reaction.

If something you eat causes an allergic reaction in your nursing baby, how long might it be before the reaction is evident? This varies. There may be a reaction after the next feeding, or two to three days later. One mother said she sees a reaction in her baby 36 hours after she eats the food; the reaction builds for 24 hours, peaks and then drops off in another 24 hours (assuming she ate the offending food just once).

If, despite a diet of breast milk only, your baby should show allergic signs, above all *do not wean*. This can only lead to further trouble, as many mothers have discovered.

Dr. E. Robbins Kimball, a pediatrician with over 30 years' experience in handling patients who are severely allergic, says:

> One can try eliminating eggs, wheat and cow's milk, the usual offenders, from the mother's diet. If allergic symptoms continue, other foods may be offenders. In 50 percent of the instances of severe allergy the offending substances in the mother's diet cannot be found. Even so, the mother should continue to breastfeed because the breast-fed child will "outgrow" his allergies faster than the non-breastfed. I have had several babies who were so allergic that they had to be hospitalized; for them, reestablishment of breastfeeding seemed to be lifesaving. One had nothing but breast milk and iron for 2½ years and three required breast milk for over 3 years. Fortunately, many severely allergic children who are breastfed become non-allergic after 10 to 16 months of breastfeeding.

Mothers who must be on a restricted diet for their babies' sakes need to supplement their own diets with adequate amounts of vitamins. However, be sure to check the label. Coloring, flavors and binders used in preparing commercial vitamins and medications are hidden sources of allergens.

Relactation for an Allergic Baby

Many mothers have been able to relactate after having weaned and then discovering that their babies were allergic to formula. Also, some mothers, not suspecting that their babies were allergic, have bottlefed from birth. When no formula was well tolerated, breast milk was tried, often with dramatic improvement in the babies' conditions. Many of these mothers have then managed to relactate and breastfeed their babies.

Joy describes the rapid improvement in her 13-month-old-son who had been weaned at 6 months:

> After Chad was weaned, his troubles began. Because of chronic diarrhea he was hospitalized for tests. For seven more months he barely survived on a diet of cereal and formula, gaining no weight and having diarrhea intermittently. Before my eyes my healthy, breastfed baby was losing the advantages he had gained by nursing. No doctor, much to my despair, could give me any concrete suggestions.
>
> In the meantime we had another baby and I was nursing him. At a friend's suggestion I expressed some milk and gave it to Chad. Later, to my surprise, he had a regular bowel movement instead of his diarrhealike stool.
>
> With only two to four ounces of breast milk Chad was able to partially digest meat, vegetables and fruit, although fat and sugar still caused him to have a burning diarrhea.
>
> When Chad was 19 months old I started attending La Leche League meetings and reading books on nutrition. I realized Chad needed more breast milk to grow properly. Still expressing my milk, I increased the amount to six to eight ounces a day. My La Leche League leader suggested I might be able to supply Chad with more milk if I could nurse him again. Although I doubted my ability to do it I decided to try. After two months I was able to nurse Chad and satisfy eight-month-old Scott, too. (11)

For information on how to reestablish your milk supply, see chapter 15, "Inducing or Reestablishing Your Milk Supply."

Starting Solids

Why Wait?

Most doctors today who are experienced with breastfed babies say that breast milk is a complete food for infants during the first months of life and advocate breast milk alone for about the first six months, with solids delayed longer for a potentially allergic infant.

The earlier solids are introduced the higher the incidence of allergies. This is true in both allergy-prone babies and in babies who do not have a family history of allergy.

Early in life, the mucous membrane lining the intestinal walls is too immature to prevent food proteins from passing through and getting into the infant's entire body via the blood. The intestines gradually "mature" if not aggravated by foreign protein so that tolerance toward foods is greatly increased.

Dr. T. Berry Brazelton, Associate Professor of Pediatrics at Harvard Medical School, and chief of the Child Development Unit at Boston Children's Hospital Medical Center, says:

> The older a child is before he shows allergic symptoms, the less severe they are likely to be and the more easily they can be treated. The child who might have had eczema all over his body had he developed it in his first year may in his second year have only a mild case in his elbow creases and the backs of his knees.

There are many cases of children who are so severely allergic that no solid foods of any kind can be added to their diet. It has been shown that good growth and development can be obtained beyond the third year on nothing but breast milk, given in adequate amounts, plus iron supplements started after six months. This is to be done only in the rare case of extreme allergy. (12)

How to Start Solid Foods

Solid foods should be introduced with extra caution for an allergic or potentially allergic child. New foods should be introduced when he is feeling well and has no symptoms which might be confused with a food reaction. A small amount of a new food should be given daily for at least two weeks before anything else is added. (It can take a week or more before a reaction such as a rash becomes evident.)

Since breast milk aids digestion, nurse first, then offer the taste of food. During this time, view suspiciously any change in health, behavior or sleep patterns. In addition, if your baby dislikes a new food, it may indicate he is allergic to it.

When a reaction does occur, give your baby plenty of time to recover before starting any new foods. A baby may refuse all solids for a while, anyway.

Many busy mothers have discovered the best way to keep track of reactions to new foods is to *write everything down.* An easy way to do this is to tape a chart to your refrigerator or on a cupboard door. Every time you give the baby something to eat, write it down. At the end of each day note any apparent symptoms. (The list in section What Are Allergies? may be helpful.) Any interferences in your new foods schedule (such as illness of the baby) should be marked on the chart. If everything is okay, put that down also so that you will know you did not forget to observe that day.

Patterns will begin to show up, things you had not realized. Some babies take a while to react to a food. Without the chart, the association could be completely missed.

Here are samples of two types of charts that many mothers have found helpful. Chart #1 works very well when you are starting on solids. Chart #2 is easier to use when the child is eating meals.

If you suspect your baby is having a reaction, be suspicious of the last few foods you have given him. Stop them immediately if the symptoms are severe and contact your doctor. When the reaction is severe, no further feedings are necessary. A mild reaction deserves repeating; the food may have to be offered again before you can be sure your child is allergic to it.

When introducing any new foods, offer only a small amount (about a quarter teaspoon), so that any allergic reaction is likely to be mild. Gradually increase the amount each day.

Many breastfeeding mothers have found that their babies like very ripe banana; it is a good, nutritious first food. Many doctors recommend that babies have meat next. One way to serve meat to your little one that is almost sure to be acceptable is to cook and slice meat such as veal or lamb into small strips,

Chart #1

Hourly Chart

Date	12	1	2	3	4	5	6	7	8	9	10	11	Comments
2-12							plum	plum					O.K.
2-13						plum				plum			diarrhea P.M.
2-14						plum		plum					diarrhea and stomach cramps

Chart #2

Daily Chart

Date	Breakfast	Lunch	Dinner	Snacks		Comments
				A.M.	P.M.	
6-12	rice orange	lamb rice bread	turkey sweet potato	apple	rice cracker pear	O.K.
6-13	rice apple	turkey potato-carrots	lamb squash-rice	soynuts	orange	wheezing
6-14	rice pear	rice bread	turkey orange	lamb	apple	asthma

wrap each in foil, and freeze. Teething babies love to gnaw on the frozen fingers of meat. Lamb and veal are good to offer as first meats because they're seldom. used in American diets— there is less chance of prior sensitizing and they are easy to eliminate if allergy develops.

Grains should be added to the diet when baby is older, as they are most likely to cause reactions. Rice may be the best grain to start with, and can be offered in various forms. Simple rice crackers or biscuits are available from health food stores.*
Since wheat is the most allergenic grain, introduce it after the other grains.

Fruits such as apples and pears are often introduced next. You will probably want to avoid the citrus fruits and berries until much later.

Vegetables are more difficult to digest so they are usually last to be introduced. Squash, carrots, artichokes, potatoes and sweet potatoes are accepted fairly easily by babies nine months to a year old.

It is very helpful to have a chart showing the botanical relationships of foods. For example, the citrus group includes lemons, oranges, grapefruits, tangerines, tangelos, and limes. Children who are allergic to one food in a food family may be allergic to the whole food group.

An allergic child may safely eat one of several foods to which he is mildly sensitive, but if he eats two at the same time, he may suffer a reaction. A limited chart can be found in *All About Allergy* by M. Coleman Harris, M.D., and Norman Shure, M.D. (13)

Before their child is a year old, many parents are especially cautious about introducing foods such as eggs, cow's milk and wheat, which have been avoided during pregnancy and lactation. Other highly allergenic foods include corn, pork, fish (especially shellfish), tomatoes, onions, cabbage, berries, nuts, condiments, orange juice, and chocolate. (14) Avoid com-

---

* Be sure to read labels. A baby may be able to tolerate only pure rice cakes. Those containing sesame seeds can cause diarrhea.

binations of foods until each food has been tried on an individual basis.

It is probably best to follow the plan for offering foods your doctor sets up for you, since there is very little agreement about which foods cause the most trouble. The foods previously mentioned are about the only ones on which there is much agreement.

In dealing with allergies, the most important thing to remember is to be open minded. You do not want to inflict any more restrictions on your child's diet or his environment than are absolutely necessary. With foods, try them in as many different forms as you can think of. Don't be afraid to retry foods several times a year.

Hospitalization

Hospitalization may create new problems for an allergic child. If your child with a food allergy must be hospitalized you may discover that the hospital dieticians really do not know much about diet management beyond the substitution of a soy formula, which may contain corn derivatives, in place of cow's milk. As in any other situation where your baby is away from home you will need to be in total charge of his diet. You may even find it necessary to bring his food with you.

Discuss the situation with your doctor; he should be able to help you. When a child is sick or injured, it is not the time to be feeding foods he has never had or to which he is known to be allergic. This is a good reason for you to go in to breastfeed, too!

Here are some further suggestions about hospitalization, from mothers of allergic children:

- Arrange for your baby to get your breast milk, rather than formula.

- Ask questions about all medications and treatments.

- Be sure special diet and other instructions are on the front of the bed or on the door to your child's room as well as on his chart.

• Remember, the nursing staff changes every eight hours, and if your child had a reaction to milk at breakfast, he may be given ice cream after dinner by someone else.

• Check any pillows on the bed to see that they are hypoallergenic.

• Make sure there are no plants in the room (they can collect mold).

Medications for an Allergic Nursing Mother

Can you continue to nurse while you are being treated with medications for your allergies? Most doctors who are familiar with breast milk and breastfed babies feel that such medications are usually safe for the nursing baby.

Dr. Glaser comments on the transmission of drugs through breast milk to a baby:

> My feeling would be to give the mother whatever medication she needs, but I would try giving it in very small doses first and if it does not disturb the baby, gradually increase it to the dosage the mother needs. Of course, the pediatrician should be kept fully informed as to what drugs the mother is taking and signs of drug intoxication carefully watched for in the infant. If a mother is temporarily taken off breastfeeding because of a drug she is taking, breast milk should be supplied from a donor if at all possible.

Dr. Robert Hamburger, of the University of California School of Medicine, San Diego, has studied many allergic mothers. Even though small amounts of allergy medications such as antihistamines, decongestants, and bronchodilators appear in milk, no special problems have appeared in the babies studied. (See also *Drugs Your Doctors May Prescribe:*

Antibiotics, in the section Drugs and the Nursing Mother, chapter 13, "When Mother Is Sick or Hospitalized.")

Your Cheering Squad

In the case of allergies, it is very important to have father's support when there are necessary restrictions. It is confusing for even a very young child if one parent allows him to eat a certain food and the other parent doesn't. Discuss the list of do's and don'ts with your husband and let him know when changes have been made. One mother found it helpful to keep current lists of each child's acceptable and banned foods for her husband. This way he was able to refer to the lists when she wasn't around.

It is important to find a sympathetic pediatrician who understands and recognizes the less common manifestations of allergies. You will need to work very closely with your baby's doctor, and having a good rapport with him will make things easier. It is also important that he share your desire for your baby to be breastfed.

As far as friends are concerned, you will be much happier if you spend time with people who understand your child's situation and try to make things as comfortable as possible for you and the baby. You will not enjoy yourself if you must spend the evening defending your position and saying such things as, "Yes, I'm sure he really is allergic," or "No, he can't have even a tiny taste of the cake."

Chapter 12

When Baby Is
Sick or Hospitalized

There is never an illness or hospitalization for which we are totally prepared. In a crisis situation most parents react from their hearts. When one member of a family is ill, all suffer in some way. The experience can tear us apart or bind us together as we reach for good health and the happiness it brings. As you read this chapter, you will see how some parents have managed their special encounters. Perhaps this will help you by providing an extra measure of confidence when you are in a difficult situation.

Breast Milk Is Best

An infant who can receive *any* nourishment has need of his mother's milk. Studies have shown that there is no food more easily digested by even tiny premature babies. Breast milk provides protection against infections that can weaken an already distressed infant by supplying antibodies which aid babies in developing their own protective mechanism. Reading Dr. John Gerrard's article "Breastfeeding: Second Thoughts" (1), may give you additional insight on the advantages of providing only untreated breast milk.

If your baby cannot nurse, you can express your milk by hand or pump using sterile techniques. (See chapter 2, "Nursing Techniques.") The fresh raw milk can be fed directly to your baby by tube, bottle, spoon, or at your breast with a nursing supplementer. Some hospitals insist on autoclaving (sterilizing) breast milk. This procedure will destroy some of the nutrients and alter the milk a bit, but it is still preferable to commercial preparations which can lead to allergies.

La Leche League leaders can be very helpful in suggesting how to stimulate a milk supply and in offering information and support to a mother who is expressing milk or who wants to relactate. There are also milk banks for special situations, which can be found listed in Appendix: Organizations to Help the Nursing Mother.

Recognizing Some
Signs of Illness

Parents soon get to know the special behavior patterns of their babies. A mother especially knows her baby better than anyone else and can detect subtle changes. Some babies sleep more or nurse less vigorously when they are sick. Some want constant nursing as if this special act can make their uncomfortable feelings go away.

Nursing mothers can rightfully be pleased about the extra protection their babies are receiving from being breastfed. Breast milk cannot be expected to prevent every illness but it is an accepted fact that the antibodies in colostrum and later in milk make it more difficult for a child to develop infections. And when breastfed babies do get colds and other illnesses, they are usually less severe than in children fed formula. (2)

Don't blame a rash, a runny nose or a temperature on teething just because a friend's baby cut a tooth at this age. If you feel something is not right, consult your baby manual for clues. Calling a doctor is a must if your baby is listless, feverish, or has a shiny look to his eyes.

Dehydration can be very serious for a baby. If your baby has six or more wet diapers a day, usually there is no need for concern about dehydration, but if he has less, check with your doctor.

Treating Illnesses at Home

Once the nature of your baby's illness has been determined, home care is often the best. A familiar place, with family members together can speed recovery. If your baby needs special care, decide where it can best be accomplished—at home or in the hospital. Often children are hospitalized because the doctor thinks it is easier on the mother, but a breastfeeding couple may be better off at home unless the special equipment available in the hospital is needed. Some equipment can be rented for home use. Sometimes it is necessary to be firm if you want to avoid a hospital stay for your baby.

Taking Care of Yourself

Your normal routines will be disrupted by time spent caring for your nursling who is ill. Worry can easily sap your energy; just remember that your good health is important to your baby. Pay special attention to your diet and fluid intake as well as your baby's during this time when he is depending on you for all his needs. Grab a nutritious snack and something to drink when settling down to nurse when meals are delayed by a fretful baby.

If let-downs don't come easily because you are tense, do everything you can to relax. A hot bath, a glass of wine or beer can help. Let your shoulders and jaw droop as you nurse. One mother listened to a favorite soothing record whenever she had to express milk. Use relaxation techniques you may have learned for a childbirth or Yoga class to help you relax. Some mothers use oxytocin nasal spray to encourage the let-down.

Dressings, Traction, Exercises

Changing dressings for burns or surgery can often be done at home. The visiting nurse may be able to come in a time or two and show you how to handle them. The same goes for long-term traction and exercises. Your doctor, Chamber of Commerce, or local Public Health Department can supply you with the phone number of the Visiting Nurse Association, or it may be listed in your phone book under "Nurses" in the yellow pages. Even though you may not be an expert, your breastfed baby will feel very secure when you are handling his care.

Many times mothers can work out their own solutions to problems. One mother found that the first few times she carefully redid her baby's finger bandages after the twice-daily soaking needed to help heal his skin grafts, he promptly pulled them off with his teeth. He was still crawling and these special fingers needed to be kept clean and protected as he explored. She decided then to cover them with a clean white sock pinned to his long-sleeved shirt. It worked as long as they settled down for a drink and a cuddle right away. By the time he was finished, he was distracted enough to forget what had just been done to his hands.

Diarrhea

Babies may appear to have diarrhea when actually it is a normal breastfed stool. Well-meaning relatives, pediatric nurses and even medical personnel who are not familiar with a breastfed baby's stool may think the baby is ill when they see the loose, curdy-looking stool. Various shades of color from mustardy yellow to green are quite normal. Also, exposure of the stool to the air can change the color if the baby is not changed immediately.

On rare occasions the frequency of bowel movements is related to something in a mother's diet. By cutting down on the offending food, the condition should improve. One mother found her baby's diarrhea cleared up as soon as she eliminated cantaloupe from her diet.

Allergic babies may have diarrhea if they receive something they are allergic to in their mothers' milk. Try eliminating certain of the more allergenic foods: milk, cheese, eggs, or chocolate. Also, one bottle of formula can trigger diarrhea.

Vitamins you or your baby are taking, especially those with fluorides, could be causing a problem. Diarrhea is also a common side-effect of antibiotics.

Some babies seem to get diarrhea from artificial sweeteners passed through the breast milk. A mother found that when she started to drink just one cup of coffee a day with a saccharin tablet, her baby got diarrhea. She stopped using the saccharin, and the diarrhea cleared up within 12 hours and never recurred.

Some mothers have been advised to stop nursing and put the baby on Jello-water and applesauce. These are both sweets which can aggravate diarrhea.

Diarrhea *can* be a symptom of a serious condition. However, La Leche League's Information Sheet on "Diarrhea in Infancy" (3) states:

> As a general rule, if the baby is able to take anything by mouth, it should be breast milk. . . . Regardless of the cause of diarrhea (if in fact it is a diarrhea and not a normal breast milk stool), our medical advisors have found that if the baby is kept on breast milk alone, he will be much more likely to make a quick recovery, without complications for either mother or baby.

Fever, Croup, Asthma

Fever is a clue that the body is fighting an illness. A cool bath and an aspirinlike medication, if prescribed by your doctor, can help keep fever under control. Fluids are important. Wake the baby to nurse if necessary or nurse him in his sleep. The same is true of croup or asthma. Fluids such as juice, water, or weak tea may be given. If your doctor says to avoid milk, he probably means cow's milk.

Rash

Rashes have various causes, including overactive sweat glands, irritation from material in the diaper or detergents, and ammonia burn. You may be told your baby's rash is caused by breastfeeding. The milk itself is not at fault. There *may* be something in your diet that is affecting the baby. Once it has been eliminated, the rash will begin to clear. When the baby is older, small amounts of the same food will probably cause no problem.

If you have been sick yourself and taking medication, and

then your baby develops a rash, you might suspect your medication. Check with your doctor. Perhaps changing to a different prescription is advisable.

It may take some real detective work to determine the cause of a rash. Some babies are sensitive to wool, and also to synthetic fabrics. Mable says she suspected the rash on her baby's face might be due to her milk until she discovered her baby was allergic to the dye in her robe. A diaper between your baby and your clothing will protect his skin if he is sensitive to the dyes or fiber content of what you wear. Some infants are also sensitive to perfumes and lotions.

Colds, Flu

A nursling who is ill from a cold or flu may have trouble feeding. A stuffy nose makes it hard to breathe while at the breast. Short, frequent feedings and some expressed breast milk or water by spoon can help. Keeping your baby upright will allow drainage of the mucus and help him breathe. Nurse sitting up. Carry your baby around on your back or front in a baby carrier while you do your housework. When you lay him down, prop him in a baby seat. Elevating the head of his bed will also help. A cool mist vaporizer will aid decongestion. Some doctors suggest nose drops be given just before feeding, but others feel they are harmful and not needed.

Some babies nurse more frequently when a cold is coming on, then stop suddenly when the milk supply is at a peak. If this has happened with your baby, keep offering to nurse. When the congestion clears, he will once again be able to breathe well and feel comfortable while nursing.

Ear Infections

The eustachian tube between the nose and ear sometimes allows fluid to pass from the nose or throat into the ear. If the fluid becomes trapped, the ear becomes infected. If your baby is fussing or pulling on one ear, see your doctor. Your baby may also have a high fever. Usually a bacterial infection is responsible and should have prompt medical attention. Antibiotics usually bring quick relief but must be taken for the prescribed length of time. Allergic children are more likely to have ear infections because their eustachian tubes swell and contain excessive mucus. Blockage occurs and bacterial growth begins. Ear infections are also common in cleft palate babies.

Mothers who have had both breastfed and bottlefed babies report that the breastfed ones had fewer ear infections. This is because breastfed infants have fewer allergies and in general have greater immunity to disease. Also, there is less irritation in the eustachian tube from breast milk than from formula.

During an ear infection, some babies may not want to nurse as long or as often as usual, while others may want to nurse longer and *more* frequently.

As your baby nurses, the warmth of your breast against his sore ear may be comforting. On the other hand, the pressure may cause him pain. Try different positions for nursing, to see which is the most comfortable. Sitting up may be better than lying down, or you may want to try the "football hold." (See chapter 18, "Nursing Twins.") Cotton in the sore ear may help if noise or air seems to bother it.

Vomiting

Vomiting may be a symptom of several conditions, including allergies, diseases, infections, and digestive problems.

However, spitting up in the early months can be normal, and is simply a condition your baby will outgrow. Many "spitters" take eight to ten *months* to clear up. What can you do while you wait for the problem to go away? Gentle handling, shorter, more frequent feedings, and holding the baby upright after feedings may help.

Although a certain amount of spitting up is normal, if your baby suddenly vomits after feeding, consider any unusual food in your diet. Or, if your baby is on solids, did you feed him anything unusual?

Usually any food you eat in moderation does not affect your baby. Chocolate, spicy foods, and vegetables in the cabbage family may cause the baby distress, especially if they bother you.

You need to pay careful attention to your baby's fluid intake, making sure that what is vomited is replaced. Frequent nursings supply this needed fluid.

If your diet has not contained anything unusual, the vomiting may be a sign of throat or ear infection or something else. If vomiting occurs more than once a day or if there is also a fever, call your doctor.

Chickenpox

Chickenpox can be a serious disease if contracted by a newborn. Mothers who have chickenpox at the time of birth are sometimes not allowed to nurse their babies for a while. However, if your baby is several weeks old and develops chickenpox, it will probably be mild and breastfeeding can continue.

Luanne's fourth son was about four weeks old when her three older boys came down with chickenpox.

> I had chickenpox as a child so I wasn't concerned for myself and I figured the baby would still be covered by the immunities he received in the colostrum at birth. The doctor warned me that the effect of the colostrum was wearing thin but wasn't worried about the baby. My baby did finally get chickenpox but he only had one pox on him and was hardly sick at all.
>
> Incidentally, my two oldest boys whom I had nursed only a short time got terrible cases of chickenpox but my third son who had nursed till he weaned had a very mild case.

Accidents

Babies who are hurt or upset because of accidents often want to nurse frequently for reassurance and to ease their discomfort. On the other hand, an accident may cause a problem for nursing.

Driving to the doctor's office or hospital is easier if someone else can drive while you comfort your baby. Once there, scary, possibly painful procedures are more tolerable inside the circle of your arms. Even if you have signed a general release, you're needed to give informed consent (see *Informed Consent* in the section, Parents' Rights and Responsibilities, chapter 14, "Working Together") and to protect your baby. In the emergency room in some hospitals, a child is taken away from the parents unless the physician gives permission for the parents to stay. Immediately ask your doctor to give this permission.

As soon as treatment is given, your baby will appreciate the comfort of being held close to you and breastfeeding can help to ease the shock of unfamiliar surroundings and care.

Hospitalization

In the book by Tine Thevenin, *The Family Bed: An Age-Old Concept in Child Rearing* (4), stress on both child and parents is explored. She writes:

> At no time must parents be made to feel less needed when their child is hospitalized for they alone will be a sign of normalcy in an abnormal situation. . . . Aside from the great benefit to the child, it is of psychological benefit to the parent to be able to care for his child during the latter's illness. Wanting to do something if only to stroke his hand is a very natural desire of a parent.

Parents need the security of knowing what is going on. Speak up; make a little scene, if necessary, to get to stay with your child if your doctor or hospital is reluctant.

Ask your doctor to *tell* the nursing staff and also write on the hospital orders that your free access to the baby at any time is part of his recommended care. When you sign the treatment consent form, add a note above your name indicating you plan to stay.

The hours spent at the hospital are long and tiring. You must take care of yourself because you are your baby's lifeline.

If you can prepare in advance, take along fruit, drinks, snacks, and some brewer's yeast for added energy. A radio, the library's longest book or a challenging piece of needlework will help during the hours that baby sleeps. A pair of comfortable shoes is a must and a baby carrier is handy for walking baby up and down the halls if he is well enough. If you must go to the hospital unexpectedly, have someone bring you what you need.

When there is also a family at home, it is hard to decide who needs you most. Sometimes there just doesn't seem to be any time or energy left over for others. Yet their needs are real, too.

Try to spare a few minutes to be with your other children to share their concerns. Can they be involved in any way with the hospitalized child, by making something for him, talking on the telephone to him, or taking a peek at him in the hospital? Maybe you can take photos of his room and other parts of the hospital to share with the family at home.

While you are with your baby in the hospital, your other children will miss you but will have the security of being in a familiar place and the comfortable feeling of knowing that if it were they who were ill, you would be with them. There are neighbors, relatives, scout troops, church youth groups, and state homemaker services to call on for help.

If possible, find a familiar person to babysit for your other children and leave lists of their routines so that their lives aren't too upset.

Husbands can be a great source of strength during times of crisis. They can keep the family at home secure and help everyone feel that in spite of the trouble, all will eventually be well. And husbands can help in the important job of taking your milk to the hospital if you are not able to stay with your hospitalized baby.

Babies are hospitalized for many reasons. During the course of his treatment or illness, a baby may have to undergo one or more unusual or uncomfortable procedures such as intravenous feeding, tracheotomy tube, spinal tap or being confined to a croup tent. Discuss the nature of the procedures with your physician and the hospital staff, along with the reason

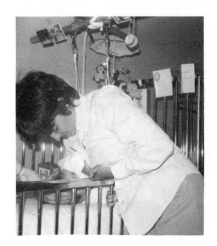

Just because a baby is in traction doesn't mean he can't nurse. Here, Margaret improvises by lowering the side of the bed and leaning over her 9-month-old baby.

they're being done. This will give you an opportunity to explain how important breastfeeding is to you and to enlist their help. The hospital staff can help to arrange special equipment to make it easier for you to nurse. Don't be afraid to improvise; crawl into bed with the baby (after checking to see that it will support the extra weight!), sit in the croup tent. Ask the nurses to arrange intravenous equipment so you don't disturb the fluid's flow while you hold your baby.* This can be hard on your back, but leaning on large pillows placed in the crib for nursing time, or sitting on a high stool while leaning over the crib may help.

Whatever makes the baby happier and more comfortable will help speed his recovery. For example, your baby can see you very well outside a croup tent so sit close and let him see and touch your face and hands through the plastic. Eventually, time out of the tent for short nursings may be permitted. Watch the baby for signs of distress and put him back if necessary.

The worry accompanying your baby's hospitalization may

---

* When children are very ill or recovering from surgery, they may receive medications and fluids intravenously. If your child is able to tolerate any fluids by mouth, you should be able to nurse during this treatment.

temporarily affect your milk supply. Darcy says:

> My fourth baby had pneumonia at six weeks of age and
> was hospitalized for six days. My doctor was all for my
> staying with Julie and nursing her every 2 hours. Although
> the hospital wasn't prepared for mothers to stay, they
> moved in a bed for me. I took over all of Julie's care ex-
> cept the technical part. What was surprising to me was
> that even with a baby this young, and not nursing for 48
> hours, I had no uncomfortable buildup of milk. I was very
> tense and worried about Julie. My body just seemed to
> "shut down production." I tried to express some milk for
> the nurses to use while I went home to see the other chil-
> dren briefly, and couldn't get more than a few drops. But
> I didn't worry about having enough; when she began to
> nurse again, I had an adequate amount of milk.

Sometimes babies must be hospitalized for emergency or
corrective surgical procedures. There are times, however, when
simple surgery can be performed on an outpatient basis, where
the baby is hospitalized for only a few hours. Hernia is a common example.

In cases of more involved surgery where the baby must
remain in the hospital overnight or longer, special arrangements
can usually be made for the breastfed baby if you request them.

Joey was ten months old when examination revealed that
he needed skull surgery as soon as possible. His mother,
Patricia, describes how she managed to nurse him:

> The neurosurgeon took it for granted that I would not
> be staying with our son. I told him my baby was nursing
> and that my husband and I felt this was not the time to
> wean. A private room was arranged at Children's Hospital.
> The night before, I was not allowed to nurse after mid-
> night, although they gave him sugar water at 6:00 A.M.
> After surgery, the doctor said all was okay, and I could re-
> sume nursing. If the breast milk stayed down, the I.V.
> would be removed. I leaned over the crib to nurse, and
> since I am 4 feet, 10 inches tall, it was just the right height.
> When the feeding had stayed down an hour, I reminded

the nurse of the doctor's order, and in half an hour the I.V. was removed.

Many mothers have used their determination and imagination to continue to nurse a baby who must be placed in traction or a body cast. Clare nursed her baby, who was in traction because of a fractured leg, for 3½ weeks. She says:

I found that I was able to nurse Craig by sliding my left arm under his shoulders and bending over him so that he could nurse from either breast. My position was awkward and uncomfortable, and in the beginning I had to nurse him at short, frequent intervals. With an electric breast pump I obtained enough milk to leave for Craig each night.

We brought an assortment of colorful toys to the hospital to entertain Craig. Since I was not able to hold him, I spent a great deal of time touching and stroking him, or putting my cheek next to his. He is a happy baby, blessed with a cheerful, friendly disposition. He seemed to tolerate the hospitalization rather well.

Looking back, I realize that nursing was *essential*— the only comfort my poor baby had! It allowed me to stay with him, gave him security and skin contact.

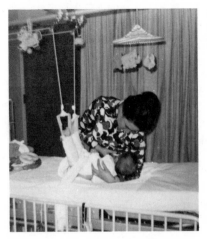

Clare nursing her 4-month-old, Craig, in traction because of a fractured leg.

The Nursing Mothers' Association of Australia publishes a booklet on the subject, "Plastered Kids." (5) The booklet is filled with suggestions, practical information and encouragement for mothers whose children are in casts.

Nursing your baby in a body brace requires special considerations. Connie, whose daughter Andrea was born with a curved spine, explains:

> Andrea could only nurse comfortably on one side because the body brace hurt her on the other. We managed okay by starting her nursings without the brace, on the side she didn't like. Then I changed diapers and braced her so she wouldn't have the brace suddenly tightened on a full stomach.

Occasionally, babies may be so ill that they require isolation from the rest of the hospital, either because of a contagious disease or because of a weakened condition, making them susceptible to infection. You can be trained to use good isolation techniques and need not be separated from your child. Breastfeeding at this time can bring reassurance, comfort and your easy-to-digest milk to assist in recovery.

Anna says that her six-month-old son was hospitalized in isolation:

> I told the doctor that I was breastfeeding Alan and that I must go with him. With the doctor's permission I spent 16 days in the room, always by his side. I was given a wash basin and ice to store expressed milk as nothing could leave the room. I filled the night stand with a large box of brewer's yeast and small cans of juice to keep up my fluids since rest was impossible with my little one so ill. At first, nursing was out because Alan was not conscious. He was put on I.V.'s and placed in the cool mist of a croup tent to keep his temperature down. A hot plate in the bathroom was the safest place to warm the milk, because oxygen was being used in the tent.

Some illnesses require long-term care and can mean frequent hospitalization. For example, heart problems can mean many hospital stays and can cause a baby to feed poorly. However, JoAnn says her baby, David, continued to thrive although he gained weight slowly and had a weak suck for the first few months.

Another mother says:

> My son was hospitalized for 100 days his first eight months and was placed in an incubator with oxygen for heart failure. We kept up our breastfeeding relationship during this time through frequent, small nursings. That way, the baby wasn't out of the oxygen long, and he was still content.

Although the medical staff was not supportive of her decision to breastfeed, Phoebe persevered in nursing her son, born with a severe congenital heart defect. She credits the nursing relationship with helping them *both* cope with repeated hospitalizations. Phoebe explains:

> One of my pediatricians told me my baby should be scientifically handled rather than breastfed. We certainly had words over *that* philosophy. Amid the tubes and I.V.'s and monitors, I put Daniel to my breast, and despite the fact that the doctors and nurses thought he was too weak to suck, he latched on the strongest of any of my babies. Daniel was in the hospital many times, and I always stayed with him. I am a firm believer that no child should be hospitalized without a parent with him at all times. Hospital personnel do many tests and procedures on the children after visiting hours when all the parents are gone. The babies are left to cry it out with no one to console them. . . . Nursing was a fantastic comfort and pleasure for us both. I think we averted many difficult periods for him by nursing, which relaxed his respiration rate. . . . Daniel is now a normal five-year-old boy with an unusually shaped heart. He has a beautiful understanding of himself and his problems, a marvelous sense of humor, and a fighting spirit to keep him going.

Hospitalized Child and Another Nursing Baby

While attending a hospitalized child, you may have another nursing baby at home who also needs you. Some mothers have managed to bring a twin or other nursling along with them. Mindy had one twin hospitalized for a hernia repair and was able to bring his brother, Scott, along. She stayed at the hospital with both six-week-old twins. Mindy kept Scott in his carriage in an empty room down the hall from brother Andy. Several weeks later Scott needed similar surgery. Andy slept in his carriage in the lobby with his four-year-old sister to "babysit." The receptionist kept an eye on them both while Mindy was in Scott's room. (6)

Some parents have been able to have the nursing baby admitted for observation so that the two babies can share a room. Others have left a hospitalized nursling with expressed milk for one or more feedings and gone home to breastfeed the other child. A few have found other nursing mothers to share their milk with the baby at home, but this is something to be carefully considered since there is always some danger of cross-infection.

When Phoebe's five-year-old son Daniel had to undergo an operation, she was nursing his three-month-old sister, Karen. Phoebe says:

> Karen and I roomed-in with Daniel for two weeks. The staff at the hospital was most cooperative. Dan was perked up considerably by Karen's presence, although at times he resented the fuss made over her by others. There were times when I needed to use Syntocinon nasal spray to help my let-down reflex, but most of the time the relaxation of nursing itself kept me going.

Home Again

Once your family is reunited, it may take some time to get everyone settled. Your baby may still have many fears. He may have nightmares for months, be terrified of anyone in white, or protest at having his picture taken if the camera reminds him of an X-ray machine. He may cry a lot and want to be held much of the time, as reassurance that all is well. He may cling desperately to you and look upon family and friends as strangers. Or, he may reject you.

Your baby may have become accustomed to the hospital routines and to having you to himself all the time. And your other children at home will need time to make up for the "eternity" you were gone.

Nursing babies bounce back quickly. Watch yours and allow room for growing. Soon your baby will have few memories of the experience (even though yours may linger). Don't hover; with the proper care and the right amount of loving, many children are able to enter into normal, active lives.

Thoughts from Other Mothers

• Milk can be pumped or nursed even if mother is not relaxed.

• Lots of liquid is vital; a little wine is helpful at times.

• A child who has been anesthetized may not nurse when you are bursting to do so after he gets out of surgery.

• Feelings of fear, guilt, and helplessness are common with parents of hospitalized children.

• If anyone jokes about your nursing inside a crib or oxygen tent, ignore it. You know you are doing what is in your child's best interest, physically and psychologically.

• If your most desperate need is for someone to talk to who will understand what you are going through, contact La Leche League and other organizations. Addresses may be found in Appendix: Organizations to Help the Nursing Mother.

Death

If your baby does not live, remember in your grief that you have given your baby the best of nourishment both physically and emotionally. Time will soften your loss but will not dim the beauty of the gift you have so willingly given your child.

The emotions you are feeling may inhibit your let-down, but you will continue to produce milk for a while. If you become uncomfortably full, a warm shower, hot compresses and a minute or two of expressing milk will help. Your doctor may prescribe "dry-up" medication. These pills can help reduce engorgement, but your body may take several weeks to stop producing milk. Wear a well-fitting bra continuously. Limiting liquids may also help. Adequate rest will help prevent breast infections, but be alert for their symptoms.

The hospital staff may be at a loss as to how to offer their sympathy, and say nothing. When you return home, the neighbors may not quite know what to say. Your friends with babies of their own may wonder if they should bring them to visit or avoid you. A well-meaning friend may pack away all the baby things in an effort to spare you. Each mother must deal with loss of her child in her own way. No one else can feel quite the same as she does about her child. No one else will remember the baby as she does.

Anna writes of her loss:

> I asked to see Cynthia after she died. A complication with the spinal anesthetic resulted in my being put to sleep before her cesarean birth. We had not met because I was unconscious when she died. I had dreamed of this baby as she wiggled inside me before her arrival. I needed to know her for a few brief moments. There would be no time in the future to hold and nourish her. My husband and I spent a little while with her after the nurse brought her in, wrapped in a soft pink blanket. I held her close and said goodbye; at least now I had someone real to remember. A dear friend sent a card and a note saying that in her religion a baby who had received only the briefest gift of life would have a special place in heaven. This

comforting thought was just what I needed to help offset the uncomfortable visits of friends and relatives, bringing gifts of flowers, clothing, and even a valuable ring. They only wanted to help, but how could possessions take my baby's place? I didn't want to offend by revealing my feelings, but it was so hard. Another comforting thought was shared with me by the Reverend George G. Swanson: "Remember to keep in mind that all the evil in the universe cannot extinguish the eternal life of the child which God gave to earth and received back safely again in a journey which we have yet to complete."

Chapter 13

When Mother Is
Sick or Hospitalized

Mothers are concerned about their families, and hardly ever consider the possibility of getting sick themselves. It's especially important for nursing mothers to stay in good health, to get the proper amount of rest (even if it's cat naps during the day and interrupted sleep at night), to eat well and to drink plenty of fluids. Most mothers can function with a cold, coping adequately with their obligations and caring for the rest of the family when they're sick.

However, a mother may develop something more serious— she may need surgery, contract a disease requiring hospitalization, or be in an accident. When this happens it disrupts the entire family. The relationship between mother and nursing baby is threatened. Father can feel overwhelmed by worrying about his wife, handling her prolonged recovery, caring for other children, and dealing with financial considerations. At this important time he also has to be prepared to assume many of his wife's responsibilities in addition to his own.

It's not an easy time for anyone. It requires a lot of love, compassion, courage and strength. It also requires an understanding of what the needs of the individuals within the family are, and the knowledge of how to go about handling these needs.

Well-meaning people, professionals, friends and relatives, sometimes feel nursing is too much of a strain on the mother under these circumstances. Actually, a mother can be on partial or even complete bedrest and still nurse her baby quite successfully since it's a lot easier than getting up to mix formula or warm bottles. With the nursling tucked in bed beside her, a box of disposable diapers and a pitcher of juice or water nearby, what could be more convenient? Nursing mothers can testify that worries and tensions seem to vanish when they snuggle in bed with their little ones. Nursing releases the hormone prolactin into the mother's body, which heightens the feeling of relaxation. Indeed, prolactin has been called "nature's tranquilizer." Contrast this to the sudden traumatic effect weaning would have on the mother: emotionally, feeling the loss of this meaningful relationship, and physically, risking a breast infection as a result of engorgement.

There are very valid reasons from baby's point of view to continue nursing. In a young baby, introduction of formula and solid foods can increase the risk of allergies, gastrointestinal disease and diarrhea. The incidence of respiratory infections like pneumonia increases as well, and these illnesses can sometimes be quite severe. Some babies may be so upset by sudden weaning that they cry inconsolably for long periods of time. Others *seem* to adjust well, but may show their grief in more subtle ways, such as by having nightmares.

Mother and baby need each other very much, especially in a crisis situation. If you are ill and require lots of rest, guard jealously the relationship with your baby. After putting things in perspective, handle only the essentials which revolve around nursing the baby and loving the rest of the family. It may be necessary to find someone to handle the housework, even if you're the type who can't stand another person fussing in your home. Your home won't know it's got a substitute, but your children will—especially your breastfeeding baby. When friends ask what they can do, *tell them.* Give them the pleasure of feeling helpful! Let them bring dinner over, do your laundry, run a vacuum or whatever you need. Switch to disposable diapers, hire a teenager to come over after school and take care of the house and older children . . . but don't let anyone convince you that nursing will be too much of a burden on you!

You may worry about the baby picking up an infection you might have through your milk. Actually, very few infections are transmitted that way. Most are passed on by direct contact (through handling the baby), or in the air (through sneezing).

By the time you know you're ill enough to require treatment, your baby has already been thoroughly exposed to whatever germs you have. Considering the immunological benefits of breast milk, nursing is definitely beneficial to the baby.

Dr. Ernest M. Solomon, a member of La Leche League's Professional Advisory Board, states: "It is almost never necessary to stop nursing the baby, whatever the illness is. However, in those rare instances when nursing must be interrupted temporarily—and this should be done only as a last resort—mother can pump her breasts and probably resume nursing within a short period of time."

Infections

W. G. Whittlestone, D.Sc., points out the importance of breastfeeding when there are infections in "The Biological Specificity of Milk." (1) He states:

> . . . the act of suckling may transfer infection into the mammary gland, which in turn responds by producing immunoglobulins locally. This mechanism is interesting because it makes it possible for the baby to survive in a highly infected environment provided that he is breastfed. The breast thus functions as a system for generating protection against infection until the baby's own immune mechanisms can come into full play—clearly a mechanism with high survival value.

Many mothers, after contracting differing kinds of infections, have continued to nurse their babies. Lori developed a bladder infection after her baby was born, but luckily she had rooming-in; her husband was allowed to hold their baby and assist her during visiting hours in caring for him. As a special treatment, she was hooked up to a machine which prevented her from moving about. Despite this hindrance, she continued nursing for the 12 days she was in the hospital. "Nursing certainly helped me from getting too depressed over my situation," she said.

Contagious Diseases

The Flu

Most mothers find that breastfeeding is a real advantage when the whole family is sick with a disease, such as the flu. Usually the nursing baby stays well or if he does become ill, it's only a mild case.

Nora says that although a temperature of 101.4° accompanied her bout with the flu, her son "nursed happily, without a trace of illness preceding, during, or after my sickness."

Fever can affect your milk supply because it uses up body fluids. If you are running a fever along with other flu symptoms, increase your fluid intake.

Chickenpox

Chickenpox is a contagious disease which can be fatal if contracted by a fetus or newborn. Nadine came down with chickenpox right before her baby was born and she was separated from her daughter, Christa, immediately after delivery. Although Nadine had the pox all over her body, even in her uterus, examination of the placenta revealed that Christa had probably not been exposed to the disease. As a protective measure, the baby was given a shot of Zoster Immune Globulin. While in the hospital, mother and baby were placed in separate rooms and kept in isolation. Once home, Nadine was not allowed to touch her baby until all the blisters were completely dried up. Meanwhile, Nadine used a hand breast pump to keep up her milk supply, and when Christa was nine days old, Nadine was finally allowed to breastfeed her baby for the first time.

Other mothers have continued to nurse their babies, even though they had chickenpox themselves. Richard Applebaum, pediatrician, author, and member of the Professional Advisory Board of La Leche League International, says: "You can nurse the infant as long as the baby has had a Zoster Immune Globulin shot. Pumped breast milk can be used for the baby, too. Breast milk would transmit immunity-building substances from mother to child, so that nursing (if baby gets ZIG shot) would be helpful in protecting baby from the disease."

If you are exposed to chickenpox a few days before your baby is born and you have never had the disease (and therefore don't have any immunities), how will the doctors handle this? It depends on several things, such as how many days before delivery you contracted the disease, and if your baby has any pox on him when he's born.

For instance, if Nadine's baby had exhibited any pox, mother and baby probably would have been isolated together, and she would probably have been allowed to nurse Christa. Since her baby showed no evidence of chickenpox, Nadine was isolated separately so Christa wouldn't get it through contact.

If you have older children at home with chickenpox, make plans so your baby won't come in contact with them while they're contagious. Let a relative (who's already had the disease!) care for the older ones outside your home or you and your new baby stay in the hospital until the "coast is clear."

If your baby gets chickenpox after he's 14 days old, he got it by exposure after he was born (as opposed to being exposed in the uterus, which is called congenital).

Doctors Remington and Klein in their book, *Infectious Diseases of the Fetus and Newborn Infant* (2), say that there is little evidence that postnatally acquired chickenpox is more serious in infants than in older children, and breastfeeding such a baby would probably be the best thing you could do for him.

Hepatitis

There are basically two types of hepatitis: infectious and serum (transmitted mostly through blood, as in transfusions). Infectious is the type most commonly referred to when talking about hepatitis. The incubation period of this disease (the period of time when you are infected but don't show any symptoms) is several weeks. During this time you've already exposed the baby to the disease; consequently, once you're diagnosed as having infectious hepatitis the "damage," if any, has already been done.

La Leche League professional advisors state:

> If the infant is going to come down with the disease, or is incubating, breast milk provides an advantage. Not only does it give optimum nutrition, but if the mother is recovering from the disease, she is doing so by action of antibodies to the disease that she has manufactured. The high probability is that small amounts of these antibodies are transmitted through the milk and are a protective factor. (3)

Although the virus may be passed in the milk, the antibodies are passed as well. The bottlefed infant is exposed to virtually as much virus from the mother by other routes and does not receive her antibodies.

Dr. Frederick C. Battaglia, Assistant Professor of Pediatrics and Obstetrics and Gynecology at the University of Colorado Medical School, feels that an expectant mother who has infectious hepatitis toward the end of her pregnancy should be permitted to take care of and to nurse her baby. (4)

The image of hepatitis sufferers lying in their beds incapacitated for months on end isn't realistic in all cases. For every person who develops a clinical case of hepatitis there are about seven subclinical cases, those whose symptoms are never evident enough to diagnose and therefore go undetected. There are probably many mothers who nurse with hepatitis and aren't aware of it.

Mononucleosis

Many mothers have nursed their babies even though they were sick with mononucleosis. One of these mothers, Ginnie, shares her experience:

> When Leah was 14 months old, my sore throat and generally run-down feeling were diagnosed as mono. The doctor told me the only cure was complete bedrest for at least two to three weeks. At this point, Leah was

still completely dependent on me for liquids; she took only a few swallows from a cup and had never had a bottle. Instead of disrupting our breastfeeding relationship, I knew enough about mono not to be concerned about passing the germs through my milk. I continued to have a healthy appetite, which helped keep my milk supply up. Only when my fever was high did I run into some trouble; I became dehydrated and soon noticed a difference in Leah's wet diapers. In order to get liquids into her, I spoon-fed her water and actually wished she would take a bottle! Once my fever came down, however, I had enough milk again.

Mumps

Mumps is not as common a disease as it once was, since children are routinely inoculated these days, and many of us had mumps as children. However, if you should develop mumps while nursing, you would most likely want to continue since the breast milk would offer some protection to the baby. Donna writes:

When Eric, our third child, was three months old, both his brother and sister came down with mumps. Two days later my glands began to swell and before the day was out I was down with a double case and high fever. On the advice of our doctor, I promptly went to bed with Eric tucked in beside me. About two days later I noticed Eric's jaw begin to swell.

The next morning I woke up to find not a sick baby, swollen and feverish, but a joyful three-month-old. To my amazement, the baby's swelling had gone down and he was fine. The doctor believed that through the nursing Eric received antibodies to the mumps and he only developed a very mild case.*

---

* Mumps for adults can be very serious, sometimes even fatal. If you are exposed to mumps and have not already had them, it is highly recommended that you get a mumps vaccine immediately. It will at least give you some protection even if exposure causes the actual disease.

Pneumonia

Can you nurse your baby even if you get viral pneumonia? Betsy contracted the disease when her daughter, Elizabeth, was four months old. Betsy was advised to wean but she knew that the baby had already been exposed to the germs. An antibiotic was prescribed and a doctor she consulted agreed this drug was safe for a nursing baby. Determined not to wean unless absolutely necessary, Betsy felt she was doing the right thing by continuing to nurse. After several days of complete bedrest, Betsy recovered, and no one else in the family contracted pneumonia. Elizabeth remained healthy and continued nursing happily.

Tuberculosis

A mother may be able to nurse with tuberculosis under certain conditions, according to doctors at the Ross Valley Medical Clinic in California. If tuberculosis is not active in the *lung* (where transmission is by close mouth and nose contact); if it can be assured that it is not in the *blood* (and therefore probably in the milk); and the medicines administered are assured to be safe for the infant, then a mother may nurse her child.

"A short separation of mother and baby may be advisable in an open, active case of TB," advises Dr. Gregory White, member of the Professional Advisory Board of La Leche League International. "Even here, with modern methods of treatment, the mother can be rendered noninfectious in a very short period of time, in most cases."

Other Contagious Diseases

Are there other contagious diseases that a mother could pass to her child through breastfeeding?

According to Dr. David Morens of the Disease Control Center, Atlanta, Georgia:

There is much that remains unknown about the transmission of disease through breastfeeding. To further complicate matters, it is difficult to sort out transmission of disease by breast milk as opposed to transmission of disease through the close mother-child contact that breastfeeding exemplifies. One thing is certain, however; as well as viruses being excreted in breast milk, so too are antibodies that may be capable of neutralizing them.

Birth Complications

Mothers have been able to nurse successfully despite complications during or after birth. Because of a severe illness, Linda was unable to be with her newborn baby. A high fever, collapsed lung, and kidney and bladder infection kept her in intensive care for several days and after the birth it was three weeks before she even saw her baby again. "I was too sick and depressed to hand express my milk," wrote Linda.

I'd heard that milk production could be stimulated even after weeks of separation from a baby—so I decided to try to breastfeed Billy. My breasts were soft and smaller than during pregnancy and I could not express any milk. For a few days I nursed Billy every 2 or 2½ hours, but my doctor told me to slow down because the uterine contractions seemed to disturb the healing process. So I nursed him every 4 hours and gave him complementary feedings. Gradually, I was able to cut down on the complementary feedings and nurse him every hour (with the doctor's permission). The result was a completely breastfed baby at six weeks of age, three weeks from the time of my homecoming. (5)

Another mother, Barbara, describes how she was successfully able to nurse following a hysterectomy:

My uterus had ruptured during the delivery and an emergency hysterectomy had been performed. The doctor couldn't promise me that my milk would still come in since he knew of no similar cases; but I was determined not to give up. In addition, "dry-up" shots had been given to me in surgery. Nonetheless, the nurses cooperated fully and brought my baby whenever I asked. I put her to the breast as often as possible and waited hopefully. By the fourth day I was having some anxious moments, but that evening I had the first sensation of my milk letting down. I made a speedy recovery and we were soon back home. (6)

Food Poisoning

When a nursing mother (or anyone else) suffers from food poisoning it's usually localized in the intestinal tract and isn't passed through the milk. The lactoferrin present in breast milk kills the bacteria. In just about all cases, breastfeeding can continue with no problems.

Skin Disease

When Mary's son, Aaron, was 14 months old, she came down with poison oak. A call to one of the doctors on La Leche League's Professional Advisory Board assured her that it was safe to continue breastfeeding, that she couldn't give her son poison oak and that she'd be more comfortable nursing him. Using a clean, white, cotton hankie to cover most of her breast, she continued to nurse Aaron. A year later, Mary reports:

Despite my precautions, I once again got poison oak; I was covered from head to toe! At this time Aaron, at age two, was still nursing occasionally each day for a few minutes. But after viewing my severely infected skin, he stopped nursing completely. Both my husband and I realized that this was no way to end a lovely and very special relationship. We put no pressure on Aaron to nurse. Instead we pointed up my gradual return to good health. I suffered some engorgement, but manual expression a few times each day helped relieve the discomfort and keep up a token milk supply. Aaron refused the breast for two full weeks and then, when only a few spots were left, he asked for some milk, and finally nursed again. (7)

Heart Disease

When Sharon was pregnant it was discovered that she had a slight heart condition (pulmonary stenosis). She wrote to La Leche League International, asking what effect this would have on nursing her newborn. "If the heart specialist feels you need medication," was the answer she received, "you can still plan to breastfeed. There are a number of drugs that can be safely taken by a nursing mother, and no doubt one can be chosen for you, if needed. Your doctor can obtain a drug sheet by contacting La Leche League International." (8)

Arthritis

If you are an expectant mother with rheumatoid arthritis and are trying to decide whether to nurse, it's important to talk this over with your doctor. Many different drugs are used to alleviate this disease. Some are safe for the nursing baby, others may not be. The drugs' side effects on the mother must be considered also.

The decision to nurse is as much a family decision as a medical one. The care of an older baby or toddler is sometimes quite exhausting and it can be difficult to pick up the child. Normal activities may at times even cause major discomfort. Breastfeeding can lighten the load of physical work a mother has to do—there's no shopping in stores for formula, no preparing bottles, or warming them—and this is something to consider. Many mothers have nursed with rheumatoid arthritis, so before making your decision, you may want to contact La Leche League International for additional information.

Carole has psoriatic arthritis, which is usually not as crippling as rheumatoid arthritis. She told me:

My arthritis tends to go away during pregnancy, because of the change in hormones at that time. I found I had no pain for six to eight months after my babies were born. I put off medication as long as possible; I took aspirin, and when I needed more, I conferred with my doctor about the safest medication I could take while nursing.

Cerebral Hemorrhage

When she was pregnant with her second child, Gail suffered a "tremendous headache" which was diagnosed as a cerebral hemorrhage. Together she and her husband made the difficult decision for her to have brain surgery. "The surgery was successful and I could lead a normal life, with no fear of another hemorrhage," explained Gail. "But I could neither read nor write; I could not walk, shop, or do anything that one takes so much for granted. I had severe aphasia, which meant that I was unable to use and understand words."

Her long and difficult road back to normalcy began while Gail was still pregnant. She was so busy with her therapy that she barely had time to think about her baby's birth. The side effects of Gail's hemorrhage had no relation to her ability to nurse her new daughter. In her own words: "I could satisfy at least one of the desperate needs I had, when usurped of all my capabilities. The care of our baby was wonderfully simple, thanks to nursing, which supplied all the baby's needs." (9)

Broken Bones

Many mothers have nursed with broken bones. Sometimes they've had to get into some unusual positions to make breast-feeding possible, but they all feel it's definitely worth it.

"Three weeks before our baby was born, I was in an automobile accident," writes Evelyn. "I had a broken left clavicle or collarbone, so a vest-type cast was put on the upper half of my torso." (10) Once the orthopedist realized how strongly Evelyn wanted to nurse her baby, he designed a yoke cast which extended down about two inches above the nipple area so that she could breastfeed. During the month spent in the cast, she continued nursing with little difficulty, only requiring several pillows under her arm while nursing from the left breast.

Another mother and her four-month-old daughter were in an automobile accident, which resulted in the baby's having a broken leg, and the mother a fractured vertebra. The mother didn't want to interrupt their nursing relationship, and since they shared the same hospital room, she was able to nurse by scooting her bed alongside her baby's crib which had no side bars. It was touch-and-go for a few days due to the awkward position they had to adopt. Although the baby was given supplementary bottles, the mother kept up her milk supply with a high-protein diet, brewer's yeast, and breast massage.

In Traction

After pulling the broad ligament which holds up the uterus, Marlene had to be put in traction. Her daughter, Bethie, was four months old at the time. Marlene has serious allergy problems and felt breastfeeding was vital for Bethie, since her daughter is potentially allergic. Her pediatric allergist suggested having a traction bed delivered to her home, so she would not have to be separated from Bethie. The medical supply company which made the delivery set it up and showed Marlene how to use it. This arrangement was convenient for mother and child; Bethie was on a makeshift bed set up right next to the traction bed, which allowed Marlene to personally care for her as much as possible.

Drugs and the Nursing Mother

Most drugs that a mother takes will show up in her breast milk, but will not affect her baby. This section discusses doctor-prescribed medications as well as those that a mother may choose to take on her own—over-the-counter preparations as well as the illegal drugs marijuana and heroin.

Does Mother Need Medication?

According to Dr. Sumner J. Yaffe, the question is not whether a medicated mother should be allowed to nurse, but whether a nursing mother really needs to be medicated.

"Breast milk is the ideal food for infants, and the answer to the question posed is usually 'No,'" said Dr. Yaffe, professor of pediatrics and pharmacology at the University of Pennsylvania School of Medicine and Children's Hospital of Philadelphia. (11)

In our society, we may be too quick to pop a pill for our problems, real or imagined. Almost any drug which is strong enough to be effective will in some way be toxic to the body; that is, there will be some undesirable side effect. Most of us become more conscious of the dangers medications can produce when we're pregnant. Past tragedies have made us very aware of these potential hazards.

The point is, do we really need to take that particular medicine? Is there some other way of dealing with the problem? Medical people are making remarkable breakthroughs using a new technique called "biofeedback," where people learn to become sensitive to their bodies and through concentration, relaxation and breathing techniques can manage without drugs or at least use smaller amounts of these drugs. (This is what many of us learn in prepared childbirth classes, with similar results.) Many doctors concerned with the overuse of drugs are investigating vitamin therapy, herbal remedies and nutritional treatments as alternatives to medication. Chiropractic, meditation, and religion are also possible means of diminishing a dependence on medications.

When Medication Is Needed

There are times when the judicious use of drugs is necessary. When your doctor decides you need medication, by all means take it. Although most medicines do come through to the milk, this is an acceptable alternative to weaning the baby. It's not uncommon for a doctor to prescribe some medication which has been thoroughly studied and found safe for the nursing baby, yet the mother is instructed to wean. Abrupt weaning can be a traumatic experience for both mother and baby. Mother may develop painfully engorged breasts, risking a breast infection and compounding the problems for which she was advised to take the medication in the first place. The whole mother-baby relationship changes. Caring for the baby and keeping him content is difficult or impossible; the baby is often utterly inconsolable. (12)

Undoubtedly the doctor who tells you to wean is concerned about the health of your baby, yet he is not taking into consideration the possible danger of formula feeding. The doctor may also be playing it safe because he is not aware how strongly you feel about continuing to breastfeed. Let him know by stating your desire to continue nursing. Ask if he can find out more about the prescribed drug and what others you could take which would be safer for your baby.

Recognize the fact that your baby is an individual, as is each situation. Factors such as how long you need to be on the medication, how strong a dosage you need, your baby's age and weight, how mature his organs are, and how much he is nursing need to be considered in each case. Some doctors instruct a mother to take her medication immediately after nursing, to buffer the drug's potency before the next nursing.

A recent professional newsletter made the following comments: "It is well established that a drug which might be dangerous to the newborn when taken by his mother may have little or no effect on the baby after the first week or so of life. Dosages, idiosyncracies, absorption factors, and other significant determinants should also be taken into consideration." (13) A drug may appear in the milk in small amounts when given orally, but may increase tenfold if given intravenously. If injected intramuscularly, it may take a long time before the drug shows up in the milk.

This same newsletter also mentions that "for every medication given to the mother which may affect the infant, there is generally another effective remedy which is harmless. Mothers should be reminded of their right to request a change of prescription from the doctor who prescribes a drug which he believes will require weaning."

When your doctor orders a medication, always make sure you remind him you're still nursing. Many doctors just don't expect mothers to continue breastfeeding past the early weeks. It's a good idea to cross-check with the baby's pediatrician, too.

Drugs Your Doctor May Prescribe

Antibiotics. Many mothers have continued to nurse while taking antibiotics. Usually, the use of antibiotics is short-term, averaging five to ten days, and the amount excreted in the milk is trivial and has no harmful effect on the baby. An exception would be a potentially allergic infant who might be sensitized to the antibiotic and have later allergic reactions to it. Your doctor may advise temporarily discontinuing breastfeeding while you are taking the antibiotic. However, consideration should be given to what will be substituted for your milk. A potentially allergic baby may be better off continuing to nurse rather than being exposed to possible allergens in other milk.

If, while you are sick and taking an antibiotic, your baby is also sick, does he need his own medication? According to an article by Dr. John A. Knowles, "Effects on the Infant of Drug Therapy in Nursing Mothers," "Antibiotics appear in mother's milk but they are in such low concentration that they cannot be considered as therapeutically beneficial to the infant." (14) In other words, each of you needs your own medicine. Any antibiotics you take will not give your baby the protection he needs if he, too, requires antibiotics.

Fluoride. "Fluoride is present in breast milk," states this same article by Dr. Knowles, "and the amount is proportional to that of the water ingested by the mother." Too much fluoride can cause problems for your baby. If it is suggested that you give your breastfed baby supplemental fluoride drops or vitamins with fluoride, first check to see if your drinking water contains it. You can call your water company or your county health department, keeping in mind that the recommended level is 1-2 ppm. Dr. Samuel Fomon states in *Nutritional Disorders of Children—Prevention, Screening and Followup* (15), that he feels babies under six months of age should not be given supplemental fluoride.

Cold Remedies.　　When a decongestant or antihistamine is needed, it's best to take a short acting one (lasting four hours or so) and take it just after your baby nurses. These drugs can decrease body fluids, and you may find some cutback in your milk supply accompanied by a somewhat fussy baby who wants to nurse more often than usual.

Oral Contraceptive.　　When Marge's daughter was six weeks old, her doctor prescribed the oral contraceptive pill. Marge writes, "I noticed my milk supply decreasing rapidly. After about a week there wasn't any milk left."

As this mother found out, the oral contraceptive pill changes the composition and amount of breast milk. "Some women using orals have produced milk containing decreased protein, fat, lactose, calcium, and phosphorus," states La Leche League International's information sheet on "Breastfeeding and the Oral Contraceptive Pill." "Besides the alteration in the basic composition of the milk, small amounts of the progestogens and/or their metabolites have been shown to be present in the milk. The long-range effects of these on the baby are still unknown." (16)

Breastfeeding itself tends to prevent pregnancies. According to La Leche League's manual, *The Womanly Art of Breastfeeding* (17):

> Studies have shown that complete breastfeeding (no solids or supplements) for the first four to six months has a definite effect on the natural spacing of children, since it usually tends to postpone the resumption of ovulation and the menstrual cycle for seven to fifteen months. The babies are then usually born about two years apart. It is

not true that you cannot become pregnant as long as you are nursing, but pregnancy is extremely unusual before the first menstrual period, if you are *completely* nursing your baby.

For further reading about breastfeeding and contraception, see the two books by Sheila Kippley listed in the Bibliography.

Drugs That Should Not Be Taken

Most drugs taken while nursing will appear in the milk, but the amount will be negligible and exert neither a harmful nor a beneficial effect. Only rarely is it necessary to interrupt or stop nursing. The question is not, "Which drugs are passed on to the infant through the milk?" but rather, "Do they affect him in any way?"

A new medical specialty, neonatal pharmacology, is just beginning to investigate drug effects on infants. There is general agreement that certain drugs should not be taken by the nursing mother. Dr. Mark Thoman, a member of the Professional Advisory Board of La Leche League International, says:

> Certain drugs that should never be taken while nursing include anticancer drugs, radioactive drugs, and most hormones. Always check with your physician before taking any drug. Drugs such as barbiturates and sleeping pills should be eliminated if a baby is not gaining weight. However, a small amount of alcohol (beer or wine) can be helpful with a poorly gaining baby if the mother then relaxes and has better let-downs.

Your doctor may have access to lists of drugs and their effects on the infant when taken by nursing mothers. However, these lists are often in direct conflict with each other. Doctors differ in their opinions on which drugs are harmful. If you are told to wean because of a drug you are taking, don't take just one doctor's word for it.

Dr. Thoman cites La Leche League International's list, "Breastfeeding and Drugs In Human Milk" (18), as the most up-to-date, comprehensive authority. This list was prepared with the advice and assistance of the Professional Advisory Board of La Leche League International. It is intended primarily for physicians desiring pertinent medical references to assist them in advising nursing mothers which of alternative medications to prescribe; whether it is necessary to discontinue breastfeeding, temporarily or permanently; or when a particular medication or diagnostic procedure is essential. The list is revised periodically and is based on the experiences of physicians who care for nursing babies.

Diagnostic Tests

If you require diagnostic testing with radioactive isotopes, it may be advisable to discontinue breastfeeding for a short period of time. Here again, it's important that you discuss your wish to continue nursing with your doctor, stressing its importance to you and your baby.

Dr. Ernest M. Solomon advises that when a mother is given a radioactive drug, its half-life should determine when it is safe to nurse again. Webster's New World Dictionary defines "half-life" as "the period required for the disintegration of half of the atoms in a sample of some specific radioactive substance."

Dr. Harold Maller, Associate Clinical Professor of Pediatrics, University of Southern California School of Medicine, believes that if the half-life is 6 hours, a minimum safe time to nurse would be 24 hours, when only 6¼ percent of the original radiation would still be present. At 48 hours it would be less than 1 percent.

If you know in advance that you will be having such diagnostic tests, you may want to hand express or pump your breast milk ahead of time, and freeze it for your baby.

X-Rays

If you need an X-ray you do not have to interrupt breastfeeding. No radiation or any other harmful substance is passed through the milk and you may nurse safely.

When You Need Additional Help

Don't try to "go it alone" where drugs are concerned. Prescribing for yourself is always a potentially dangerous practice, especially when you're nursing. Always talk it over with your doctor. Sometimes he may suggest weaning because he just doesn't have any idea whether a drug is safe for a lactating mother or not. You may feel frustrated and upset, but it's important to try to discuss the matter with him.

La Leche League offers these guidelines:

- Does the doctor know that you are nursing—and just how much you want to continue?

- Have you checked with the baby's doctor for his opinion?

- If the doctor recommends discontinuation of nursing, have you asked if there is another drug or treatment which would also be effective while allowing you to continue?

- Have you considered getting a second opinion from another doctor?

You can contact your local La Leche League leader who can put you in touch with a professional person who has information from La Leche League International on drugs excreted in human milk.

Licit Drugs

How many of us consume coffee, alcoholic beverages, cola drinks and smoke cigarettes . . . without being aware that we're using drugs, and perhaps affecting our nurslings? Caffeine and nicotine are just two drugs that many of us take daily and may even be addicted to, without realizing it.

Cigarettes.   Cigarette smoking presents more of a hazard to the fetus than to the nursing baby. Doctors strongly recommend that a pregnant woman quit or cut down on her smoking.

Heavy smokers experience a higher incidence of stillbirths, premature babies and babies of low birth weights.

Nicotine is found in the milk of smoking mothers and researchers suspect that it will adversely affect the nursling. Also, according to the American Lung Association, children whose parents smoke in the home suffer from twice as much respiratory disease as do children of nonsmokers. Children whose parents smoke are more likely to become smokers themselves. By not smoking, you will be protecting yourself and your baby.

In an article, "Drug Excretion in Breast Milk" (19), Helmuth Vorrheur states: "There is somewhat more risk involved with heavy smoking (more than 20 to 30 cigarettes a day); this may decrease the milk yield significantly and (albeit rarely) cause symptoms like nausea, vomiting, abdominal cramping and diarrhea in the infant."

Dr. Harold Maller reports: "If a mother smokes a pack a day, the baby gets about 10 percent of the minimum lethal dose of nicotine; if she smokes two packs a day, the baby receives 20 percent of this dose, and so on." Also, Dr. Maller points out that a child can die from *eating* one cigarette.

The nursing mother who wants to quit smoking altogether might find this is an ideal time to do it. The hormone prolactin which is released in the mother's bloodstream during breast-feeding helps her remain calmer and more even-tempered. The mother's need for a cigarette might not be as strong as before she began nursing.

In a study of "Infant Admissions to Hospital and Maternal Smoking" by Susan Harlap and A. Michael Davies (20), it was found that "The infants of mothers who smoked had significantly more admissions for bronchitis or pneumonia, especially in the winter, and more injuries. . . . The excess of bronchitis and pneumonia in the group exposed to smoke increased with increasing number of cigarettes smoked by the mother. . . . The findings support the hypothesis that atmospheric pollution with tobacco smoke endangers the health of nonsmokers."

Even if you don't smoke, your baby can be affected just by being in the same room with a smoker, and by being exposed to the sidestream smoke which goes into the air from the cigarette. You are certainly well within your rights to ask smokers to step outside for a cigarette or to remove the baby from the area where people are smoking. It's not uncommon for babies to exhibit allergies to the gases released by a burning cigarette.

Caffeine.   Caffeine is found in various concentrations in cola drinks, coffee and tea. Too much caffeine can cause nervousness, insomnia, irritability, loss of appetite and other unpleasant side effects in nursing mothers—and babies. If a baby exhibits these characteristics, he is often considered "colicky." If your breastfed baby seems to be colicky, start becoming more aware of your caffeine intake. Many mothers have found that cutting caffeine intake way down has helped. If hot coffee or tea relaxes you and improves your let-down, perhaps some other hot liquid, such as soup, will be just as effective.

Alcohol.   Many books about breastfeeding suggest moderate use of beer or wine for a nursing mother. A small amount of alcohol in the evening may help a nervous first-time mother relax, which in turn helps condition the let-down reflex. However, in her book, *Nursing Your Baby* (21), Karen Pryor tells about "a mother who drank a quart of port at a sitting: both she and her baby passed out." So . . . if a glass of wine or beer helps, fine, but remember to keep it in moderation.

Illicit Drugs

Illicit, or illegal, drugs such as marijuana, LSD, heroin, methadone, uppers, downers, and speed are best avoided by the nursing mother.

Marijuana.   Is it safe to smoke marijuana while breastfeeding? This is an important question because millions of people today smoke grass as a social intoxicant. To date no research has been completed and it's not known what effects marijuana can have on the nursing baby.

An article published in 1971 by *California Medicine* (22)

reported that "in studies in which rats, hamsters, and rabbits received large parenteral (injected) doses of marijuana extract during early gestation, there was an increased incidence of fetal malformation and rejection." The article goes on to warn that "it appears reasonable to caution women specifically against the use of marijuana during pregnancy."

There are other things you may want to consider. The side effects of the drug include reality distortion (which may make it hard to cope in an emergency situation), difficulty in performing small motor activity (such as pinning a diaper), and after the high wears off, a desire for sleep, usually quite deep, in which a mother may be unresponsive to her baby's needs. As for the baby, an important point is that marijuana's active agent, THC, being fat soluble, is concentrated in breast milk.

As mentioned previously concerning cigarettes, anyone in the room where a joint is being smoked will undoubtedly be exposed to the sidestream smoke which goes into the air. It would be wise to remove your baby from the room no matter what's being smoked.

No one can say for sure whether smoking marijuana during breastfeeding will or will not harm your baby. By smoking it you are taking a risk. The best advice seems to be: don't.

Heroin.   If a pregnant mother is using heroin, her newborn baby will probably be addicted to the drug, and will suffer the same withdrawal symptoms as an adult. These include jitteriness, convulsions and even death, depending on how much heroin the mother regularly takes.

Heroin can also affect your baby through your milk by making him sleepy and by decreasing his appetite so that he is not eating enough.

Whether a mother on heroin breastfeeds or not, her newborn must taper off slowly, so if you are pregnant and using heroin *please* tell your doctor, for your baby's sake.

Methadone.   Dr. James Good, a La Leche League International Professional Advisory Board member, speaking at a

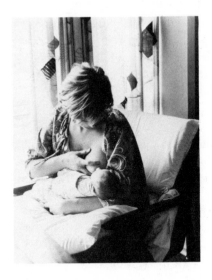

Rooming-in should be considered when mother is hospitalized, as an alternative to separation. Both mother and baby are spared the trauma of such a separation, and breastfeeding may continue, if mother's condition allows.

recent La Leche League International Conference, said, "Small amounts of methadone have been found in breast milk, but no harmful effects on nursing babies have been noted." Since only trace amounts of the drug are reported in a mother's milk, virtually none of it reaches the baby. Based on these findings, Dr. Good concludes that breastfeeding is permitted.

However, long-range problems caused by methadone have yet to be determined. So, if you are pregnant and on a methadone maintenance program, coming off the program slowly during your pregnancy would avoid potential risks to you and your newborn.

When Mother Requires Surgery

When a mother needs surgery, many arrangements need to be made. In some instances you may have days, weeks or even months to plan a hospital stay, but when an emergency situation arises, you simply have to do the best you can at short notice. Reading how other women have coped may help if you are ever faced with surgery during the time you are breastfeeding.

Doctors have long been aware that a patient's emotional

and mental health are as crucial to successful surgical recovery as her physical health. Keeping the nursing relationship intact following surgery can lift a mother's spirits while giving her a feeling of usefulness and purpose.

When You Have Time to Plan

La Leche League International's professional advisors suggest that in cases of elective surgery the mother ask her doctor if it could be postponed until a time when her baby could handle separation more comfortably. If he says no, she is certainly within her rights to seek another medical opinion. Separation of a nursing mother and child, even under the best of conditions, is difficult for them.

One of the best ways to handle the hospital stay for mother and nursling is for the baby to room-in with the mother. Some hospitals will admit them together.

· If you are going to nurse after surgery, this should be discussed ahead of time so the surgeon can take your needs into consideration. Charlene's doctor planned her anesthesia to suit her needs.

She was hospitalized to have an inguinal hernia repaired when her baby, John, was three months old. The doctor estimated her stay at four days, and when Charlene expressed her desire to continue nursing during this time, he agreed. He selected spinal anesthetic as the best method for a nursing mother and promised to get Charlene out of the hospital as soon as possible.

Her baby nursed an hour before the operation, and later that afternoon following surgery. Although Charlene was on her back and not allowed to move, when her husband brought John in three times a day, she was able to hold him up at her side to nurse. She also saved what milk she pumped in between to be given in a bottle. Within two days she was released and back home nursing her son.

Because Jill had time to plan her surgery (a small nodule in the right breast required a biopsy under general anesthetic), she selected a hospital 40 miles away. Its family-centered care made up for the distance, and was the determining factor in her decision to have the surgery performed there.

Since she did not plan to wean her nine-month-old son, Jill's doctor suggested that she "board" the baby in her room, a policy the hospital followed with nursing babies.

> My husband was there during the surgery and afterward to help me when I nursed Eric. Coming out of sedation I was too groggy to hold him and nurse him at the same time, so my husband put him beside me and stayed to make sure he didn't fall off the bed. The hospital had assigned a nurse to Eric for that day, in case my husband had not been there. She would have watched and fed Eric while I was in surgery and while recovering from sedation.

If the hospital doesn't provide a nurse to help with rooming-in the first day or two following the operation, have a relative or close friend there. If necessary you can hire a trained nurse.

Take Time to Plan, Even in an Emergency

Janice's major concern before being rushed to the hospital for an emergency appendectomy was her five-month-old allergic baby. Janice said, "Sarah had difficulty digesting even breast milk so when I was told to wean her, I refused." Her doctor allowed Sarah to be admitted to pediatrics and she was brought periodically to Janice to nurse. She nursed just before the operation and then eight hours after, and in between Sarah had a bottle of Janice's milk which she had frozen for such emergencies. Although sleepy from the maternal medication for one day, Sarah nursed happily throughout the hospital stay.

Determination Can Make a Difference

Wendy was not as fortunate as Janice; her request to keep her nursing daughter in the hospital met opposition every step of the way.

Wendy was told by her doctor that the lump she had discovered in her breast had to be removed. At first, her surgeon refused to consider the possibility of her continuing to breastfeed. She argued her case, citing multiple night nursings needed with a bottle, colic (which would worsen on formula or be aggravated by air bubbles from a rubber nipple), and her state of mind entering and coming out of surgery if she was worrying about her daughter. Also, an incision in an engorged breast could not heal properly, and the baby would ensure against engorgement. Wendy further pointed out that a breast pump would be rougher on a sore breast than the baby would. Her surgeon relented, and after much arguing Wendy also got permission from the hospital staff for rooming-in.

"I arranged to dispense with preoperative medication so I could nurse my daughter immediately before surgery and then sent her home until the anesthetic had worn off. We only missed two feedings."

Following surgery, Wendy's surgeon told her she could not resume nursing for a week to ten days because the lump had been infected.* Backed by reference sources from La Leche League, she continued nursing, and the breast healed completely.

When a nursing mother is adamant about her desires and convictions, a doctor often will go along with her wishes—and learn some things as a result. When Pam had to be hospitalized for a week, and rooming-in was not available, her husband was able to arrange special visiting privileges for their baby. She was brought in each evening and on the second day after the operation she was brought in twice during the day. On the third day, at Pam's request, when the baby was brought to her at 10:00 A.M. she was allowed to stay until 2:00 P.M., and this was continued the rest of the week, along with the evening visits. This arrangement worked out to the benefit of parents and baby and surprised the obstetrician, whose experience had been that hospitalized patients

---

* The "lump" was not actually a lump but a passive infection which had become encased in scar tissue.

invariably lose their milk even though efforts are made to express it to keep up the supply.

Because of their strong convictions and their polite but firm approach, Becky and her husband were able to accomplish what had never been done before at their local hospital. Becky entered as an emergency patient and her stay was extended for two weeks. She didn't want to stop nursing her eight-month-old, Alisa, so she asked the doctor if she could continue, at least until he received her test results. Both doctor and hospital staff agreed, with the stipulation that she be completely responsible for her daughter. Since Alisa was already eating solids and drinking from a cup, Becky felt she could get by with nursing once in the morning and once at night. With the help of the nursing staff, she was also able to pump her breasts and send milk home for Alisa. Becky said, "Alisa and I became even closer during this time. She knew I had not suddenly abandoned her, and I was able to relax after nursing, knowing that she was happy and content."

When Baby Can't Go Along

It is not always possible to take your baby with you to the hospital. Even when you have the time to make plans beforehand, sometimes the hospital just will not allow the baby to board in. Other times, especially in an emergency situation, you have to make the best arrangements from limited choices. How can you make the best decisions for all concerned?

First of all, it's important to maintain the breastfeeding relationship if this is possible under the circumstances. This implies not only keeping up the milk supply, but also keeping mother and baby together. This relationship is deep and vital to the emotional well-being of both members of the team. Indeed, mourning takes place after separation of any significant duration; for the young baby this can mean just two days away from his mother. The separation should be as short as possible and the nursing relationship should be reestablished as quickly as possible.

Surgery As an Outpatient

When Shirley learned that surgery could restore her hearing in one ear, she had several months to make arrangements for the operation. All attempts to set up a rooming-in situation for her small baby in area hospitals were futile. "Finally I hit on the idea of doing it as an outpatient," she explained. "I called the ear doctor and told him of my plan and he said he'd never done that surgery on an outpatient basis but if the hospital agreed to it, it was okay with him." The hospital consented, and her surgical procedure, a stapedectomy, was done when her son was 4½ months old. "I was away from him for about five hours altogether. I had made arrangements for an ambulance ride home just to be on the safe side and I nursed him on the way. He was at an age where I could easily take care of him in bed for a day or so while I recuperated." An extended separation was avoided because Shirley took the initiative to come up with an alternative plan; both she and her baby benefited.

Your Husband's Attitude Is Important

Even when conditions are far from ideal and you are faced with an uncooperative doctor and/or hospital, your husband's support can overcome a lot of obstacles.

Marcia needed emergency abdominal surgery when her son, Gage, was almost two years old. With her husband's help she was able to keep the nursing relationship intact. Still happily nursing four or five times a day, Gage was just not interested in being weaned. During her ten-day hospital stay, Marcia's husband brought her down to the lobby several times a day to visit with her family and to nurse their youngest. (23) This is a good arrangement when mother can manage it physically. Baby's activity is not hampered and seeing mother seated in a chair is less upsetting than seeing her lying in a hospital bed. Other family members being around also adds to the atmosphere of normalcy.

A husband can also have a negative effect on the outcome

of the nursing relationship. After her second hospitalization within ten days, Joanne was physically and emotionally exhausted and yielded to advice to wean her two-month-old baby, Lisa. Two weeks later, she attempted to nurse again and would have succeeded if her husband had not pleaded with her that she had been through enough. This advice, though well intentioned, was not in the best interest of either mother or baby; it was discovered later that Lisa had a severe cow's milk allergy. Joanne regrets having stopped nursing, and is determined to let nothing discourage her from nursing another child in the future.

Reestablishing Your Milk Supply

If your baby isn't allowed to room-in with you and nurse as freely as he is able to at home, you will probably notice a decrease in your milk supply. How much your supply decreases and how long it takes you to get back to "normal" depends on several factors: your overall condition, what you do to keep your supply up, how long you're away from your baby, your fluid intake, and your baby's eagerness to nurse.

A mother needs lots of support and encouragement when trying to build her milk supply again. Ann found La Leche League to be very helpful and reassuring. Her baby, Aaron, was barely three months old when persistent gall bladder attacks necessitated surgery for Ann. A La Leche League leader located an electric breast pump, which enabled Ann to pump milk before and after her surgery. She pumped her milk for two days until special permission was secured to allow the baby to be brought to her once or twice a day. (Any discomfort in holding Aaron was eased by putting a pillow over the stitches.) Ann writes:

> The following Monday (a week after surgery) I was released. That first day home was harrowing. My baby nursed every other hour and was never satisfied. I felt as though I was going completely dry. Frightened and dismayed, I called my La Leche League leader to ask if I

should give him a supplementary feeding. She calmly explained that his frequent nursing was Nature's way of stimulating my milk to return. The only supplement needed was for me to drink plenty of fluids. I relaxed, let him nurse and forced myself to drink as much as possible. By the end of the next day, my appetite had increased and my milk supply was normal. (24)

Even after weeks of not nursing it's possible to reestablish a good milk supply. It may not happen as quickly as you'd like, but you will be able to totally breastfeed your baby if you nurse him frequently, drink plenty of fluids and get lots of rest. Until your supply is reestablished, your baby can be kept satisfied with contributions from other nursing mothers as well as any previously stored frozen breast milk.

Reestablishing a milk supply at the same level as before the hospitalization may not be as important a *nutritional* need with a toddler as with a "breast milk only" infant. The toddler nurses primarily for the emotional closeness, the love relationship, and nutrition is secondary in most cases. He will often settle for a lot less milk since being reunited with mother and being able to nurse again is so important to him.

For further discussion on milk supply, see chapter 2, "Nursing Techniques" and chapter 15, "Inducing or Reestablishing Your Milk Supply."

Foster Nursing

Every so often we hear of a nursing mother who becomes a temporary "foster mother" for the baby of a friend or a relative caught up in an emergency situation. Unfortunately, modern formulas are looked upon as satisfactory substitutes and generally make foster nursing seem unnecessary.

Nursing someone else's baby is not being recommended here as a convenient way to arrange babysitting for planned periods of separation. Each mother's milk is designed specifically for her baby, and no other mother's milk will be quite the same. For example, according to La Leche League Professional Advisory Board Member Dr. Lawrence Gartner, there is a theoretical possibility that a baby's body may eventually reject antibodies received through another mother's milk. Therefore, at this time, he feels it is much safer to use a mother's own milk for her baby.

Foster nursing also runs the risk of cross-infection. And there is another and perhaps greater risk—that of interfering with maternal-infant bonding, so necessary for baby's emotional security.

However, when truly necessary, foster nursing can help make a difficult situation much easier for the young nursling, and in the case of a severely allergic child there may be no alternative except to secure another mother's milk. While her baby's needs are being met, the hospitalized mother must handle the physical problem of engorgement which results when she stops nursing for any length of time, and the problem of maintaining her supply so she can resume breastfeeding when conditions permit.

The fewer the number of mothers involved in nursing your baby, the better. It's best if only *one* need be involved. In Olivia's case, her sister was the one who provided foster nursing. When Olivia's daughter, Eve, was just a little over 2 months old, Olivia was admitted for surgery to remove an IUD which had penetrated the uterus. Olivia's sister, who was still nursing her 13-month-old daughter, began nursing Eve also. Olivia wrote:

> The IUD was removed and I returned home two days later. Before surgery they gave me an injection to dry up my body fluids. This shot and the two days of no nursing had almost dried me up. Eve and I stayed in bed, and she nursed constantly. In the evenings, my sister would give her an auxiliary nursing which put her to sleep for a few hours at least. After 1½ weeks I was nursing on my own.

Olivia's choice of her sister as a substitute was a wise one. Her older children were familiar with their aunt and cousins, and no doubt little Eve benefited from being with relatives and in an environment very similar to the one she was used to.

When You Nurse Another Mother's Baby

Mothers have found nursing another mother's baby in a crisis situation to be a very satisfying and rewarding experience.

Dorothy offered to nurse her friend Jean's six-day-old baby along with her own, when Jean was rushed to the hospital for an emergency operation. Dorothy says, "The part that amazed me was that I had an ample supply of milk for both babies. Nursing this baby was a new experience of love and I felt very important to the baby and her family. I only had her for a few days, but I couldn't help thinking how easy it was to care for her along with my own four children. The fact that I had no formula or sterilizing to bother with was a wonderful time-saver and convenience." (25)

How the Baby May React

Each hospitalization experience will dictate its own specific solutions. Each baby is an individual and what might work well for one might make another miserable.

Norma Jane required surgery when her daughter was eight weeks old.

> I left her with a mother who was eager to nurse her for the 24 hours before she was allowed in the hospital with me. I've felt since that my baby would have been happier with grandma or daddy and frozen bottles of breast milk, since she was extremely upset by strangers, even at that age. A year later, however, I kept and nursed a baby for almost a week while the mother underwent surgery. In this case, the baby seemed to do much better because of being able to nurse. It's what we always say, all babies are different.

Accepting a substitute mother seems to be easier for a very young infant, or for a baby who is familiar with his substitute. However, older babies and children have their own ways of adjusting to a stressful and difficult situation, as the story of Eleanor points out.

Eleanor was 17 months old when her mother, Lada, was hospitalized. Eleanor was born totally allergic to all foods except breast milk, white rice and honey, which constituted her entire diet. Her life depended on being able to get enough breast milk to survive while separated from her mother, and being so old she needed a great deal. Lada said:

> I was told I would be hospitalized a week to six months. I pumped milk all the time I was in the hospital and sent it home, but it tended to sour since mother's milk is very difficult to keep fresh. Also, while I was in the hospital she developed diarrhea. My husband started taking her to Weena's house to be nursed. Even though her father was holding her, Eleanor would cover her eyes with her arm while she nursed, so she wouldn't have to look at the lady who was nursing her.

The nursing relationship is much more than just breast milk to a child Eleanor's age. Although saddened by her mother's absence and missing the intimate, unique love relationship they shared, Eleanor showed great courage in accepting breast milk from another mother.

Babies seem very adaptable to nursing from their own mothers, however, and often will find their own unique solutions to gaining access to mother's breasts. A mother who had breast surgery found afterwards that her daughter held the bandage up with her right hand so her nose would fit and wasn't bothered by her mother's prominent red medication markings.

It's hard to realize the effects that separation from mother can have on a baby or young child. They can't verbalize their feelings as adults can; however, they do express how they feel through body language and behavior. A 1976 newsletter published by the organization Children in Hospitals contained excerpts from a study which helps explain the reactions of babies and toddlers when separated from their mothers:

For the very young child the mother is not only a loved object, she has many functions besides. The mother stands as a buffer between her young child and the environment, mediating its stress and demands so that they remain within his tolerance. She arranges life around her young child, helping him to master as much as he can but always ready to protect him when necessary. She is responsive to his cues and understands his meagre language as no one else does.

So the behavior of the separated young child is not determined only by the loss of the mother as a loved person. It is influenced by the extent to which his new caretaker(s) are able to maintain her functions—by the extent to which they understand and respond to the cues he offers, can keep life running in familiar ways, and can protect him from stressful impingements of the environment. (26)

Chris was seven months old when his mother, Fran, was hospitalized for an inner ear infection. The eight-day separation took its toll. She managed to reestablish her milk with little difficulty but found that Chris had developed some emotional problems because of the sudden separation. He had begun to suck his thumb and cried loudly and fearfully whenever Fran was out of sight. Chris is now over a year old, still nursing, and seems to have recovered his trust that his mother won't abandon him again. Fran feels that being able to nurse him helped him over the emotional hurdle. (27)

One mother was sent to the hospital for an emergency operation when her daughter, Sarah, was 11 months old. When she returned home after three days, the reunion was the opposite of what she expected. Sarah looked at her mother and began to cry, seeming very confused, nearly hysterical. It was breastfeeding that united them again. Once her father calmed Sarah, mother and daughter settled down to nurse, and by the end of the session, Sarah had accepted her mother again. (28)

Chapter 14

Working Together:
Doctor, Hospital, Parents*

Many of the situations described in this book involve some contact with a doctor and a hospital. How can you most effectively communicate your needs and desires to your doctor or hospital? How can you, your doctor, and your hospital work together with your baby to make the best of a difficult situation? Should you try to stay with your baby in the hospital? Can you breastfeed him there? What if *you* must go to the hospital while you have a nursing baby? What are your rights? What are your responsibilities? This chapter contains information, ideas, references, and examples you might adapt to your own situation.

Your Presence Does
Make a Difference

You're not an odd, overprotective parent if you want to stay with your sick child. It's a natural urge, and it's best for him, too. The first American hospital to have a pediatric ward where parents are permitted to take over responsibilities usually assumed by professional personnel was the University of Kentucky's Medical Center. In the center's Care-by-Parent Ward doctors have found that children get well faster when their parents are on the scene as part of the team. (1)

Any hospitalization is an emotionally traumatic experience.

---

* Part of this chapter has been adapted from La Leche League International publication no. 143, "In Hospital, The Child and The Family," by Betty Ann Countryman, M.N., R.N.

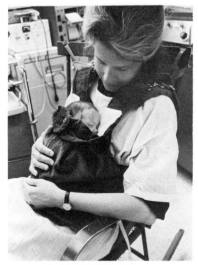

In a premature ward, a mother gives her baby plenty of attention by stroking and rocking.

The Children's Hospital, Denver
Snugli Cottage Industries

As one doctor has written, "The age of the child who must be hospitalized may influence the kind of concerns he has. For children under five or six, separation from home and parents is an even more terrifying aspect of the experience than the pain or illness he must endure." (2)

A baby or little child doesn't really understand about hospitals, doctors, treatments, and pain, even if you have explained them to him ahead of time. People wear masks and strange clothing, and may subject him to frightening and painful procedures. Breastfeeding your baby can give him considerable comfort during such upsetting times.

Father's presence is reassuring, too. One mother of a premature baby weighing a little over three pounds reported that when the baby's father stroked him and held him in his large hands in the Isolette, the baby moved more vigorously than at any other time. The nursery staff even commented favorably about this on the baby's chart.

Nurses rarely have the time to give each child the kind of attention a parent can give. Babies need lots of cuddling, holding, rocking, and skin-to-skin contact, especially when they are distressed. Loving parents and babies have a special feeling for each other which no nurse or doctor, however dedicated, could be expected to have.

But aren't babies better behaved when their parents are not around? Dr. John Bowlby (3) (4), Dr. James Robertson (5) (6), and Dr. Vernon L. James (7), the founder and director of the Care-By-Parent Ward, point out the stages of protest, despair, and detachment through which a lonely little person passes when the day-to-day closeness with his mother is interrupted. Dr. James describes it this way:

> A child separated from his mother is likely to rebel. He may scream and yell until he is exhausted. Then, when he finally gives up, he's apt to go into his shell and become very depressed. Though a casual visitor to a children's ward might think the docile child lying quietly in his bed is well adjusted to his plight, the opposite is more often true.

An older child may revert to infant patterns of sleeping, eating, and bed wetting; thumb sucking may reappear or intensify as the child attempts to mother himself. (See also Home Again, in chapter 12, "When Baby Is Sick or Hospitalized."

Some of this behavior is lessened or avoided when the parent lives in with the child during hospitalization or spends most of the time in the hospital with him. Don't expect to avoid *all* problems, however. Some children express anger when hospitalized even if mother is there full time. This is especially true when surgery is involved. Hospitalization is very upsetting for mother and child. Yet it's certainly better if you are there to be aware of procedures and medications and to encourage regular habits as much as possible.

The younger the child, the greater the need for his mother's presence while he is hospitalized. Whether you are allowed to help with his physical care or not, your presence is valuable support at this frightening time.

Finding a Supportive General
Practitioner, Obstetrician, Pediatrician

With a doctor and hospital staff who are in favor of breastfeeding, your chances of successfully nursing through a problem situation are high.

You may already have a doctor that you like. If his usual breastfeeding policies are different from what you want, should you look for another doctor? Not necessarily. Good rapport is very important. Is he willing to consider information and studies which support your requests? Just by asking many parents have found out that what seemed to be a "rule" with their doctors was actually only a "preference." There is an element of flexibility in preferences.

If you do not have a doctor and you're looking for one who is already knowledgeable and enthusiastic about breast-feeding, how do you find him? You might ask any of these people for recommendations: friends who have had good experiences; other breastfeeding mothers such as those you might meet at La Leche League meetings; Medical Associates of La Leche League in the area (if they cannot specifically help you, they can recommend other physicians); childbirth class leaders who have had experience dealing with local doctors. Select a few of the doctors, and ask to meet with them or talk with them on the telephone.

What do you say when you want to learn a doctor's views about breastfeeding? First of all, inform yourself as completely as possible about all aspects of breastfeeding. Read and take to the interview information such as *The Womanly Art of Breastfeeding* (8), La Leche League Information Sheet no. 20, "Together, and Nursing, from Birth" (9), and La Leche League Information Sheet no. 158, "White Paper on Infant Feeding Practices." (10) Information should be multisourced, recent, and documented.

Here are some questions you might include in your initial interview with a doctor:

General Questions

How many of your patients are breastfed children or breast-feeding mothers? (The attitude with which this is answered is as important as the actual answer!)

What do you consider some of the most important reasons for breastfeeding?

Obstetrician

I've read about the many benefits of early nursing and want very much to nurse my baby soon after delivery. Do you have any objections?

What do you recommend in case of a breast infection?

Do you have patients who were permitted to have their nursing babies with them while hospitalized?

Do you prescribe the oral contraceptive pill? (If so, refer to *Oral Contraceptives* in the section, Drugs and the Nursing Mother, chapter 13, "When Mother Is Sick or Hospitalized.")

Pediatrician

Which can you arrange for us after the baby is born: rooming-in, demand feedings, or having my baby brought to me on a three-hour schedule?

How do you gauge whether a breastfed baby is doing well? (Does he judge mainly by the weight gain, or consider the individual baby's own health and development?)

I'm concerned about having enough milk. How can I tell that the baby is getting enough? (Again, notice the attitude and positive suggestions.)

Do you feel a baby needs to have supplements while breast-feeding?

I've read that breastfed babies can do very well without solids for six months or even longer if allergic. Are many of your patients nourished this way?

How long do most of the mothers in your practice breastfeed?

Do you advise weaning the nursing baby at a certain age?

If Your Baby Is Going to Be Hospitalized

What arrangements can be made for mothers to stay with their nursing babies? (Including food and some provision for rest and cleaning up.)

How close to surgery, both before and after, can I breastfeed my baby?

You can listen to a doctor's response to your questions and judge whether you want him to be your doctor. You may get a variety of opinions if you talk to several doctors. There is leeway for doing things differently. If a doctor says, "Well, yes, I hadn't thought of it that way. Yes, that might be true," when you present an idea that he is not accustomed to, this may indicate a satisfactory, open-minded attitude.

Finding a Supportive Specialist

Your child's doctor may be able to direct you to a specialist who is supportive of breastfeeding. Some problems such as a heart defect or cleft palate require care which only a limited number of physicians in your area may be able to provide. You may have no choice but to go to the only one available. On the other hand, for a more common problem such as tonsillectomy, there may be several ear-nose-and-throat specialists practicing in your area.

You may choose a specialist whose knowledge of nursing is important for your child's care, as with a digestive problem. In other circumstances, the doctor's expertise in his special field may be the overriding consideration.

Distance may be a consideration for you, too. Some parents are able to commute great distances to see a specialist who is both skillful in his field and knowledgeable about breastfeeding. However, you may want to consider the difficulties which may result from being far away from home and family support at a time of stress. It may be more desirable to choose the best physician available locally. As parents together, you can present your feelings about breastfeeding to the doctor and possibly offer to give him information on breastfeeding of which he may be unaware.

If you are working with more than one doctor, one may be able to intercede on your behalf with another doctor who may not think breastfeeding is important.

A mother whose child has had kidney problems since birth said that when the child was 12 months old and had to go to the hospital for surgery, the urologist did not want her to stay with her child, even though she was breastfeeding. He was very cutting and demoralizing in his remarks, saying she was "smothering" the child. "She can have a bottle in the hospital. She'll only be there three or four days," he said. The mother, very upset, was referred with her daughter to see Dr. Justin Call, an international authority on mental health problems of infants and head of the Department of Child and Adolescent Psychiatry at the University of California at Irvine.

Dr. Call verified the strength and significance of the mother-child relationship, the importance of breastfeeding in sustaining that relationship, and the positive mental health implications of the bond between mother and child. He also explained to the urologist the deleterious effect on both mother and infant which abrupt unplanned weaning from the breast to the bottle could have at that age, stressing the fact that by 12 months of age infants have begun to endow the bond with the mother with very strong feelings and complex meanings. The urologist then called the mother and arrangements were made for her to be with her daughter in the hospital.

Dr. John D. Michael, pediatrician at the Ross Valley Medical Clinic in Greenbrae, California, says that if the child's physician does feel strongly that breastfeeding can be accomplished in specific situations and has had experience in dealing with the situation, then he can alert other professionals who are dealing with the child and the mother about breastfeeding. Nevertheless, Dr. Michael points out, this does not mean that the other professionals will take to heart what the child's doctor tells them, but it is still worth communicating, not only for the particular mother and child, but also for others who follow them.

Routine Medical Care

In the months that follow your baby's birth, the relationship that you develop with your doctor during periodic checkups and minor illnesses will set the tone for dealing with any problems that may arise.

You should feel free to ask questions. Many times there are alternatives, if you just ask. For example, when our twins were about three months old, our pediatrician said, "You can start solids now." When I asked why start them, he said, "So they'll get used to a spoon." "Is it okay if I give them *breast milk* from a spoon?" I asked. "Oh yes, that's fine," he replied.

Learn as much as you can about different approaches to parenting. Read books. Discuss parenting with others. Then you will be able to state your preferences to your doctor calmly and with confidence.

When there is illness, report accurately to your doctor. Carefully follow his instructions for administering medication. A responsible attitude builds good rapport.

Sometimes it may seem that your doctor doesn't have the time to talk, but if you have questions, keep asking. You are paying for his care. Answering your questions is an important aspect of this service.

If your relationship with your doctor is strong and positive during routine care, he will respect your ideas and feelings and will accept you as part of the "team" during a crisis.

Selecting a Hospital

You may have no choice of hospital if a need for hospitalization arises. Your circumstance may require special care which the staff at only one hospital is prepared to give. However, if you have a choice, check into various hospitals in your area to see which ones are more "family centered," meaning in favor of breastfeeding and parents being with their children.

Doctors are often amenable to switching a patient to another hospital besides the one they usually refer patients to. Talk to the head nurse on the pediatric ward about established policies. Inquire about visiting hours. (Twenty-four-hour visitation is especially desirable if *your* schedule is limited.) Ask about the hospital's policy on parents staying overnight, or a baby staying or visiting mother, if *you* are the hospitalized one. Ask how your milk will be used for your hospitalized baby, if you will not be breastfeeding directly during part of baby's stay. Attend the hospital's orientation program for parents.

If you want to make special arrangements, check with your doctor or, if necessary, with the hospital administrator(s). Many hospitals are willing to consider special requests. They are in business to attract you to their hospitals—in a nutshell, *they* need *you*.

Letters Preceding Hospitalization

When hospital procedures take into consideration the importance of breastfeeding, newborn babies can enjoy the full benefits of early and frequent nursing, and older babies can continue the breastfeeding relationship during hospitalization.

A letter can pave the way when you know ahead of time that you or your baby will be entering a hospital. If your doctor's orders are different from the usual hospital policy, it helps to take along copies of a letter signed by your doctor, noting his orders in your case. Some of the points in the following example may help you compose the letter.

Doctor's Instructions for Patient _____

1. No water or formula. Baby being breastfed.
2. Mother allowed to stay with baby during all treatments and tests.
3. Mother allowed to stay in room with baby at all times.
4. A cot to be provided in baby's room for mother.
5. Mother to accompany baby to entrance to surgery suite.
6. Mother to be allowed in the recovery room after baby returns from surgery.
7. Mother allowed to breastfeed baby _____ hours before surgery and _____ hours after surgery. (Provided there are no complications.)
8. Mother may stay with baby as long as she wishes.
9. Mother and father allowed 24-hour visiting permission.
10. One of these procedures, for newborn in hospital with mother:
    Baby brought to mother on demand
    Baby brought to mother every 3 hours
    Baby to room-in with mother
11. If there are no complications, breastfeeding to begin _____ hours after birth.
12. See checklist Dr. _____ submitted.

_____   _____
Date   Physician

Joleen, who was expecting twins, wrote to a hospital, inquiring about their policies on rooming-in, nursing on the delivery table or within an hour after birth, and having her husband participate in the entire process. She asked that the hospital reply in writing, and received the following letter:

Our rooming-in policy has been changed since your last admission.
You may breastfeed in the delivery room:
    a. Baby full term
    b. Wrapped with blankets
    c. No more than three minutes

Our rooming-in policy is the following:
  a. Baby must have stable temp, pulse, respirations, and pink color.
  b. Baby must have had first sterile water feeding.
  c. Baby must not be mucousy, gagging, or choking.
  d. O.K. from floor nurse as to mother's condition.
  e. O.K. from nursery nurse as to baby's condition.

We will be looking forward to having you visit us again. If you have any further questions before or during your stay, please feel free to call.

Thank you,
O.B. Coordinator

Joleen sent a copy of this letter to her obstetrician, and put a copy in her suitcase. When new nurses were not familiar with this policy, she showed them the letter, which brought immediate results. Although the hospital required a sterile water feeding as a general policy, Joleen's pediatrician wrote a request for withholding sterile water. Should a nursery nurse insist on a sterile water feeding, Joleen had the following note prepared, for the nurse to sign:

I hereby accept full responsibility for administering sterile water. I am aware that I do this against the wishes of the parents.

An alternate approach would be for a mother to sign a similar note accepting full responsibility for *not* giving the water feeding.

If hospital staff raise objections to procedures previously agreed upon by your doctor or the hospital, ask if there is a patient advocate on the staff whose job is to act on your behalf. Ask your doctor to intervene. Call the hospital administrator if necessary. It's your baby and it will be your bill. As a *last resort*, it is sometimes necessary to seek legal assistance. However, usually your own firm, reasonable approach will accomplish a great deal.

Here are some further suggestions for writing a letter to a hospital:

• Say something nice about the hospital, even if it is only that they seem to be open to hearing the needs of clients.

• Tell why the letter is being written: "I expect to be using your facility on Oct. 12, to give birth to my baby," or "My baby will be hospitalized on Feb. 8 for . . ."

• Ask questions: "How many minutes must elapse between delivery and nursing, or may my doctor decide?"

• Be specific about what you are asking to do or have done: "I wish to room-in, 24 hours a day, with my baby."

• Give reasons for your request: "Colostrum, available right after delivery, is easy for baby to digest and rich in immunity factors." "Frequent, short nursing periods contribute to an abundant milk supply." "Research shows that fresh, raw breast milk is even better than that which has been frozen and sterilized, since valuable nutrients and immune factors are preserved. Even frozen or sterilized, breast milk is better than formula." (11)

• Report some kind of support, such as "My doctor will cooperate" or "My husband and I feel . . ."

• Thank the hospital for its concern for your needs.

After the experience, write to the hospital about what happened. Encourage them to help other families. Let them know your likes and dislikes. This is one of the major ways hospitals institute changes. James Staton, director of Boston Hospital for Women, says he considers three letters on a particular subject a *trend* and appropriate measures are made to provide for it!

A letter to the hospital should be sent to the hospital administrator, with copies sent to the chief of pediatrics (or other department), the director of nursing, and your own physician. Nancy Cohen, co-founder of C/SEC (Cesareans/Support, Education, Concern), makes this additional suggestion: "If a hospital or doctor is not supportive, it is important to write a *cordial* but effective letter as to why you are not satisfied. For example: 'I would sincerely like to use your facilities when your policy has been changed, as your hospital is close to me geographically.' "

Staying with Your Hospitalized Baby

If you feel strongly that you and your baby need to be together during hospitalization, it is usually possible to find at least one hospital which, to a large extent, understands and goes along with your point of view. In a 1974 survey, Carol Hardgrove of the University of California School of Nursing found that 54 percent of general hospitals with pediatric wards and 83 percent of children's hospitals now offer parents the option of rooming-in. However, the number of hospitals that actually encourage and systematically inform parents about the advisability of rooming-in is relatively low. You and your physician may have to take the initiative and make any necessary special arrangements. (12)

It is sometimes possible to initiate changes in official policies or at least reach a compromise. When Sheri was told she couldn't stay with her hospitalized baby, she talked to the floor nurse to find out why they preferred she didn't stay. When the nurse told her there was a staph infection on the pediatrics floor, Sheri replied:

> Okay, I understand that, but I feel very strongly about mother and baby being together and I cannot bring my baby in and leave her for a week. Some other person taking care of Lisa just will not be able to fill my baby's need for her own mother. I am willing to do whatever is necessary to avoid contamination. If I am not allowed to be with my baby, I will not bring her to the hospital.

Sheri reminded the nurse about the surgery and the fact that the doctor did not want her baby to cry *at all*, because of the stitches. "The nurses don't have time to stay with Lisa all the time, as I do," she said. A compromise was reached: There was a small anteroom where Sheri could be with her baby, after scrubbing up. She had to wear a sterile gown and use a "sterile" (wiped with a disinfectant) rocking chair. "It was uncomfortable," she says. "There was no place to lie down, but we were together."

Sheri's baby had to return to the same hospital several times for further surgery. There was no problem about Sheri's staying on these subsequent visits.

If you are not able to stay with your baby full time, try to arrange to take turns with your husband or some other relative or friend your baby is familiar with, so that someone is with your child all the time. Consider using vacation time or sick leave or working part-time. Such arrangements, even when complicated, are worth it.

If you need money to tide you over during this time, look into welfare provisions. A note from your doctor recommending or requiring your presence with your hospitalized baby may be helpful when applying.

Important Times to Be Present

Every child, even an older one, needs his mother's presence in varying degrees when he is hospitalized, and the younger the child, the greater the need. The baby and preschooler almost certainly require the comfort which only full-time mothering can provide. Even a short hospital stay can be terrifying for a small child. Yet, what if you are not able to room-in because of other children at home or some other reason? What are the most important times for you to be present?

You'll want to be with your child during regular visiting hours. His loneliness will be emphasized if he is aware that other parents are visiting, but not his own. Your husband may be able to be with your baby at times when you cannot be there. A visit from a favorite relative or friend occasionally may be an acceptable substitute for you.

Your baby will surely need you the first night in the hospital. The nights before and after surgery or other painful or frightening treatments are also important. If special arrangements are made with the hospital, you may be permitted to bring your child in on the morning of surgery, rather than on the preceding day. However, even at home, it is important to follow your doctor's instructions about no eating or drinking prior to surgery. See section N.P.O. (Nothing by Mouth) in this chapter.

Try to be at the hospital when your baby awakens in the morning, and when he settles down at night.

Many children are particularly frightened when anesthetic is being administered and when they are awakening from it. Fortunately, some hospitals and doctors recognize your importance and cooperate with parents who wish to be with their children at these critical times. (13)

Leaving Baby at the Hospital

If you must leave your baby, it is a good idea to tape a card to the bed. List his name, favorite toy or game and any other suggestions for the play lady or parents of other patients. They will often lend a hand, as in the case of a child who couldn't wind his favorite music box with his bandaged hands.

If your baby gets breast milk only, a note to this effect is in order. Even though these needs are on file at the nurses' station, an unusual practice like feeding frozen breast milk may be overlooked until after formula has been used. In an allergy-prone baby this may cause a needless risk.

One mother brought a bottle of scent and put a dab on the pillow as a reminder of her, when she had to leave. If your child cries when you go, that is healthier than if he ignores you or seems resigned to your leaving.

Tell your child where you are going and when you will return. Tell his nurse also so that she can check on him frequently in your absence and comfort and reassure him that you'll be back.

Privacy

Feeling at ease with breastfeeding while your child is being treated is something that seems to be easier for some women than for others. The attitude of the nurse or doctor can make a big difference in how comfortable you feel. Sometimes *their* sense of modesty is at fault. Whatever their feelings, it is reasonable to expect that no one will put unnecessary obstacles in the way of breastfeeding your little one, especially following a painful procedure. For privacy, usually a chair turned to the wall is sufficient.

N.P.O. (Nothing by Mouth)

If your baby is scheduled for surgery, the following comments by Betty Ann Countryman, Assistant Professor of Maternal and Child Health Nursing at Indiana University— Purdue University, are of value:

> Prior to surgery or to the application of a cast, and even before certain tests, it is routine in many hospitals to place all patients, even small children and nursing babies, on N.P.O. (nothing by mouth) after midnight. Although the operation may be scheduled for 8:00 A.M. the following day, delays of several hours can and do occur. Even if the procedure begins promptly, eight hours is often much too long for a little baby to go without nourishment.

> Vomiting while under anesthesia can be dangerous, since stomach contents may enter the lungs and cause a serious pneumonia. The purpose of the prolonged fasting period prior to anesthesia is to ensure complete emptying of the stomach. Since breast milk is much more quickly and completely digested than formula, it seems reasonable that the period of fasting could be considerably shorter for the nursing baby. If your baby's feeding is to be restricted, you will probably want to discuss his nursing pattern with the doctor and ask if the time of fasting might be shortened for your breastfed baby. We know of mothers whose babies were permitted to nurse up to two hours before surgery without ill effects.

The chances of a baby's vomiting are fewer today than formerly, since many of the newer anesthetics are less prone to cause nausea and vomiting. If vomiting should occur and the baby is awake, or can be turned on his side, it may be an unpleasant, but not dangerous, experience. Since it is commonly accepted that vomiting is increased by anxiety and crying, if you are with your baby he will be less apt to vomit because of the security he finds in your presence.

One thing is certain: whatever his condition, your nursing baby needs the comfort which you and your breast can best provide. (14)

The wait before surgery is much easier on parents and child if surgery is scheduled for early in the morning. You can request this.

Some mothers whose babies nurse frequently, even during the night, have best been able to handle the N.P.O. ruling when the doctor recommends a mild sedative so that the baby will be less likely to wake and want to nurse. Other mothers have nursed the baby very frequently all day and evening, before the surgery. Some have given the baby a big meal at midnight, so that he will be full at that time and will sleep through.

If you ordinarily have the baby sleeping with you (and nursing) during the night, before his hospitalization you might try having the baby sleep only with your husband—and you sleep in another room.

One mother told me that rearranging her baby's schedule worked well for her. Marla's 16-month-old daughter, Brooke, was severely burned. For her first surgery, Brooke was in the hospital the night before, with her mother. When Brooke awoke and Marla had to refuse to nurse her because of the N.P.O. ruling, Brooke cried and pounded on her mother's chest. Brooke would not be comforted by anyone else. Says Marla:

> It was a miserable experience, and I was really dreading her next operation. I called several other mothers who had had babies hospitalized and asked for their suggestions. My baby is fairly open to change, so trying to

rearrange her day seemed the best suggestion for us. Brooke normally took a late morning and a late afternoon nap, and went to bed about 7:00 P.M. The day before the surgery we skipped the morning nap. I kept her awake until about 4:00 P.M. When I put her down I made her room dark. She thought it was night. She slept until 8:00 P.M. I was going to try to keep her up until midnight and nurse her a lot during the evening. She didn't seem interested in extra nursings, but during the last half hour she did take a teaspoonful now and then of a mixture of cream and egg yolk. I hoped this would keep her stomach full and help her to sleep through the night.

I played with Brooke a lot that evening, to keep her awake. Finally, she nursed to sleep about 11:30 P.M.— about five minutes of nursing.

She didn't wake up during the night! At 6:00 A.M. I woke her. We were occupied with getting dressed and getting to the hospital by 7:30 A.M. (the scheduled time of the surgery) and Brooke didn't ask to nurse. Unfortunately, the surgery was delayed. About 8:00 A.M. she started to ask to nurse. I kept her busy as best I could playing hide and seek, and playing with toys. I couldn't pick her up or she'd ask to nurse. Finally they took her for surgery about 8:30 A.M.

Some babies are not adaptable to any changes in their schedules. Try getting the baby very tired before putting him to bed at his usual time. Maybe then he will sleep an hour or two longer than he normally does. And when he wakes, it may be best if father is the one to rock him or play with him, while you remain out of sight.

Parents' Rights and Responsibilities

Informed Consent

Whenever your child needs treatment you should be there, for you must be able to give informed consent. This means that after your doctor explains the planned treatment and all the possible complications which may result, you may then ask what the alternatives are. It is up to you, the parents, to make the final decision.

Consultation

If your doctor's advice seems to be in conflict with your information about breastfeeding, discuss this with him. There are often alternatives which are better suited to a breastfed baby's care.

Instant weaning may be suggested or even insisted upon. This can be very upsetting to a baby at *any* time. When he is ill or hospitalized he especially needs the comfort of nursing.

Some parents have found it necessary to change doctors when they could not work together. However, it is wise to discuss differences and ask questions to develop better understanding with the doctor.

Doctors frequently consult each other and you need not feel embarrassed to ask for another opinion. For example, you may want another opinion if formula is proposed for a sick baby who is not gaining weight. You can go to another doctor, on a one-time basis, and still stay with your regular doctor. If you do get a different opinion, talk it over with your doctor. Most doctors do not object to your doing this. It is your right. If you get a second opinion which differs from your doctor's and you're still undecided about what to do, you might want to get a third opinion.

Medical Views

As parents we are now in a better position than ever before to bring our own needs and those of our children to the attention of hospital personnel. Statements from the nation's outstanding professional health care organizations affirm our rights.

Here are selections from the Patient's Bill of Rights, approved by the House of Delegates of the American Hospital Association in February, 1973. (Complete copies of the Bill are available from most hospitals.)

The American Hospital Association presents a Patient's Bill of Rights with the expectation that observance of these rights will contribute to more effective patient care and greater satisfaction for the patient, his physician, and the hospital organization. Further, the Association presents these rights in the expectation that they will be supported by the hospital on behalf of its patients, as an integral part of the healing process. It is recognized that a personal relationship between the physician and the patient is essential for the provision of proper medical care. The traditional physician-patient relationship takes on a new dimension when care is rendered within an organizational structure. Legal precedent has established that the institution itself also has a responsibility to the patient. It is in recognition of these factors that these rights are affirmed.

The patient has the right to considerate and respectful care.

The patient has the right to obtain from his physician complete current information concerning his diagnosis, treatment, and prognosis in terms the patient can be reasonably expected to understand. . . . He has the right to know by name, the physician responsible for coordinating his care.

The patient has the right to receive from his physician information necessary to give informed consent prior to the start of any procedure and/or treatment. Except in emergencies, such information for informed consent should include but not necessarily be limited to the specific procedure and/or treatment, the medically significant risks involved, and the probable duration of incapacitation. Where medically significant alternatives for care or treatment exist, or when the patient requests information concerning medical alternatives, the patient has the right to such information. The patient also has the right to know the name of the person responsible for the procedures and/or treatment.

The patient has the right to refuse treatment to the extent permitted by law, and to be informed of the medical consequences of his action.

The patient has the right to expect that within its capacity a hospital must make reasonable response to the request of a patient for services.

The patient has the right to know what hospital rules and regulations apply to his conduct as a patient.

The statement concludes:

No catalogue of rights can guarantee for the patient the kind of treatment he has a right to expect. A hospital has many functions to perform, including the prevention and treatment of disease, the education of both health professionals and patients, and the conduct of clinical research. All these activities must be conducted with an overriding concern for the patient, and, above all, the recognition of his dignity as a human being. Success in achieving this recognition assures success in the defense of the rights of the patient.

Recently the National League for Nursing defined and published its beliefs about the nurse-patient relationship. The following points, in particular, should have considerable impact upon care of the hospitalized mother or baby. These are:

That nursing personnel caring for a patient be sensitive to his feelings and responsive to his needs.

That . . . the patient and his family will be taught about his illness so that . . . the family can understand and help him.

That efforts will be made by nursing personnel to adjust the surroundings of the patient so as to help him maintain or recover his health.

Your right to stay with your child in the hospital is explained this way by George Annas in his book, *The Rights of Hospital Patients* (15):

> In general, if the law or the hospital requires the parent's consent for treatment of the child, the hospital cannot prevent or restrict parents from being with their children while in the hospital.

> The legal right to be with one's children derives from the doctrine of informed consent. Parents may not be able to give fully informed consent for their children if they are not able to be with them constantly to monitor their reactions (which they can interpret better than anyone else because of their experience with their children).

And finally, from the Massachusetts Children in Hospitals pamphlet there are the following statements:

> Based on the experiences of many parents and the advice of medical advisors and legal consultants we advise parents to: *Trust your instincts.* You know your child better than anyone else does. If you feel he needs you, stay with him as much time as you can. You have the right to stay with your child whatever hours you wish to stay no matter what hours are stated for visiting by the hospital. This is true whether you are a clinic patient or a private patient.

Along with hospital rights come responsibilities. Some hospitals have been, and some still are, hesitant about involving parents when children are hospitalized. As parents show a cooperative, helpful attitude, as children recover faster and are less upset by hospitalization, and as hospital personnel receive assistance with some of their duties, hospitals begin to encourage parents to stay with their hospitalized children as much as possible. How can you contribute to a more beneficial hospital stay for your child?

Preparing for Hospitalization

If you know in advance that your baby will be hospitalized, it is certainly a good idea to prepare yourself and your baby. In most pediatric units there are booklets for parents that give details about procedures that can be expected. Many hospitals give parents a preview of intensive care units before their children's surgery so that they can become familiar with the many pieces of equipment that may be needed to monitor their children's progress. Some hospitals have study groups for parents to attend while their children are hospitalized. Find out what programs your hospital provides and take advantage of them.

Talking with other parents whose children have been hospitalized will help you get a realistic idea of what you might expect, especially if *their* children have been through similar procedures. You might ask your doctor to recommend someone with whom it would be helpful to discuss your concern about your hospitalized child. You can also check with a La Leche League group or a self-help group.

It may be difficult for you to discuss the coming hospitalization with your child, but if he is able to understand even part of what you are saying it will be helpful. Dr. T. Berry Brazelton, Associate Professor of Pediatrics at Harvard University Medical School, studied the results when parents were urged to read a booklet to their children explaining a hospital and its procedures. He says:

> The value to each of the children after they were on the ward was so obvious to us that we have continued to press parents to prepare their children in this way. With such preparation children do not become as frightened or as withdrawn; they eat, sleep and recover better from their illnesses, both in the hospital and after they return home. (16)

If you can, arrange to introduce your child a week ahead of time to the people he will see during his hospitalization.

It's the unknown that frightens people—children *and* adults.

What Is Expected of You

Hospitals have established routines which they have found satisfactory in the past. Many of these are based on concern about infection. Expect to be required to take certain precautions, such as washing your hands and putting on a sterile gown.

Your calm reaction to hospital procedures is necessary. A doctor told me, "Fear is contagious. A fearful mother can make her child afraid, creating an impossible situation. Experience in air raid shelters in England revealed that if the parent remained calm, the children responded in kind." Make sure that you are disciplined enough to give the support you want to give.

"Know Thyself" is an important concept to keep in mind. Some parents faint or vomit just from seeing a drop of blood. Preparing as much as possible for the hospitalization helps to alleviate fears. If you feel you need support, ask a relative, a friend, a nurse, or someone from an organization interested in your child's problem to go with you to the hospital. If the person is familiar with hospital routines, so much the better. Being in the hospital will be hard for you, but remember, even the calmest person is never totally unafraid. Your presence during examinations will be reassuring to your baby. During blood tests or any other procedures that may be upsetting to you, you can quietly remove yourself from the scene. Tell your child, "I'm going to talk to the nurse," or "I'm going to get a drink of water. I'll be right back." Being with your child most of the time is better than staying away the entire time.

One of your responsibilities when you stay with your hospitalized child is to see what is happening and question anything that seems amiss. Anyone can make mistakes, including hospital personnel. If your doctor discusses a planned procedure with you and you notice later that the nurses are not doing it, *it's not only your right but your responsibility to question this.* You are not interfering.

A lot depends, of course, on how you approach the doctor

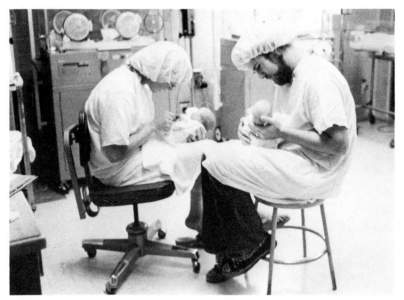

Parents of newborn twins (hospitalized for 4 weeks because of hyaline membrane disease) visit each day to hold and caress their babies and talk to them.

and nurses. For example, you might say, "I spoke with Doctor
_____ a while ago and he said he wanted to do
_____ (procedure). I noticed that this has not been done and I wonder if you could check the chart again."

It is also a good idea to be aware of what medicines your child is getting, and why.

Parents who stay with their children in the hospital need to arrange a cooperative working relationship with the nurses. You will probably be sharing in the care of your child, at least by giving him drinks of water and changing his diapers. It is your responsibility as well as the nurses' to establish this working relationship. I heard of one mother who complained that she had to seek out a nurse to request more diapers for her child. The particular nurse, on the other hand, felt that the mother, being present so much, would naturally have let her know when more diapers were needed.

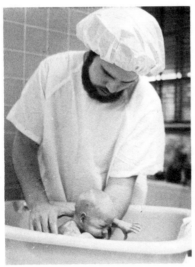

*Father gets involved by helping
with the bathing.*

St. Francis Hospital, Lynwood, Calif.
Sandra C. Wallace

You may be asked to give your child medicine. As one nurse commented, parents usually do a much better job of giving medicine to their children, since they are more familiar with the methods and particular habits.

More Ways You Can Help

You may be fortunate enough to be in a hospital that welcomes active participation by parents in the care of their children and even teaches them skills they do not already know. One such facility is the Parent Care Unit of Riley Hospital for Children in Indianapolis, where parents learn to care for their sick children under the safe supervision of a knowledgeable staff. Dr. Brazelton describes the advantages of such a setup:

> There's obvious value to the ill child not only in having parents nearby, but also in having them in the familiar role of taking care of him. He may even be able to see himself in his old healthy image rather than the new, sick one. And there is obvious value to the hospital—not only have costs of hospital care at Riley been cut in half

as a result of parents' participation, but children improve more quickly. (17)

If you are not allowed at first to perform more than the basic routine care for your baby, just quietly watch what the nurses are doing, and see if there is something *you* could do.

There are many other things you can do to make your child's hospital stay more bearable. How about brightening his surroundings with colorful pictures or a mobile? If your baby is old enough to understand, encourage friends and family members to telephone and send tape recorded messages, drawings, or get-well cards. The drawings and cards can be taped on bulletin boards or the crib or hung from traction hardware. You can bring pictures of the family to the hospital, and together paste them into a scrapbook. Bring your baby's own toys (well labeled), a radio, or a music box. Talk to him, read to him, and play games. You may find some ideas for things that you and your toddler will enjoy together in the book *What to Do When There's Nothing to Do*. (18)

Special Situations for Mother

If *you* are the one hospitalized, you may want to get an allergist's recommendation or a psychiatric or pediatric recommendation that it is inadvisable for your nursing baby to be without you during your hospital stay. Actually your nursing baby is not a visitor, but an extension of yourself.

Sometimes, hospitalization for a mother can be deferred until the baby is older or is no longer nursing. However, if you think your baby still will be nursing in a few months you may not wish to wait. It may take some persuasion to have your baby stay with you in the hospital, but it has been done. See Determination Can Make a Difference, in chapter 13, "When Mother Is Sick or Hospitalized."

If your physician is hesitant about your breastfeeding in a certain situation, such as after breast surgery, you can offer to sign a release. It's usually called an "Against Advice" form.

Cesarean Birth

Mothers who have cesarean births are sometimes talked out of nursing by doctors or nurses who are not aware of the advantages of breastfeeding and how rewarding it can be to a mother in this situation. As one mother said, "After months of preparation for natural childbirth, especially in a psychological sense, I felt somewhat cheated on an aspect of motherhood when I had to have a cesarean birth. Nursing helped restore my confidence in my mothering ability and in my functioning as a woman." In talking with your doctor, it may help to show him the list in chapter 5, "Nursing after a Cesarean Childbirth," of procedures that are possible with a cesarean birth and breastfeeding.

What about your children at home? According to Nancy Cohen, co-founder of C/SEC, "Seven days is a long time to be separated and this is very difficult for mother *and* her other children. Sibling visitation is *essential* with cesarean births."

Blind Mother

When a blind mother has a baby, nurses are often at a loss as to what to do. Some may avoid mentioning anything about your blindness. Others may give you too much help and offer you too much unasked-for advice. Talk to your doctor ahead of time and be *sure* he puts it in writing on your records that you intend to breastfeed, you *must* have the baby on demand and you *can* be left alone with the baby.

Kristin offers these suggestions for other blind mothers, based on her experience:

> When you're in the hospital, ask enough questions so that the nurses realize they *can* leave you alone. Don't make them feel that you're too proud to ask; they really do care about you. Let them know you really appreciate their concern and interest. I ask for a few things I really need and then they're less likely to bother me with things I don't need. And keep in mind that you have to educate *each shift* of nurses.

Rooming-in is a really vital learning experience, especially with a first child, and is well worth any aggravation you might have to go through to get it. A blind mother should not back away from it because she's afraid of too much solicitous help from the medical staff.

"Role playing" with a friend at home, before going to the hospital, can be very helpful. Practice what you're going to say in response to what *they* might say. For example:

Mother: I'll change the baby's diaper after I nurse him. I know where everything is, so you don't need to stay.

Nurse: Well, no dear, we can't leave you alone with the baby.

Mother: In just a few days I'm going to be home alone with the baby. I really need to build my confidence while I'm here. I need to know what I'm doing. You're helping me most by helping me to be comfortable in being alone with my baby. The call button's right here. I'll sing out if I need anything.

Kristin adds these further suggestions:

Prior to your admission to the hospital, it is a good idea to tell them you're coming in and that you're blind. Call the O.B. supervisor and make an appointment with her. When you go in, tell her some of the things you'd like to have— such as your baby in recovery. Later, if there is any question about the things you've discussed, you might say, "The supervisor was very concerned about this and she told me to call her." Also ask the supervisor for the names of key staff members who might be the most helpful, like the nursery nurse, and the charge nurse. Arm yourself ahead of time with the names of people you can contact for help if you have a problem.

Attitudes and Dialogue

Having your desires heeded by your doctor and hospital is often directly related to both the firmness with which you stand up for what you believe and the friendly respect you show in promoting your point of view. Attitude *does* count. (19)

One mother whose four-year-old child has been hospital-ized seven times told me:

> In dealing with medical people over the years, I have found that the parents' attitude is the single most impor-tant factor in being well-informed and in getting the non-medical cooperation that is necessary to continue the breastfeeding experience. A parent must be aware of her rights and willing to be firm in her insistence. This doesn't mean that bad feelings and cross words must pass between the doctor and mother—in fact, most of my relationships with doctors and nurses have been very friendly. They have always been aware that I will question quite thoroughly everything that is told to me. I am not afraid to ask questions if I don't understand something. My greatest feeling of pride came when I asked a resident at Boston Children's Hospital if the rules had changed in re-gard to nurses giving out detailed information on my child's condition. I had no difficulty in obtaining any information that I asked for. He said, "Don't you know that your child's surgeon has left specific instructions that *you* be told anything that you want to know?"

When faced with negative options, explore *various* types of procedures. For example, with your doctor's approval you may be able to shorten your hospital stay. A mother who has stayed in the hospital several times with her baby who has spina bifida said:

> When Michael was operated on at eight months of age, we stayed in the hospital five days. We were supposed to stay two weeks, but we found the hospital to be a dis-ruptive place for family life. I told the doctor I would come to his office each day if we could just leave. Since that time, Michael has had two other surgeries, and we were able to do them on what I call an "in and out"—the child is not admitted to the hospital but taken directly to the operating room. Both times my husband and I went into the recovery room immediately following surgery and

I nursed Michael as soon as they would let me, and then we left.

NOTE: If you are considering an "in and out" operation, check first to see if your health insurance will still pay. If instead you decide to be *admitted* to the hospital, it might still be possible to be operated on, go to recovery, and be out of the hospital in just a few hours.

So much of what you do is the way you do it. If you feel strongly about a certain policy, ask politely why your doctor or hospital has that policy. Be prepared to back up your reasons for wanting a deviation from the standard procedure with specific reference sources. Use phrases like, "I feel very strongly about this," or "This really means a great deal to me." It's important to let the doctor know that these things really matter to you. Then he can see that it's not just a passing whim.

You may encounter some negative attitudes about breastfeeding, or about your staying in the hospital. Be persistent about *your* needs. Try to remain calm (that's the hard part). One mother who felt she received no help or encouragement from anyone on the staff said, "Each day I had to give myself little speeches about their attitude, realizing it was from lack of education and experience. Also if I didn't remain cool, the next woman that wanted to breastfeed would have an even harder time." Indeed, some time later she and the baby did return to the same hospital for surgery, and found that one doctor was now responsive to their needs. At another hospital their experience was completely different. There the doctor's accepting attitude towards rooming-in and a breastfeeding couple seemed to permeate the whole unit.

It can be quite a challenge to balance the needs of doctor, hospital, parents, and child. A calm, reasonable approach in making your requests, together with an understanding of the hospital point of view, can get you far in obtaining nonstandard considerations at a hospital. Be tactful. Plan ahead of time what you are going to say. Work on compromises where parents, doctor, and hospital can be satisfied. You might say, "If I cannot nurse on the delivery table, how about in the recovery room after my baby is cleaned and wrapped (leaving delivery room free for another possible delivery)?"

Ask in a positive way. Saying confidently, "I'm planning on staying the night. What kind of arrangements are usually made?" nets better results than asking, "Can I stay with my baby?" (which is easier for a doctor to flatly refuse). If the hospital tells you that you can't stay because they can't provide the accommodations you'd like, you might say, "Do you have a little cot for me to sleep on?" or "Can I bring my own cot, roll-away bed, air mattress or sleeping bag?", or "Can you bring me a chair?" Maybe being in a chair all night is your best solution if there simply is no cot available. Parents can share the night shift, with each staying half the night. As a last resort you might want to say very nicely, "It probably would be best for us to transfer our child to a hospital that allows parents to stay."

If your doctor forbids nursing because of a drug he is prescribing for you, inquire about alternative drugs that would still allow you to nurse. Asking for a change in prescription will let your doctor know how much nursing means to you. For a further discussion of drugs and their effect on the nursing baby, see Drugs That Should Not Be Taken, chapter 13, "When Mother Is Sick or Hospitalized."

An informed and involved husband can give you valuable support. Sometimes doctors and nurses feel that breastfeeding mothers are rather "peculiar" about their babies. Somehow the doctors and hospital staff seem more agreeable when the couple is a unit and when they know what they want.

Some parents have found it helpful to talk with the chief of psychiatry at their hospital, having him understand the importance they place on the psychological implications of having baby and mother together, and sometimes father, too. If what you are requesting is against policy, there's always a first time.

Hospitals That Care

Several hospitals throughout the country now have a

family-centered philosophy where family unity and the total well-being of the patient is considered. At Children's Hospital in Los Angeles, for example, parents are permitted to stay overnight, without charge, when their children are hospitalized. Couches are provided in many of the patient rooms as well as in parent rooms. In the intensive care unit, where there is no room for parents to sleep, a separate room is available which has couches that open into beds. Parents who are sleeping there are welcome in the intensive care unit to visit with their children. In the neonatal unit parents are encouraged to begin taking care of their babies—changing diapers, giving medication, bathing, and any special feeding that may be required. Janice Mayes, R.N., a specialist in the Neonatology Division, says:

> We encourage parents to get as involved in their baby's care as possible. It is not uncommon for parents to be hesitant about handling their small infant. It may take a good deal of support to convince them that they are as capable as the nurses. For example, sometimes at discharge an infant will require suctioning (to remove secretions) at home. We teach the parents how to do it, and they do beautifully, surprising themselves and often providing better care than the nurses. We ask all parents to spend one or more full days here with their babies, before their babies go home. Shortly after admission, the feeding preference of the mother is determined. Those mothers who express an interest in breastfeeding are offered information and assistance in breastfeeding, in pumping their breasts and in collecting and storing their milk.

At the St. Francis Premature and High Risk Nursery Center in Peoria, Illinois, Dr. Tim Miller, the neonatologist, is also very much in favor of breastfeeding and breast milk. If a mother is not going to breastfeed, he asks for permission to use another mother's milk. (Nursing mothers in the community go to the hospital and pump their milk there, using the hospital's electric breast pump.) Breastfeeding mothers either hand express milk at home for their hospitalized babies, or rent the hospital's electric breast pump, and take in milk either frozen or fresh. A baby may be fed breast milk by gavage (tube) at first, then by bottle, then alternate feedings of breast and bottle. Finally the baby is totally breastfed.

Dr. Miller is especially insistent on breast milk if a baby is very small, has respiratory problems, anoxia, cold stress, or if labor and delivery were difficult. (For more on this center, see Support of Doctor and Hospital Staff in chapter 6, "Nursing a Premature Baby.")

In the Care-By-Parent Ward mentioned at the beginning of this chapter, one wing of the fourth-floor pediatric ward was redesigned and refurnished with the goal of eliminating "the hospital look." The staff shares its knowledge and duties with the parents, according to the complexity and seriousness of the child's case and his parents' ability to understand and perform necessary tasks. Parents have learned to help, even with serious conditions. This ward, begun on an experimental basis, has more than proved its worth; it has eliminated the chief fear children have about going to the hospital—the anxiety about being separated from their parents. It has also helped to prepare parents naturally and effectively for the home care necessary after the children are discharged. Noting the program's success, other hospitals are creating similar units. (20)

Parent Support Groups

Hospitals have begun to change drastically—to treat the total child rather than just his disease, and organizations have been formed to encourage these changes. Twenty years ago N.A.W.C.H. (National Association for the Welfare of Children in Hospitals), began working in London to implement a government report which officially recommended open visiting by parents. With reinforcement from the organization and its thousands of members, mothers and fathers find the problems of staying with the hospitalized child considerably lessened in most hospitals in England. (21)

There are several active organizations in the United States. One of the most vocal and successful is the Massachusetts C.I.H. (Children in Hospitals). Lay and professional people have been working together to avoid separation of parent and hospitalized child and have met with considerable success and cooperation from hospitals in the Boston area.

Another organization, Parents Concerned for Hospitalized Children, states in its brochure that "One of our major goals is to help parents to develop a greater understanding of the needs of hospitalized children, the reactions of the child and his family to the hospital situation and ways in which parents can help make the hospital stay a more positive, less traumatic experience for child and family."

See Appendix: Organizations to Help the Nursing Mother, for information on how to contact these organizations as well as groups dealing with specific situations such as cystic fibrosis, prematurity, or cleft palate.

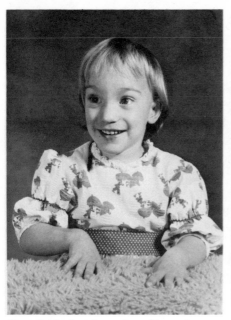

Mari Kay's daughter, Amanda, at 3 years of age.

"Mandy was born nearly 3 months early and she survived! She weighed just 1 pound, 12 ounces at birth and measured 13 inches. Expressing milk gave me something to do to help Mandy, making me feel less helpless. When she was 2 months old, she reached 3 pounds and she actually started nursing."

Mari Kay
(Nursing a Premature Baby,
Chapter 6)

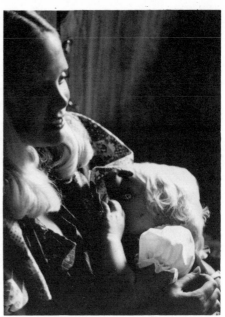

Anne Chapman Tullar

Vicki nursing Danika, while pregnant.

"At times I get irritated by the nursing, but I think it's part of being pregnant and tending to want to wean more at this time than I would normally. Most of the time we both enjoy our nursings."

Vicki
(Nursing While Pregnant,
Chapter 16)

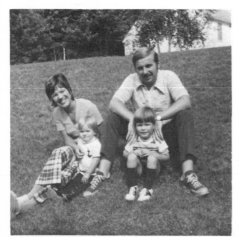

Wendy and Richard with their 2 children, Stacy and Michael.

"When I was to be hospitalized for 3 days to have a benign tumor removed, I was determined to take Stacy to the hospital with me. It took 2 hours of arguing and waiting, presenting my case to 4 or 5 people, but it was worth it because we finally got the okay."

Wendy
(Working Together,
Chapter 14)

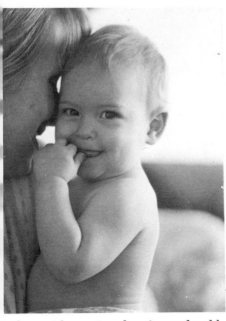

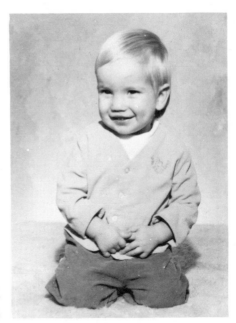

Alice, with son Brendon, 9 months old.

Pat's son, Joey, 2 years old.

"We have a family with genetic allergic tendencies. Jody, my first son, developed an allergy to cow's milk during a hospitalization at 3 weeks. He was fed formula despite my efforts to avoid it. His rashes and loose bowel movements disappeared after we resumed breast-feeding. Brendon, my younger son, has never had formula and has been practically free of the problems that Jody had."

Alice

"At 10 months of age, Joey required skull surgery. The surgeon took it for granted that I would not be staying with our son in the hospital, but I found that once the doctors and staff understood my desire to nurse, they cooperated. I have learned that if you explain the reason behind why you believe something, you may get more cooperation."

Pat
(When Baby Is Sick or
Hospitalized, Chapter 12)

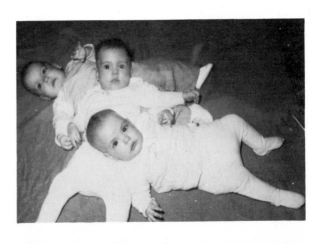

Shirley's 6-month-old nursing triplets, Jacky, Madye and Danny.

"When an X-ray showed triplets were expected, the doctor asked, 'How do you expect to breastfeed 3 babies with only 2 breasts?' I replied, 'One at a time!'"

Shirley
(Nursing Twins,
Chapter 18)

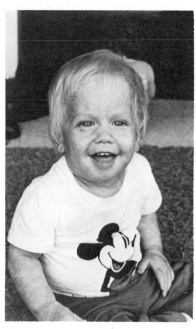

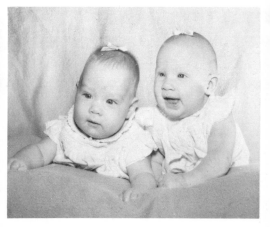

Author's twins, Karen (left), and Sharon, 4½ months old.

"With my twins, I found it's fun to cuddle and nurse 2 babies together. Neither had received anything but breast milk when this picture was taken."

Pat Brewster
(Nursing Twins, Chapter 18)

Anne Chapman Tullar

Laurie's son, Jake, 13 months old.

"Jake suffers from a congenital skin disease. I wasn't allowed to touch him for 7 days after birth, due to the danger of his developing an infection. Using a breast pump was tremendously important. I was able to provide him with my milk, and in effect breastfeed him, even though we were separated."

Laurie
(Newborn and Infant Problems, Chapter 7)

Neva's son, Jarret, at 2½ months of age.

"Jarret was 2 months premature and weighed 3 pounds, 5 ounces at birth. He was fed by tube for 22 days, then by bottle. We were finally allowed to try nursing when he was 27 days old. Now at 5 months, he is a happy, healthy, totally breastfed baby, and has more than tripled his weight since birth."

Neva
(Nursing a Premature Baby, Chapter 6)

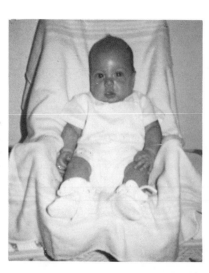

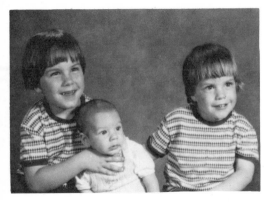

Paula's trio, left to right: Robb (5 years old), Michael (3 months old), Bradd (3 years old).

"Bradd has some special speech and perceptual problems. For a long time, nursing was our only form of communication. At 2½ years, he began to speak, and his first word was 'num'—the word I had repeated every time he wanted to nurse!"

Paula

Marti's 7-month-old son, Andy.

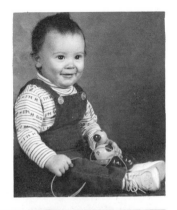

"Andy has PKU, an inherited disorder, affecting protein metabolism. We are very pleased with his progress and his physician's approach to the diet management, where as much breastfeeding as possible is allowed. We feel this approach is responsive to his needs as an individual and our needs as a family. This has enhanced our enjoyment of our special baby."

Marti
(Problems Related to Baby's
Altered Body Chemistry,
Chapter 9)

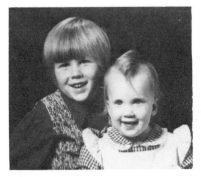

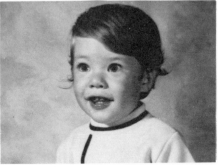

Jenny's son Bob (3½ years) with sister Renée (1 year).

"Renée has cystic fibrosis. It took us about 2 months to realize that while Renée needs special help, Bob must be included in our love and attention."

Jenny
(Problems Related to Baby's
Altered Body Chemistry,
Chapter 9)

Jeri's son, David, 1 year old.

"David was an unhappy baby who cried constantly except when nursing. He rebelled against being held, yet he desperately needed the tactile stimulation. It wasn't until he was 4 years old that he finally was diagnosed as having minimal brain dysfunction with some hyperactivity."

Jeri
(Nursing a Baby with Special
Developmental Conditions,
Chapter 10)

Chapter 15

Inducing or Reestablishing Your Milk Supply: For Natural Born or Adopted Baby

If you or your nursing baby has been hospitalized and your milk supply is low, can you build it up again? If you have taken "dry-up" medication or have never nursed your baby, but are having trouble finding a formula he can tolerate, can you still start to nurse now? If you have an adopted or a foster baby, can you nurse him?

Many mothers *have* nursed their babies under such circumstances. Situations like these are discussed in this chapter, along with questions such as: Does it matter how old the baby is? What problems might you expect? What techniques are helpful? How much milk might you expect? What are the reasons why mothers do this?

Keep in mind that no nursing couple is exactly like any other. Babies react differently, and what "works" with one baby will not necessarily produce the same result with another—even if they have the same mother. The information and examples in this chapter are meant as a guide to give you ideas for finding a satisfactory approach to your own situation.

What Is Meant by Inducing and Reestablishing?

Lactation is the secretion of milk by the breasts; inducing lactation means initiating milk production (which is then increased and established) in a woman who has not recently given birth, or perhaps has never been pregnant.

The reestablishment of milk production after an interruption in lactation is called relactation. It can mean beginning again after a complete break in breastfeeding or after a separation of mother and baby. It can also describe induced lactation by a woman who nursed previously, even if it was several years earlier. Sometimes the term is mistakenly applied to women who've never nursed, thus being used interchangeably with induced lactation.

Clinical Obstetrics and Gynecology (1) offers this description of human and other mammalian lactation which differ from the usual procedure:

> The paramount importance of sucking stimulation is shown by the fact that lactation can be initiated by this alone. Selye and McKeown demonstrated this in both rats and mice. They allowed litters to suck females who were not their mothers and who had not recently been pregnant. First, the milk glands enlarged as they do in pregnancy. Then the foster mothers started to produce milk. The litters began to grow as well as if they had their own mothers.
>
> There are ample and well-documented reports that this phenomenon also occurs in women. Mead described the Mundugumor tribe in New Guinea, who customarily gave away one of each set of twins. The foster mother put the adopted baby constantly to her breast, and within a few weeks she had a good supply of milk. Similar examples have been reported from Asia, Africa and Europe, where women who have not been pregnant for years have adopted and suckled babies successfully. Even today in remote rural areas of the United States, this phenomenon is not unknown. Recently we received a well-documented report of a 60-year-old Mississippi grandmother who decided to adopt and nurse her grandchild when her daughter died. The milk appeared as expected, and the child was breastfed until he was able to walk.

Why Is Lactation Induced or Reestablished?

Mothers induce lactation to feed their children human milk. For all human babies, human milk is the species-specific food just as cow's milk is species-specific for calves.

Adoptive mothers, foster mothers, even grandmothers, aunts or friends may induce lactation to feed babies in their care, in order to provide the nutritional and emotional benefits of breastfeeding. It is especially beneficial for allergic or ill babies who sometimes cannot thrive, or even survive, on substitutes.

One allergic baby, David, could not tolerate formula and went through 15 formula changes before he began nursing. His mother Jean Ann describes the situation:

> When we brought David home from the hospital on Friday he had a slight rash. I thought it was just a redhead's skin rash. By Monday we had decided he was allergic to his formula. The doctor ordered a formula change, but the new formula didn't agree with David. We kept changing formulas, but each change of formula only resulted in a change of reaction, ranging from blood clots in his bowel movements to hives, open sores at his waist, and vomiting. I considered nursing, but the pediatrician said no— "David's problem is digestive." Formula changes and bottle changes continued. In all, David's formula was changed 15 times, using 11 formulas and repeating 4.
>
> When David was almost three months old, in desperation I called La Leche League, to ask if I could buy breast milk. They told me I couldn't buy it, but that I could bring in my own milk.
>
> Several women were willing to nurse David and express milk for him, while I worked to bring in my own milk by hand expressing. The breast milk stayed in his stomach—no vomiting—and the sores went away. However, I found hand expression a very slow, drop-by-drop process. I tripled my fluid intake, and hand expressed at least once an hour from 6:00 A.M. to midnight. After three weeks I could express three ounces a day. But I lacked the stimulation of my baby's sucking. He'd nurse from any woman with a plentiful milk supply, but never from me. We tried everything. I put honey on the nipple so he would suck, and he'd lick it off. At one point I nursed one woman's baby who was younger than David, and she

nursed mine. We took David's pacifier away. Finally, when he was about 4 months old, he decided I had milk and began nursing. He weaned at 22 months, having mostly outgrown his allergies by then.

Jean Ann is one of countless mothers who have nursed adopted and foster babies and babies they had weaned and ones they hadn't planned to nurse at all. Throughout the world, throughout history, the law of demand has created the supply which has satisfied babies and the women who nursed them.

Techniques for Inducing Lactation

Nursing your baby is the best stimulus for lactation. Other techniques are suckling by another baby, electric and mechanical breast pumps, breast massage, and hand expression. Back rubs are helpful, too.

Your intense desire to nurse your baby can be as important as nipple stimulation in initiating milk production. Some chemicals and drugs have been used and will be described later. Good nutrition and rest are also significant.

First, Prepare Your Mind

Consider why you are inducing lactation. If you're relactating to give essential nourishment to an allergic or sick baby you probably have little uncertainty about your motives, but you may have doubts about your ability to produce milk. You can be comforted by the knowledge that mothers with desperately ill babies seem to have the best success in induced lactation. If your milk supply still needs to be supplemented, there's human milk available from milk banks or donors.

If you are planning to nurse an adopted or foster baby, do stop to think through what you are expecting from the experience. It is helpful to prepare yourself emotionally as well as physically.

While no adoptive nursing mother would ever suggest that another woman lightly undertake adoptive nursing, it's not inappropriate to do it on a tentative basis. Some adopted babies are "lazy nursers" and are uncooperative about learning to breastfeed. If totally breastfeeding your baby doesn't work out, breastfeeding with supplemental feeding may be an alternative.

Nipple Preparation

Your nipples will probably be getting unaccustomed stimulation from the extensive breastfeeding time needed to initiate and build up a milk supply. To prevent soreness, the nipples can be introduced to stimulation gradually. Advice on nipple preparation is found in chapter 1, "What's Normal?" Be sure to read this to prepare yourself as much as possible. However, one adoptive mother reports, "My nipples were really sore for the first two months of nursing, even though I had done months of nipple preparation before my son arrived."

Nursing Time with Your Baby (or Another)

If you're trying to increase your milk for your natural born* baby who's ill or if you've been ill and separated from him, try to spend as much time together as possible. If you're home, let your family and friends tend to your other responsibilities while you concentrate on mothering and nursing. No one else can do that for you.

If your baby is hospitalized, you may have to assert your legal right to be with your minor dependent at all times. You'll find that while hospital staff may tell you to leave, they won't force you if you're calm and polite, but insistent. They know (but don't tell you) that if they try to remove you bodily they are liable to charges of assault. Being with your baby is a comfort to both of you; mere hospital routine should not separate a nursing mother and child.

Try to get an early start when establishing a nursing relationship with an adopted baby. Encourage the agency to

---

* "Natural born" is being used to distinguish from adopted.

arrange early placement, and if possible, arrange to nurse the newborn baby. Visit and nurse the baby in the foster home before placement with you. Perhaps your home can be the foster home. Basically, your goal is to get together with your baby as soon as possible and begin breastfeeding and mothering.

If you have a toddler who is currently nursing, he can help you prepare for your adopted baby by keeping up your milk supply and keeping your nipples toughened.

How do you go about preparing by nursing another baby? Regina Carlson, in an article in *Redbook* magazine (2) said:

> In order to prepare for nursing my adopted child, I sought out mothers who had babies they would let me nurse.
>
> It is hardly something one does through the Yellow Pages. The sources I tried were La Leche League, pediatricians who had a breastfed clientele, local childbirth instructors who might have new mothers in the area, and friends of friends. This searching produced a few names, so I screwed up my courage and called some women, explained my situation and asked if they'd let me nurse their babies.
>
> My first several contacts refused my request, but luckily the next three mothers I called said yes. They were enthusiastic about my plans, happy for a little relief for their tender nipples and willing to share their babies with me.
>
> Washing my hands and my breasts before each nursing was the only precaution suggested by La Leche League to protect the babies, and I adhered to that advice. The week's intensive nursing increased my milk supply appreciably.

Tandem nursing with another nursing couple could work for you, once your baby is home. (Tandem nursing is nursing more than one baby or child at a time. It can be twins, triplets, infant and older sibling or your own baby and another baby.) In tandem nursing for relactation purposes, you and another mother (who has a well-established milk supply) nurse each other's babies. Your baby nurses as much as he will from you, and also nurses from the other mother. This way, he is getting supplemental milk and the idea that milk can be obtained from nursing. And hopefully, the other mother's baby will be happy to nurse from you "just for fun," thereby giving you necessary stimulation.

Switching babies should never be done casually, since problems may arise. Infections can be passed from baby to baby via a mother's breast. Also, a baby may become confused by the situation.

La Leche League cautions that if you do nurse another mother's baby you should wash your hands with soap and water. Your breasts need to be washed between nursings of different babies, but avoid soap on the nipples since this is drying and encourages cracked nipples.

Besides suckling a baby, there are other methods to stimulate your breasts. You can perform hand expression by first massaging your breasts, then squeezing gently with your fingers and thumb on opposite sides of the breasts. (See chapter 2, "Nursing Techniques," for further description and pictures of breast massage and hand expression.) One mother described a locomotivelike rotation of her arms which she found fruitful. Begin by placing your hands on your shoulders (right hand on right shoulder, left hand on left shoulder), then rotate your arms forward, down, and upward, rubbing against the outer surface of the breasts. This massage may be done prior to expressing. If you feel you need further instruction in hand expressing, ask an experienced friend or a La Leche League leader. You may not express any visible fluids at first. Keep trying.

Electric breast pumps can be helpful and often can be rented through a La Leche League group or a supplier. You can also try a mechanical-suction pump. There are simple rubber bulb pumps available at low cost in drugstores. (For further discussion of breast pumps, see chapter 2, "Nursing Techniques.")

Back rubs between the shoulder blades (where nerves to the breast tissue radiate) can increase circulation to the breast to ease expressing, according to Elizabeth Hormann, author of

"Relactation: A Guide to Breastfeeding the Adopted Baby." (3)

How often you follow these suggestions depends on you. You can base your decision on how your body is responding and when you expect your baby. One approach is to get a good head start, then aim at maintaining a consistent program. But time spent in preparation can become burdensome if you're waiting for a baby who doesn't seem to be coming. To simulate a nursing schedule, you would "nurse" (whatever equivalent or approximation you settle on) three to five minutes at each breast every couple of hours. Set up regular, convenient intervals for preparation. For instance, every time you go to the bathroom, take three to five minutes for routine preparation. It might help to wear nursing clothes during this preparation period. Otherwise, the inconvenience of baring the breast may cause preparations to be skipped.

On the other hand, some mothers have begun induced lactation "cold turkey" when presented with a baby. They have had various degrees of success.

Can a Mother Nurse Who Has Never Been Pregnant?

This is a different situation in which to induce lactation. Childbirth (or miscarriage) triggers milk production, and even mothers who have not nursed for months (or years) can often produce a drop if they try. However, if you have never been pregnant, you don't have this advantage of having even a drop of milk from which to start building your supply. But if you have a cooperative baby, it *can* be done. It may take several months to build an adequate milk supply, and maybe you will never have a *full* supply. Yet even if you do not completely breastfeed, you can still have a complete nursing relationship.

A suckling baby at your breast and a strong desire to breastfeed can produce lactation outside of the normal course of pregnancy and nursing. Both baby and desire trigger the production of the hormone prolactin, which stimulates milk production.

345

Charmaine had never been pregnant when she adopted her baby. She says:

> I used hand expression, a hand breast pump, an electric breast pump, and nursing of other infants in order to prepare myself for nursing our adopted baby.
>
> The first technique I tried was hand expression. After my first few attempts at this I found, to my surprise, that I was experiencing uterine contractions concurrently with these exercises. Then my breasts became firmer and increased one cup size.
>
> About three months later I had the opportunity to nurse several babies, ranging in age from two weeks to six months. Some seemed content just to suck without getting any milk. Others would have nothing to do with such an arrangement.
>
> Several months after I started hand expression I began using a hand breast pump, and that was when I found I was able to extract sizable drops of a yellowish fluid . . . colostrum? We eventually rented an electric breast pump to further stimulate my breasts.
>
> Our daughter Sandra was released to us when she was 3½ weeks old. From my first attempt at breastfeeding, she proved to be a very active nurser.
>
> In order for Sandra to associate suckling not only with pacification but also with a source of food, I tried several things. First, a friend with a newborn baby volunteered to breastfeed Sandra once daily so she would be encouraged to nurse when she become hungry. I also experimented with various formula strengths (ratio of formula to water), but found the technique of allowing her to nurse part way through her feeding with no supplementation, then adding formula for the rest of the session to work the best.*
>
> The true double-feeding technique I practiced during the first few weeks (a total separation of breast- versus

---

* Diluting formula must be done only under a doctor's supervision. An infant might lose too much weight with this method.

bottlefeeding) caused Sandra to separate the source of readily available food (bottle) and the source of slower arriving food (breast). The natural result was that she began to equate the bottle with food and the breast with pacification. About that time another mother who nursed an adopted infant sent us a valuable suggestion to associate suckling with both pacification and a source of food. Lady Clairol has five-ounce tint and toner bottles with long, hard plastic tips, which are sold empty in most dime stores or beauty supply stores. Use new ones, of course. The tip can be inserted into the corner of the infant's mouth while nursing, thus dispensing breast milk or formula. This proved to be a fairly easy method of dual-feeding, allowing for my control as well as the infant's control, since the tip and bottle could be removed and replaced easily. It was a long time before the baby realized some of the food came from the black tip.*

Arranging to Nurse Another Baby

How do you ask to nurse someone else's baby, if one is not "volunteered"? If you're talking with a nursing friend or relative about the baby you're expecting to adopt, for example, you might weave into your conversation some comments about how mothers' milk has been used for other babies in the past, and mothers have nursed babies who were not their own. There are examples in this chapter you can describe, and there is an interesting section in Karen Pryor's book, *Nursing Your Baby* (4), under the section "Wet Nurses and Milk Banks."

It might take two or three conversations to reach the point where you decide your friend is ready to be asked. Or, she may offer on her own. Once you have asked and your friend is agreeable, you can then discuss the arrangements of when and where you will nurse her child. If you can, try to duplicate a nursing schedule.

---

* Whenever a device is used to feed extra milk to a baby, care must be exercised so that the flow is not too fast for the baby to handle comfortably, without tongue thrust or choking.

On the other hand, if your friend is at all hesitant, you can offer to lend her a book or pamphlet, and say you'd be interested in hearing what she thinks about it. Then, hopefully, your next conversation will lead to your friend's agreeing to let you nurse her baby.

Changes You Might Notice in Your Body

Some women inducing lactation report an increase in breast size or greater firmness. Your appetite may increase. Uterine contractions and a milk let-down (tingling feeling which normally signals the release of milk) are other changes experienced. Some women have diminished menses. However, if your menstrual periods stop, do check with your doctor; you may need a pregnancy test.

You may experience sexual arousal or pleasure from some preparation activities just as some nursing mothers do. You may observe pleasurable response in the baby you're suckling, including erection of the penis in male babies. It is a natural part of nursing.

How Long before Your Milk Comes In?

Expressing several times a day may produce anything from drops to several streams within one to six weeks.

Alice's natural born son, Cameron, at three months was being fed intravenously, because he was unable to tolerate any kind of formula. Human milk was suggested, and after three days of receiving donated breast milk, he was well on the road to recovery. A La Leche League leader helped Alice bring in her own milk, and other mothers furnished supplemental breast milk temporarily. In two months Alice was completely breastfeeding Cameron, and he was totally breastfed until he was able to start solids at about nine months.

Claire was nursing her 17-month-old about once a week

when she received news to expect their newly adopted daughter from Korea in a month. Claire pumped five minutes on each breast four times a day the first week, eight times the second week, hourly during the next ten days and then five minutes each breast every two hours around the clock the last three days. When her four-month-old arrived there was plenty of milk.

Fern, after giving birth to twin premies, and losing one, was given "dry-up" pills. However, through La Leche League she learned she could still attempt nursing. When her baby was almost two months old, she began by using an electric breast pump. The first day she obtained 6 cc's (30 cc's equal one ounce), and in a few days she was increasing by an ounce a day. The baby was small and colicky and Fern wondered if she had enough milk. It took a while for her to realize that she actually had more than enough milk!

Karen nursed two adopted babies simultaneously. They were both older than the babies usually seen in cases of successful relactation. Brian was 5½ months old when he was adopted, and it had been three months since Karen had nursed her 2½-year-old son. The first day Karen had one "bead" of milk on the left side, none on the right side. Karen used the Lact-Aid supplementer to give Brian extra milk, while maintaining the nursing relationship. She expressed milk after and between feedings. She also tried diluting the supplemental milk. After two months she was able to produce about one-third to one-half the milk that Brian needed. When he was 12½ months old (and still nursing, with the help of the Lact-Aid), the family adopted a daughter, Shannon, 3½ months old. Karen continued nursing with the supplementer for several months and eventually was able to nurse both babies naturally. Brian weaned at 34 months. Shannon was still nursing at 27 months.

How long will it take for your milk to come in? As these examples indicate, it varies greatly, depending on the circumstance, the mothers, and the babies. You can gauge your progress if you see droplets, then dribbles, then streams of whitish liquid.

If No Visible Milk Appears

Suppose you're doing all the right things on a regular basis and there is still no milk to show for it. That may mean you'll just have a longer wait. You might want to check your techniques with an experienced person. Remember that while visible milk production is a sign of success, lack of expressed milk does not necessarily signal failure.

Also, you may not let down as easily to anything other than a baby in your arms, nuzzling at your breast. Niles Newton has demonstrated that most nursing women in normal situations who don't secrete enough milk to entirely feed their babies, have trouble not with milk production, but with milk ejection. Through the use of the drug oxytocin, these women let down enough milk. (5) Oxytocin is available as a nasal spray or in tablet form. If you'd like to try it, check with your physician. One mother used it but reported she was soon conditioned and only had to reach for the bottle to stimulate her let-down reflex.

Various tranquilizers, taken in large doses, seem to stimulate milk production. Some women, working with their doctors, have tried to simulate pregnancy with birth control pills. However, neither drug is necessary, nor does either guarantee success and both are potentially dangerous. So why not do it the natural way?

Some women have conditioned themselves to let down with a warm, wet cloth on their breasts, a glass of wine, a drink of water before each pumping, a back rub, or nipple stimulation. See also How to Insure a Good Milk Supply in chapter 2, "Nursing Techniques."

Your Diet

Lactating women have high nutritional and caloric needs. You need fluid, protein and B vitamins to produce milk. Milk is a good source of all of these but you don't need to drink milk *as such* to produce milk, as long as your nutritional requirements are met in other ways.

Surprising numbers of people don't drink milk and yet thrive. Many people don't tolerate it well, especially people of Negro or Asian descent. If you are black or Asian (or the baby you're nursing is), you will want to keep this in mind regarding milk.

A good rule, while you're concentrating on relactating, is to enjoy a glass of some form of liquid with each pumping or nursing. Psychologically it says, "I'm drinking so much that I must be making milk."

Most mothers notice or report no problem foods. Most foods in moderation are fine.

Important People in Your Life

An admiring, supportive husband is your best asset in relactation. Ideally, his love for you and the baby will mean he will do everything he can to help. Your own thoughtfulness will lead you to be specific in your requests or directions as well as understanding his limits in helping.

A husband totally opposed to breastfeeding may be a good reason to choose another feeding method. However, you may feel so strongly about your baby's need for mother's milk that this is not possible for you. Talk with other nursing mothers, to see how they have handled "touchy" situations where there is a difference of opinion. A La Leche League leader may be able to put you in touch with another mother or two.

Your doctor may be familiar only with lactation following birth. If you're trying to reinitiate lactation after you and your baby have been separated, he may not be aware of good management techniques. If you're planning to nurse an adopted or foster baby, your physician may be in totally new territory, so it's especially important for you to be informed. Then you can share your desires and information with him and ask for medical guidance. Remember: a physician is supposed to be a trained counselor whose job is to inform you so you can decide what *you* want to do.

Some mothers have been able to educate doctors who

were at first skeptical so that they became supportive and eventually, even enthusiastic.

A mother who miscarried at four months reports her doctor encouraged her to pump her milk, which came in three days later, to freeze for use with premature infants. That way she kept her milk supply in and nursed an adopted baby for a year.

The best advice may be to find a supportive doctor before, not after, your baby is born.

The reaction of relatives and friends will be as varied as they are, but expect a high level of skepticism. Trying to explain about nursing your baby to some people is like trying to explain the joys of parenthood to confirmed childless people.

Ongoing support from one other person can mean a great deal. Probably the people who will be the most enthusiastic, understanding, and appreciative of your efforts are those who've done it and know how nice nursing is.

Your Chances of Success

La Leche League's medical advisors maintain that fully 90 percent of all women can produce milk if they want to, even without having been pregnant. However, they caution that some mothers have been very successful in nursing one adopted baby, but have been less successful in nursing another adopted one.

No nursing couple is like any other. Factors that influence success are: prior history of lactation and mothering; physical well-being; emotional climate; age of baby; and willingness of baby to nurse. None of these seem to guarantee or forestall success.

How much of your baby's need for milk might you expect to supply? It varies, from about 25 to 100 percent. Usually, the younger the baby, the better. If you've miscarried or delivered within the last three months, even if you haven't been nursing, you have an advantage. Mothers of severely ill infants generally manage to produce 75 to 100 percent of the milk needed. However, there is really no way of predicting milk production since babies and mothers and situations vary greatly. How long can you expect production of a full milk supply to take? Elizabeth Hormann reports some adoptive mothers attain full supplies within three months; some take eight months.

How Much Milk Does a Baby Need?

All the foregoing information has been directed primarily at you as the nursing mother. But a good provider needs a good consumer. Ideally, baby will nurse happily every 1½ or 2 hours, for five minutes or so per breast (if your nipples are up to it). While your milk supply is still growing, he will be "topped off" with breast milk which you have expressed (or which has been donated), formula or solids.

Generally, the younger the baby, the better induced lactation will proceed. A baby who is a premie needs less milk and inducing lactation may be easier. But then again a premie may not be robust yet or developed enough to nurse well.

Very young infants usually need close to 2½ ounces per pound of body weight every 24 hours. Thus, a one-month-old, seven-pound baby needs about 17 ounces of milk a day, slightly more in very hot weather. The amount needed gradually decreases to about 2 ounces per pound by six months and continues decreasing after that. The addition of solid foods further decreases the amount of milk needed.

Supplemental Food

Basically, you want to nurse your baby and then give him enough supplemental food to tide him over comfortably for a couple of hours. Don't overfeed him because he may not be hungry again for three or four hours, and you won't get the frequent stimulation needed to increase your milk. Be sure to feed him only enough to take care of his hunger;

some babies will eat anything offered, whether they need it or not.

Some babies will resist nursing at first from a mother with little milk. If so, you might try some supplement to satisfy your baby's initial intense hunger, then try nursing. As you nurse, switch from one breast to the other several times. This provides more stimulation for your breasts and more milk for baby. Then, if necessary, finish off the feeding with some more supplement.

Reluctant Nursers

Sucking at a breast not freely flowing with milk can make some babies wonder if it's worth the bother, even though other babies think it's lots of fun. Mothers coax babies to nurse from a dry breast by various methods. Here are some of their suggestions:

Start to nurse before the baby is extremely hungry.

Initiate nursing by picking the baby up while he's still sleeping and putting him to your breast.

Walk the baby while nursing.

Express dribbles of breast milk into his mouth.

Put drops of formula on the nipple.

Slip some formula into the corner of baby's mouth with an eyedropper or small spoon.

Put a drop of honey on the nipple.

Use a nursing supplementer device (see Lact-Aid, later in this chapter).

If your baby is fussing a lot and doesn't seem to want to nurse, maybe it's not your milk supply that is the problem. Jean Ann discovered while she was relactating to nurse five-month-old David that his painful crying and irritation were due to a urinary tract infection.

On the other hand, your child's illness may make him more willing to nurse. Lena says:

> Kimberly was 9 months old and had almost weaned when the doctor diagnosed an allergy to cow's milk and recommended she be put back on breast milk if at all possible. Kimberly wasn't too interested in nursing until she became ill with an ear infection. She was miserable, and she nursed frequently, increasing my milk supply. Then at 10½ months Kimberly had the flu and couldn't keep anything down but breast milk, so she started nursing again. After the flu was over, Kimberly continued nursing and I was able to nurse her three times a day until I became pregnant.

Trying to nurse a baby who balks, worrying about him and your milk supply, coping with tender nipples, to say nothing of having to neglect everything else in your life for a while can be overwhelming, discouraging and frustrating. Dale describes her situation with her adopted baby:

> Relactation had become an all-consuming activity. I was literally feeding her nearly all of her waking hours. There were many times when my daughter's fussiness and frustrations made me wonder if I was really doing the best thing for her. When my nipples were incredibly sore and bleeding, knowing I had to feed her again in just 15 or 20 minutes, I wondered what it was doing for me. And when my husband's whole view of life at home was extra chores and the back of his baby's head, he began to wonder, too. But our pediatrician's encouragement spurred us on. He was willing to try all sorts of options. Following his directions, we diluted her bottles and gave them only when her diapers seemed dry for a long time. Cereal and fruit provided her with some nutrition not requiring sucking, so we could save the sucking for nursing. I also expressed milk, used a breast pump, had 12 brewer's yeast tablets every day and so many fluids I thought I would burst. Eventually, we were nursing completely, without any bottles!

If you're in a nursing situation of choice (foster or adopted baby who can tolerate formula or relactating to nurse your natural born child for nonmedical reasons), the roughest times will probably prompt you to reconsider how much this matters to you, your nursing baby, and your family.

If you're in a situation of necessity, such as relactating to feed your baby who is allergic, remember that in such cases the success rate is the highest.

Reducing Supplement

There can be signs in mother and baby which indicate that supplement can be reduced. You may see signs of increased milk production in yourself: spurts can be expressed, your breasts may feel full; you may feel a milk let-down; you may leak between feedings. Baby may show these signs: greater satisfaction at the breast; milk running around the corner of his mouth; longer periods between feedings; not needing as much supplement after nursing; gulping sounds.

One way to reduce supplement is to cut the amount offered by ½ ounce or 1 ounce. If baby was taking seven daily feedings of 2½ ounces, for example, offer 2 ounces at each of the seven feedings. The baby may want to nurse again sooner. If your baby can go at least an hour and a half between nursings, you are probably doing fine (that's an hour and a half from the beginning of one feeding to the *beginning* of the next). When baby shows signs of being satisfied, you may want to again reduce the amount of supplement.

Of course, progress may not be orderly. You may find the baby needs more food in the evenings when you're tired or not letting down as well. Or you may have a bad day. This is normal.

Diluting formula is another way to reduce supplement, although this method is seriously questioned by some authorities. It should be attempted only under a doctor's supervision since formula which is too dilute can mask a baby's hunger and result in starvation. Some mothers have diluted formula with a half ounce of water, rather than reduce the formula by half an ounce. The baby may not quite finish all the formula-plus-water offered, but is left feeling immediately full despite the decreased feeding. He will then want to nurse sooner and this in turn will stimulate your supply. If he doesn't want to nurse sooner, then he probably didn't need that half ounce. You may then want to check with your doctor about offering slightly less formula at the feedings.

Make Sure Baby Gets Enough Food

This is crucial, especially since a baby in an induced lactation situation may already be ill or in a weakened condition when you get him. How can you tell if your baby is getting enough food? He should be producing six or more wet diapers a day, sleeping comfortably between feedings, gaining well, and should be alert and generally happy when awake.

Watch the baby's skin. It should not become slack and doughy in consistency. This can be an early sign of dehydration. Consult your doctor on what to watch for. Basically you are in a special situation, and special caution is appropriate.

A baby should not be kept hungry to encourage nursing. Your purpose is to feed the baby, not to starve him. Keeping a baby hungry is counterproductive because once a baby gradually slips into dehydration or starvation, he nurses less effectively.

A normal breastfed baby produces a yellow green, soft stool. Formula-fed babies eliminate darker, more formed, adultlike feces, which are smellier. If you're supplementing with formula (rather than human milk), the baby's bowel movements will tell you whether he's receiving mostly formula or mostly breast milk. Solid foods will also affect the appearance of the bowel movements; they will be more formed, and may vary in color according to what your baby has eaten.

Delivering Supplement

Parents have used eyedroppers at the corner of the nursing baby's mouth, spoons, small cups, even turkey basters extended with cocktail straws to give supplement. Some mothers, like Charmaine, have even resorted to Lady Clairol bottles (see section, Can a Mother Nurse Who Has Never Been Pregnant? in this chapter).

These unusual methods were used to prevent getting the baby accustomed to a bottle and nipple, which requires a different action than nursing; while much easier to suck, bottle and nipple tend to discourage nursing.

But your baby may already be a "bottle-addict." Here's Harriet's experience trying to relactate for her allergic, natural born baby Vicki, then 15 weeks old:

> We started our project realizing that we had a "bottle-hooked" baby, and we would have to "wean" her from the bottle to the breast. At first, we were so anxious to have Vicki totally breastfed that after a three-week period, we were all very discouraged when she was still taking bottles. We contemplated throwing them all away. Then a La Leche League Area Coordinator reminded us that weaning is a process that often takes years—yet we were trying to rush it into a three-week period! With that in mind, we successfully accomplished our project with more patience and understanding.

If you're going to supplement by bottle, a conservative approach would be to use the Nuk orthodontic nipple or a blind (holeless) nipple in which you make your own very small hole. Hold baby against your bare breast with the bottle nipple near your nipple so he has to turn to the breast to feed; this helps maintain his rooting response better than feeding him facing out at the world.

Supplementing at the Breast: The Lact-Aid

The Lact-Aid* consists of a presterilized plastic bag to hold

---

* For more information, see address listed in Appendix.

supplemental formula or breast milk, and a length of tubing which carries the supplement to the baby's mouth. The baby suckles both the mother's nipple and the tip of the tube at the same time. In this way, a baby is encouraged to nurse from a dry breast and the sucking stimulation can help increase the mother's milk supply.

Milk Banks and Donor Milk

Human milk banks generally make milk available on doctor's prescription only, reserving it for babies with a medical need. If you're failing to produce an adequate milk supply for your baby who must have human milk, investigate these banks. For additional information, see Milk Banks in chapter 2, "Nursing Techniques." A list of milk banks may be found in Appendix: Organizations to Help the Nursing Mother.

Donor milk from mothers in your area may be available informally or through La Leche League. La Leche League has a policy of only "formally" providing milk for three weeks, although in cases where a mother is trying hard to relactate and the baby is desperately in need, La Leche League mothers sometimes donate milk for a longer period of time. It is not fair to impose on other nursing mothers for an extended period unless the mother receiving the donated milk is willing to relactate. When such milk is donated, it is up to the family receiving it to collect the milk unless someone else volunteers.

Unconventional Supplements

If you're a breastfeeding mother who is not lucky enough to be getting human milk for supplementing, you needn't regard commercial cow's milk formulas as the only other alternative. There are, of course, commercial formulas based on meats or soybeans. And there are also goat's milk and yogurt made from goat's milk.

Working with a pediatrician or nutritionist, some parents have devised special nutritious formulas as supplements for their babies.

Solid foods might be an appropriate supplement, although they are unnecessary and discouraged for normal nursing babies for the first half year. If you adopt a baby who is already used to them, you may want to continue the solids as a supplement as well as to maintain a familiar routine.

If Your Baby's Mother Was a Drug Addict

Babies born of mothers on potent drugs can have serious problems. Try to get all the information you can about the mother's drug habits so you and your physician can nurse the baby along. Anna, a foster mother, tells of one baby she cared for whose situation was relatively mild:

> Mark hated to be awake and needed lots of close body contact, nursing, pacifiers, baby carriers, stroking, rocking, and nights in our bed to make life bearable. Eventually, we discovered he was having withdrawal symptoms from a drug his mother had been using. One day he woke up smiling and all was well. Within two more weeks he was much more content, and at three months went off to a new home, happy with the world.

If you encounter such a problem, get the best medical advice you can. Seek physicians who work with drug-addicted pregnant women or medical advisors working for an adoption or foster placement agency.

Special Considerations in Adoption

Uncooperative adoption agencies can sabotage adoptive nursing by placing an older baby, or refusing placement when they hear about a mother's plans for adoptive nursing. You'll have to play it by ear about letting the agency in on your plans, balancing their potential to help you against their power to undermine you.

You're not a freak. You only want your child to have the

same gift nature intended for *all* children. Your job, if you reveal your plans, is to convince the agency that the baby's welfare is more important to you than success in a breast-feeding experiment. If the baby needs human milk for medical reasons, of course they'll be on your side. Or, you might make a point of offering to take an allergic baby or one with a family history of allergies, since pediatricians especially recommend breastfeeding for these babies.

Adoptive nursing is becoming more common now and more is known about it. Hopefully, you'll be able to educate the agency if necessary, and they'll be supportive. You might want to discuss with the social worker some of the experiences described in this chapter, as well as Regina Carlson's article and other references listed in the Bibliography.

What if you adopt a baby while pregnant? Can you still nurse the adopted baby? This was Jan's experience:

I found out I was pregnant with my third child the day before we received the call saying our adopted child was awaiting us. Jessica was ten days old when we brought her home, and for the first week I fed her with a bottle and used the breast as a pacifier. I then decided to try the Lact-Aid, and despite the gadget and the artificial milk, I felt that I was nursing my baby.

I was not worried about my milk coming in, since I knew that to hope for milk before the baby was born was like trying to fool mother nature. Sometimes my breasts felt full and I wondered if I was getting a supply of colostrum. Sometimes Jessica's bowel movements reflected that something other than formula was going through. I worried, as Jessie grew older and became less patient with the slow-flowing Lact-Aid, that I might not be able to keep her nursing till the baby was born. I switched to regular nursing bags which held more than the four-ounce Lact-Aid bags. Then there was the problem of my enlarging shape. The last month, when Jessica was seven months old, I was big and uncomfortable, not to mention crabby. I didn't nurse her for that month. We used only the Nuk nipple with warmed formula, and even though it was not

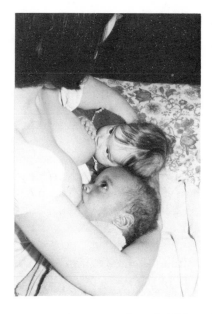

Jan with Jessica (right breast), 14 months old and Rachel (left breast), 6 months old.

easy for me to do, I held her close and never allowed her to hold her own bottle.

Rachel was born at home in mid-October. When the milk came in, I tried again to nurse Jessica. Thinking there was nothing there, Jessica resisted heartily. I tried putting honey on my nipples; the result was two sticky, frustrated people. The next day I offered her the breast (no honey this time) and she took it. From that moment on I had my nursing baby again.

Special Considerations in Nursing during Foster Care

Like adoptive mothers who nurse, as a foster mother you may encounter lack of knowledge and animosity from the placement agency responsible for the baby, or you may encounter enthusiasm.

Foster nursing just seems to come naturally to some foster mothers, though actually it may have taken them a while to realize its desirability. And foster nursing suits some babies but not others. Carol says:

As foster parents, we mainly had newborn babies waiting for adoption. It had not occurred to me to nurse them, though I had nursed my own three. One of my first attempts at nursing a newborn foster baby wasn't a success, because she was not terribly interested and it did not seem to be the natural and needed thing at the time. A year later, however, we had a foster baby who liked to nurse. She came at three days old and ate eight or nine times a day. I nursed her at each feeding; before a bottle if she was willing for as long as she wanted, or after if she seemed not to want to wait for the bottle. My milk came in beginning the third day. From three to twelve weeks she had a bout with colic, and although medication was some help, nursing was a real comfort. About the time the colic was over, my milk supply had reached a stable amount, but did not seem to be increasing. I was nursing before each feeding (five times a day) and she was taking a four-ounce bottle as well, or part of one. Looking back on it, I realize that I was going by the standard bottlefed baby schedules in my expectations, and that if I had been seriously trying to get her completely on the breast, I would have had to cut down or eliminate the bottles and nurse much more frequently.

To people nursing foster or adoptive babies, I'd say that it is important to remember that all babies are different. Some are easier to nurse because they like to suck, and eat frequently. Perhaps the ideal approach would be to nurse as often as possible, enjoying the baby and not getting "uptight" if milk is not produced. Then, any milk production could be welcomed as a "bonus." Nursing (even without milk) is a way of giving some extra sucking that is warmer and more natural than a pacifier.

Nursing foster babies differs from nursing adoptive babies in one obvious way—it is only a temporary relationship. A foster mother has to be able to enter fully into the relationship with the baby and yet be able to let go when it is time for the baby to move on to his permanent home. Her role is not only to give him love, but to prepare him for someone else's love. This relationship has difficult aspects, but for me the more I put into the relationship, the easier the giving up is. If I know I have done all I can for the baby, I feel I have gotten him off to a good start. I feel having the most intimate, loving relationship possible with his foster mother is the best preparation for whatever life will bring him.

Looking at foster nursing from the viewpoint of the permanent parents, full foster loving, including nursing, is valued. Foster parents seem very special to most people, while others can't imagine being able to relinquish a child, especially after nursing. Sometimes it *can* be very difficult. Marge says:

> Our foster baby, Matthew, came to us from the hospital at four days, weighing 6 pounds, 11 ounces. I had nursed all of my babies, so I decided to nurse Matthew, too. Because I was in the weaning phase with my three-year-old, I still had some milk. I nursed Matthew almost completely for the first two or three weeks, but I felt it would be grossly unfair to him to wean him from the breast *and* from me at the same time, so I gave a few bottles.
>
> When he was three weeks old, I called the agency to say that if the family he was to go to didn't want him for some reason, could we *please* keep him? However, a placement date had already been set. Knowing when he would be leaving, I cut down on nursing time. During his last week with us, I only nursed him two or three times a day and at night, because if I nursed him more often he'd balk at the bottle. He clearly preferred nursing. The tapering off was easy on both of us, plus my three-year-old was still nursing sometimes. Being responsible dictates giving bottles, so that along with the trauma of going from the only mother he has known to strangers, the baby doesn't also have to face sudden weaning.

How Intensive Nursing
May Affect Your Routine

Many mothers inducing lactation nurse for 20 minutes every hour and a half; that's over 5 hours a day. Spending that much time with your nursling means your family will have less of your attention. You'll all need to be prepared for that. On the other hand, when you're nursing, rather than bottlefeeding, you do have one hand free for another child.

What if any of your other children are also nursing? Gwen reports that her 23-month-old Robert, nursing about once a week for two minutes, showed an interest in nursing only twice when she was inducing lactation for her adopted daughter. After that it was "baby's milk."

In Oklahoma, one nursing mother got her adoptee off supplements within one week and her success was partly attributable to her older child, who nursed more frequently for a while, which helped build the supply.

Sound advice from one adoptive mother is to pretend you delivered that baby (if he's adopted) and realize you wouldn't be zipping around if you had. She curtailed almost all outside-the-home activities for about three months.

One adoptive mother, who took a leave of absence from her job to induce lactation and be with her new baby, also thought she'd use the time at home for putting in a garden and finishing some work she had stacked up. Well, it just didn't happen, she said.

Sleeping with Baby

One area of maternal behavior in which nursing mothers differ markedly from nonnursing mothers is sleeping with baby. There's a threefold difference: 26 percent of nonnursing mothers report they sometimes sleep or rest in bed with baby while 71 percent of nursing mothers share beds with their babies regularly.

Since it's an easy way to increase your baby's time to nurse and your time to rest, it's especially appropriate for intensive nursing situations and sick babies. So, if you feel inclined, do it. Prevent a possible fall by putting your baby's side of the bed against the wall or putting a pillow or bolster behind him. Or, put your mattress on the floor. During the day, if you have other little ones to tend to and find it difficult to nap, you can all lie together on the bed. As you rest and nurse, a child can snuggle in and pat baby's head or stroke him, while you talk quietly together or sing. Books, quiet toys, and nonmessy snacks are other pleasant diversions for older children at this time.

Mothering the Mother

In one society, a mother with a new nursling has no other responsibilities except her own toileting; she is literally spoon fed. Dana Raphael reports this and other behaviors toward nursing mothers in her book, *The Tender Gift: Breastfeeding.* (6) She suggests a modern equivalent to pregnant women: find another friendly expectant mother, due about three months from your due date and make a partnership. The first to deliver is helped by the second while she's initiating nursing. Then she, with her settled-in infant, will help the second during the initial nursing.

As a woman inducing lactation or relactating, you're going to need even more mothering. Ask for it. Make a bargain with a pregnant friend. Let your mother or father move in and fuss over you. Spend some of your savings for household help or child tending for your other children while you establish a nursing relationship with your baby. Your husband should have far less reason than the average new father to feel left out, unless you're being too heroic. How about asking your neighbor for an hour's help daily for a month and suggesting in return you'll take her kids for a weekend later on or paint her kitchen. Baby yourself for the sake of the baby.

One mother had friends bring bottles of their milk several times a day when she was lactating for her foster child. They were not in a position to be foster mothers themselves, but they wanted to be a part of it. You will find your friends appreciate being able to help; they want to support you as a friend and want to participate in your loving act.

Your Response to the Situation

Success is what you say it is in these situations. Don't let other people write the definition for you.

If your baby is ill and needs human milk, your focus on

milk production will be inevitable. But your willingness to try relactation counts for something, too. You're doing your best. Actually, by relactating *you'll* benefit as well as the baby; it's a comfort to have something to do rather than pace the floor and it's a reason for lots of bodily contact with your baby.

Adoptive and foster parents whose children can tolerate cow's milk or other formulas can have a more relaxed perspective on milk production. For them, the happy bond of mothering is what counts and any milk that is produced is a bonus to the relationship.

If you had experienced nursing before this special situation, you'll no doubt find that the word perseverance takes on new meaning. But you probably have intensely positive feelings about nursing to undertake induced lactation or relactation.

If this is your first nursing experience, you may be surprised at how you have responded. One mother began what she expected to be a normal nursing relationship with her newborn. She returned the La Leche League manual which she had borrowed, feeling, as she put it, "I was really doing fine and did not need the help of a group of fanatics." But she became ill and was hospitalized, which threatened her nursing relationship with her son. She says, "I had not realized how very strongly I had become attached to nursing until threatened with its termination."

Niles Newton, professional psychologist and author, says:

> The survival of the human race, long before any concept of duty evolved, depended upon the pleasures of two voluntary acts—coitus and breastfeeding. Were these acts not so pleasurable that humans sought their repetition, man would have joined the dinosaurs in extinction ages ago. (7)

So, you're not just involved in an extraordinary act by inducing lactation or relactating; you're performing a primal behavior. You can expect the experience to be powerful, even disturbing, and most probably, deeply pleasurable.

Chapter 16

Nursing While Pregnant

They say pregnant is beautiful. Obviously "They" have never been pregnant. Let me tell you what it's really like.

Pregnant is trying to wash dishes or hug your husband from two feet away.

Pregnant is a handy shelf to rest your drink on—until the baby kicks.

Pregnant is feeling relatively slim until someone comments "My, you're getting BIG!"

Pregnant is turning around and knocking your toddler off balance because you couldn't see him down there.

Pregnant is a glamorous wardrobe of stretch panels and pup tent blouses.

Pregnant is trying to hide your bulging tummy while your toddler nurses.

Pregnant is having to be a contortionist to paint your toenails.

Pregnant is the knowledge that you are nurturing a totally unique individual.

Pregnant is planning to give your child the very best, starting with your milk.

Pregnant is feeling privileged because you carry within you a precious new life.

Pregnant is preparing for that thrilling moment of birth.

Maybe after all, pregnant IS beautiful; maybe pregnant IS radiant; maybe pregnant IS blossoming. But just once why couldn't pregnant be SLIM?

Reflections of a Pregnant Mother
by Rose A. Sodergren

This verse reflects some of the aspects of pregnancy, a time of mixed emotions. If you are nursing your baby and also are pregnant, you may wonder whether to continue nursing and perhaps question whether it's safe.

The Advantages of Nursing

Weaning one child while pregnant with another may seem a "natural" thing for a nursing mother to do. It requires a certain commitment to continue nursing one baby while your body also devotes itself to nurturing another baby within. There *are* many mothers, though, who have nursed through pregnancy and are happy they did. Reading about the experiences of other mothers may help you make *your* decision.

Most of us have mixed feelings at the beginning of a pregnancy, even when the new baby is planned. While there is joy and eagerness and curiosity about the coming baby, there are usually some doubts and fears, too. These feelings tend to be compounded when you have a small child, or other children, already. This may be especially true when you are expecting your second child. Not having been mother to more than one before, it is hard to know how your love can be multiplied by your children and that it doesn't have to be divided among them. At some time you, like most mothers, will probably experience concern that the new baby will steal your love from the child you already know and hold so dear. On the other hand, you may fear you can never love your expected baby as much as you love the one you already have.

While these perfectly normal feelings are running their course, it may be helpful to know that you can continue breastfeeding your little one if you choose. Many mothers who have nursed through pregnancy comment on the satisfaction they gained from being able to meet the needs of both the baby and the toddler and what little conflict there was between the siblings when the older one had opportunities to satisfy his needs with mother, too.

One mother, Jan, says:

> I learned that we were expecting our second child when our son David was about 16 months old. Nursing had been an important part of his life. I sensed that David was not ready to wean. I felt very healthy and did not believe I would cause any harm to myself or either baby if I continued nursing David. Nursing through my pregnancy was natural and uneventful. My husband and I feel that David's good adjustment to the baby was partly the result of his being allowed to nurse as long as he needed to. Being free of the problem of sibling jealousy proved to be a great advantage.

Even when a child initiates weaning during pregnancy a mother may occasionally wish nursing had continued. Karyn reports being "somewhat regretful that my youngest did wean herself during my pregnancy. She still needs to be cuddled and rocked. She weaned herself to a pattern of sucking her thumb as a substitute which, although it doesn't bother me, is obviously less beneficial to her than continued nursing would have been."

There are extraordinary things that happen, too. Some mothers who have weaned early in a pregnancy have been heartsick later when the pregnancy ended in miscarriage. Mothers whose newborns have been too ill to nurse for a while have wished that the weaned toddler were still nursing to relieve the mother's engorgement and help maintain her milk supply. Rose, whose baby died a few days after birth, says, "My breasts were achingly full of milk, and I had no baby. You can imagine how thankful I was that my daughter Mary was still nursing. I desperately needed both the physical and emotional release that breastfeeding offered."

Is It Safe to Nurse?

One of the questions that nursing mothers sometimes have when they become pregnant is whether continued nursing will stimulate labor and cause a miscarriage. Mary White, a founding mother of La Leche League, is tremendously reassuring on this point. In a reply to a letter from a mother whose baby died when she was five months pregnant, and nursing a two-year-old, Mary said:

I know just how hard it is to lose a baby this far along in the pregnancy. It happened to me once, many years ago. In fact, it was our first baby, and at about five months along, we learned that the baby had died in utero. I have, over the ensuing years, given birth to eleven fine, healthy babies. During those years, however, I had three more miscarriages. The interesting thing is that while I nursed all of our children (many of them through the whole of the next pregnancy), not one of these three miscarriages occurred while I was nursing a baby. In other words, the pregnancies which I carried to term, and which ended in healthy babies, most often coincided with a time when I was nursing a toddler. However, the miscarriages occurred, without exception, after the previous child had weaned.

We have many times been asked if there is any relationship between miscarriages and breastfeeding during pregnancy. Our doctors feel, from experience in their own practices as well as from the experiences of the thousands of mothers who have been in touch with La Leche League, that there really is no connection at all. If anything, the percentages would seem to be in the other direction. That's probably coincidence, though, based on the fact that the nursing mother keeps herself in good health generally, and leads a happy and well-adjusted life. These factors, of course, would contribute to a healthy and uneventful pregnancy. The number of mothers we know personally who have nursed their little ones all the way through the next pregnancy is great, and to all appearances, neither the new nor the "old" baby, nor the mother, seem to have suffered any deprivation at all.

I think then that we can be pretty sure that breast-feeding during a pregnancy is not itself an adverse influence on that pregnancy. The percentages just don't seem to bear this out and there are no studies that we know of relating to breastfeeding during pregnancy and miscarriages.

Milk Supply

Most women observe a decrease in milk supply during pregnancy. It's possible that this is partly due to the hormones of pregnancy. Some babies seem to wean as though in protest to the decreased milk supply. Others continue nursing despite the decreased amount.

It seems quite possible that frequency of nursing influences milk supply in pregnancy, just as it does at other times. A baby whose mother conceives within five or six months following his birth has probably spent a somewhat reduced time at the breast, by sleeping all night, sucking a pacifier, or by receiving supplements or solids. It has been proven over and over that completely nursing your baby will almost always keep you from ovulating for six months or longer. There are, of course, exceptions. (1)(2) If a pattern of limited sucking is continued after conception, a diminished milk supply is very likely.

However, nursing seems to mean much more than milk to many babies. In La Leche League's Information Sheet, "Nursing Siblings Who Are Not Twins" (3), a mother explains:

> By the time I was six months pregnant and Elizabeth was 10 months old, she was nursing at naptime, and once during the night. It was apparent she was getting only a token amount of milk at each nursing, and yet those periods seemed to be as important to her as if they were her only source of nourishment. At that point she weighed between 18 and 20 pounds, was eating three large meals a day, and was drinking about a pint of milk from a cup.

You may not notice any decrease at all in your milk supply, especially if your baby is "older." In fact, if he should become ill, frequent nursing at that time might even lead to an *overabundance* of milk, even though you are pregnant.

As you continue nursing during your pregnancy, watch your baby to determine if any extra feeding is necessary.

Some time toward the last month of pregnancy most nursing toddlers indicate their awareness of a change in the milk. Some mothers notice that the milk seems to contain mostly colostrum. Some babies seem not to like the taste of this and they gradually wean themselves.

Incidentally, there is no danger of depriving your new baby of colostrum because your toddler is nursing. Some mothers express colostrum while they are pregnant, as a possibly helpful means of opening up the milk ducts in preparation for nursing. Their experience is that, if anything, their supply of colostrum is more copious than before. And mothers who have nursed their toddlers throughout their pregnancy have reported similar findings. (4)

Sore Nipples

There is much variation in mothers' reports about discomfort, especially nipple tenderness, during pregnancy. Some mothers find it becomes extremely painful to nurse during pregnancy, while others have no tenderness at all. For some mothers nipple pain passes after a month or so, while others have some degree of pain throughout pregnancy. How your own nipples feel and how well you can deal with any discomfort you may have will be one factor in how you proceed—continuing to nurse on demand during your pregnancy, nursing on a limited basis, or perhaps not nursing at all.

Nipple pain during pregnancy is not caused by the same kinds of irritations that lead to sore nipples in the newborn period. Soreness is your body's individual reaction to the hormonal changes of pregnancy and probably will not respond to lanolin-and-air treatment.

The degree and duration of nipple tenderness varies

greatly from mother to mother. You may experience less discomfort as long as you are nursing frequently and your milk supply is ample. Jan says, "In the last months of my pregnancy, my nipples were tender enough that they caused discomfort when David nursed—not the whole nursing period but for a moment when he took hold of the nipple. I found no way to relieve this, and since it was minor, I just put up with it."

Some mothers find that this nipple pain becomes more acute as pregnancy advances. Occasionally, just anticipating the feeling before starting to nurse can cause a mother to cry. Many mothers find that the pain later diminishes.

One mother had sore nipples during pregnancy and even when she nursed during labor. After delivery, she nursed on the delivery table and the soreness was gone!

It may be worthwhile at times of nipple pain to practice some of the routines that enhance the let-down reflex. (See chapter 2, "Nursing Techniques.") And don't overlook the possibility of infection as a cause of the discomfort.

Ask other mothers who have nursed through pregnancy for suggestions on what they have found helpful for sore nipples. One mother said lanolin *did* help her; another mother suggested nursing in different positions (such as the "football hold"). One woman describes two things she found helpful:

> When I took my full complement of vitamins, especially brewer's yeast, the soreness decreased a lot, and when I discovered glycerine and used it five or six times a day liberally, topically applied to the nipples, the pain and soreness went away entirely. I experimented, going two days without glycerin, then back to it, and there was a definite cause-and-effect relationship.

One thing for sure, is that you won't be nursing with sore nipples forever. And, if you continue nursing throughout your pregnancy, think how much better prepared your nipples will be for nursing when your new baby arrives! However, it is well to keep in mind that a newborn nurses very differently from a toddler and nipples can become sore, even though you have nursed all through your pregnancy. Therefore, some nipple preparation during pregnancy is recommended.

Irritability

Some pregnant mothers experience restlessness or irritability while nursing. These feelings are normal and are by no means confined to nursing during pregnancy. As a nursing toddler grows older, mothers begin to feel such changes also. This gradual change in the pleasure of nursing prepares us to be content when total weaning occurs.

Lynne describes her mixed feelings on continuing nursing during pregnancy:

> These feelings surprised me; I never expected to feel that way. At times I wished Jason would not ask to nurse any more. I found it physically irritating to be touched. My nipples were sore. My sex drive was gone. My whole body seemed to need a rest. I wanted to concentrate *only* on *being pregnant.* Jason would nurse a couple of minutes and then I'd say, "That's enough. Mommy's nipples are sore," and he'd stop. Sometimes he'd accept a glass of water or milk instead of nursing and gradually, by the time I was five or six months pregnant, he'd completely weaned.
>
> I think mothers can feel guilty about weaning their babies, and they can feel guilty about not weaning them. I did feel guilty about even this gentle process of weaning Jason, because *I* initiated it. But I don't feel guilty now. It wasn't traumatic for either of us. Jason did chew on his fingers for a few weeks, and tried nursing once or twice more. But he soon was content with life as a nonnurser. A little push in this direction seemed to be what he needed. My philosophy now is—let the child nurse until *he* is ready to quit or until he is able to understand that *I* don't want to nurse anymore.

Comments from Other People

What do you do if you're in public and your toddler wants to nurse? How do you handle comments at home, from

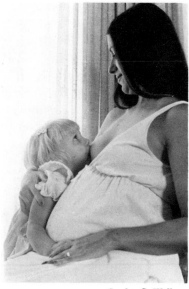

"The most important thing to remember is not to let friends, relatives or doctors discourage you from continued nursing while pregnant. Let the baby wean at his or her own speed—you won't regret it in the long run."
Debbie

Sandra C. Wallace

a well-meaning friend or relative who nevertheless disapproves of nursing in general and is flabbergasted at the thought of nursing while pregnant? What if you're warned that your unborn child will be malnourished and harmed in all sorts of ways? Helena says, "I continued to nurse my baby amidst the dire predictions. . . . As a perfect squelch for those people who had predicted a malnourished baby because of my 'indulgence' of Matthew's needs, Randolph was a solid 9½ pounds, and according to the nurse, 'Just about the healthiest baby I've ever seen in here!'" (5)

You might try avoiding nursing around people who may disapprove. This may work well for you if your nursing baby is old enough to be satisfied with other distractions or will accept your suggestion of "We'll nurse when we get home." If these don't work, you can try to find a secluded, quiet place to nurse your baby. Of course, wearing clothing especially suitable for inconspicuous nursing helps. (See Clothing for Discreet Nursing, chapter 2, "Nursing Techniques.")

However, sometimes you just may not be able to avoid

nursing "in public" or be able to do it inconspicuously. Carol, eight months pregnant, was attending a big family reunion in a park when her two-year-old came down the slide head first and hit the ground. She says:

> There was blood spurting out of Jared's nose. We had blood all over both of us. He was screaming and I knew he wanted to nurse. I didn't want to nurse him in front of all those people, but it just came to the point where nothing was comforting him and I said, "I'm sorry. I just have to nurse my baby." He calmed down immediately.
>
> The reactions to seeing this very obviously pregnant woman nursing a two-year-old were varied. I can't blame people for their reactions. Culturally we're not prepared for a sight like that. One woman said, "Well, for crying out loud, why didn't you do that in the first place?" Another was somewhat accepting, and said, "Well, if that's your thing, go ahead. You have a right to do whatever you want to do." A third was just devastated. She came up to me and said, "Do you mean to tell me you still let that child *suck* on you?" I really felt sorry for her. It was obvious it had ruined her day. The whole incident does point out that people really do have different reactions to seeing breastfeeding.

Criticism and misinformation may be the most troublesome obstacles you face in nursing through pregnancy. It helps to have answers ready such as, "My baby still needs to nurse, we enjoy it, it's best for us, and it's not harmful to the new baby." You might mention that most (if not all) mothers who have nursed siblings have found that doing so greatly minimized any feelings of resentment or jealousy that the older child might feel towards the new baby. Relating the experiences of other mothers, such as those in this book, may help. Quotes from reference sources may be useful. For example, after urging rest and a good diet for mother, *The Womanly Art of Breastfeeding* (6) states, "Nature sees to it that both babies are getting what they need."

But even though you explain, you may be limited by other

people's ability to really *understand* what you are saying. Often, it's easier just to keep smiling knowingly. No one except your baby has a right to pressure you to continue nursing during your pregnancy or to pressure you to wean. It's up to you.

Weaning

As you know by now, there are pros and cons to nursing through pregnancy. Whether *you* decide to continue or not, your baby may have other ideas.

It is not uncommon for a toddler to wean during pregnancy. Perhaps it is when he reaches his natural weaning time, or out of sympathy for mother's discomfort, or because of the change in the milk. But be careful not to assume that a temporary lack of interest in nursing means your baby has decided to wean. Look to your baby. Could there be some other reason, tension or teething, for example?

On the other hand, some toddlers nurse all during the pregnancy, then stop when the new baby arrives. Edith describes the different reactions of her nursing twins: "Both twins nursed while I was pregnant with Erik. Kendal weaned when Erik was born. She just never asked to nurse after I came home from the hospital, even though I was in the hospital only 24 hours. The other twin, Andrea, continued to nurse about once every two or three days."

Many toddlers are delighted by the renewed milk supply after the new baby's birth; however, some wean when they find themselves flooded with milk. And, as if things don't seem unpredictable enough already, some toddlers who wean during pregnancy want to resume nursing when the new baby and new milk supply arrive.

One little girl looked up at her three-months-pregnant mother during a nursing and said, "The baby took all your milk away, Mommy, isn't that sad?" "But surprisingly she really didn't seem to mind too much," said her mother, "She weaned, but just temporarily. I assured her that once the baby came there would be plenty of milk for both of them and she was free to choose to resume nursing if she wanted to."

If *you* initiate the weaning, proceed as you would if you weren't pregnant, gradually omitting one feeding every week or so. Look for other activities to substitute for nursing. Cuddle and rock, sing, read, go for a walk, play games. Offer something else to drink. How about a tea party for the two of you?

It can be a difficult decision to stop nursing. Maybe we feel guilty because of our determination to do everything that is best for our children, and because we won't let ourselves believe that doing something for *ourselves* is sometimes the best thing for our children. Perhaps we have been brought up to believe that concern for ourselves is selfish and therefore always wrong. Surely, if something is continuously unpleasant or uncomfortable, there is good reason to consider a change in the situation. If nursing has become miserable, consider the possibility of stopping. Being sensitive to your child, you can tell whether he is ready. If he isn't, and makes that clear to you, you can go back to nursing with strong motivation. Now you will *know* that it is best for your child.

Helpful Hints

Your Husband

This is a time when negative emotions are quite normal. When you're able to discuss them with your husband they seem to diminish and you're better able to deal with them.

One mother said that nighttime started to become a real problem after she became pregnant. She said:

> Before, when Matthew woke and nursed, I would relax and go right back to sleep with him in my arms. Later on, I found myself awake and becoming more and more tense as Matthew nursed on. This resulted in my being very irritated with him when he awoke, and in my husband's being angry with me for being snappish with Matthew.

I finally had a talk with my husband about my feelings and how they were influenced by physical changes in my body. He suggested that perhaps if he were to rub my back when Matthew nursed at night, this might relieve my tension. He only had to do this two or three times during the rest of my pregnancy. I think the greatest comfort was in knowing that if I needed him he would understand and help. (7)

One Day at a Time

Nursing during pregnancy is something you need to take day by day. Vicki described her experience this way:

I encouraged Shanna to wean. But when I'd suggest something else to do instead, she'd often say, "Gee, I really *want* to nurse." I finally adjusted to the fact that I'd be nursing two. But about the time I adjusted, Shanna weaned.

She was twenty months old when her sister, Danika, was born. About a week later, Shanna tried to nurse again. At first she didn't like it with all that milk. For the next few weeks she asked to nurse about once a week, but would only put her mouth on. She didn't suck.

Suddenly, one day Shanna actually nursed. I asked her why she was nursing now and wouldn't earlier. She said she'd decided the milk tasted good. From then on, Shanna nursed about once every other day, for six months. This was another adjustment for me, after having become used to the idea that she'd weaned. It was hard for me to accept emotionally. I wished then she had not weaned during the pregnancy. The nursings dwindled to about once a month, and then Shanna finally weaned herself. (8)

Chapter 17

Nursing Siblings*

Making the Decision

Nursing siblings can be a joyful, beautiful thing. It can pose problems, and is not for everyone, but for many mothers these problems are more than outweighed by the advantages. As one mother said, "Nursing siblings hasn't turned out to be the difficult and unpleasant experience that I'd heard it would be. As a matter of fact it's lovely and feels quite natural to nurse both of them. It's kind of nice to nurse the infant knowing she will grow big someday like her sister, and then nurse her sister remembering how it was to nurse her as an infant."

Another mother, Vicki, says:

> Nursing siblings is one of the most difficult things I have done while childbearing. If my children had weaned easily before a new baby was born I would have been pleased. But they obviously needed the continued nursing. I found nursing siblings especially difficult in the early weeks after the new baby came, because the toddler wants to nurse most then—for reassurance, and the new baby, of course, needs to nurse most frequently then, too. Yet I'm really convinced that it's worth it to nurse siblings. Nursing my toddler reminded me that she is still a baby. Sometimes we talked together about how good it is that she can be a baby *and* be a big sister, too. When I nursed

---

* This chapter is concerned with nursing siblings who are not twins.

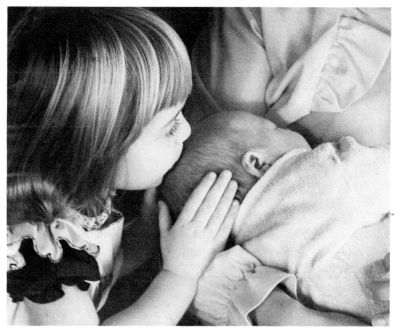

Sandra C. Wallace

Nursing a baby and an older child can foster a closeness between the two, as well as between each child and mother.

simultaneously, the toddler put her arms around the baby. It was nice to see my children relating to each other so lovingly.

Nursing siblings is much more than just a question of having enough milk for both. Nursing a toddler and a newborn is quite a challenge. Your older baby can be just as demanding as the newborn and for a while, may seem to require as much time and attention. Whether or not you are nursing the older child, he may act "babyish." This may be annoying, but it's to be expected. In nursing both your children, you are placing the emotional needs of your infant and young child high on your scale of values. You are letting your toddler outgrow his baby ways at his own pace. It may require certain sacrifices, but you can also expect to reap great benefits.

Ann Horne says in "Observations and Reflections on Nursing Siblings Who Are Not Twins" (1):

> In order to respond sympathetically to the needs of your infant and older baby, it is imperative that you assess the emotional needs of the two children accurately. This can be done by honestly looking at the children from their point of view and not your own. For instance, it is absolutely impossible for a busy mother to take time to sit down with a whining 18-month-old for a genuinely responsive nursing session if all she sees is a demanding toddler who is keeping her from finishing the kitchen cleanup. On the other hand, it is not at all difficult to take a welcome respite from the housework by fulfilling the obvious need for physical contact of a youngster who is just beginning to learn how to give and receive love.
>
> . . . It is necessary to accept wholeheartedly the philosophy that nursing at the breast provides a youngster with far more than nourishment . . . remind yourself of it repeatedly, and most especially just after your two-year-old has charmed the milkman into all sorts of remarks about how grown up she is, then broken your best bottle of perfume, then awakened the five-month-old baby from a sound sleep, and then crawled into your lap and demanded in a most ungrateful way a midmorning nursing that she hasn't asked for in three weeks. You either give yourself over to the proposition that nursing provides a child a wealth of values besides milk or forget the whole matter.

If you anticipate nursing siblings as a problem, it may be one. You might consider gently and gradually encouraging your child to wean before the new baby is born. (Abrupt weaning can be upsetting for you both and it should be avoided.)

Milk Supply:
Enough for Baby?

The most common question asked when considering whether or not to nurse siblings is, "Will I be able to produce an adequate milk supply?" Once again the law of supply and demand takes over. The amount of stimulation your breasts receive affects the amount of milk they produce. There may even be *more* milk than you need at first. (This often happens after birth, even if a mother is nursing only a newborn.) Some mothers find that the extra stimulation and increased supply caused by nursing two makes the milk flow too fast for their tiny babies. If this happens, you can nurse your newborn from the breast which is least full and your toddler from the fuller breast.

If your newborn coughs or fusses or sputters occasionally while nursing, sit him up or lay him across your shoulder. Gently pat his back and help him to catch his breath, then resume nursing. He may sometimes become overly full and spit up more than he normally would, so don't be alarmed. (See Overabundant Milk Supply in chapter 7, "Newborn and Infant Problems.")

When siblings are nursing, generally the older child nurses for the emotional closeness and gets some of his nutrition from family meals and snacks. It is important to make sure that your baby gets first chance at the breast. This can be done by nursing the younger baby first for as long as he wants on both breasts. Or, nurse the baby first on one breast, then let the toddler have that side while the baby nurses from the other side. The toddler can then finish this second side. Another method is to nurse each child on only one side—that way the supply will equal the needs of each.

For the baby who wants lots of sucking but not a lot of milk, offer the breast which the toddler has just nursed.

For more information on milk supply when nursing two, see Milk Supply in chapter 18, "Nursing Twins."

Baby's Arrival

Emotions

The separation of a child from his mother when a new baby is born at the hospital can sometimes be a traumatic period, especially if the child is nursing. More mothers today avoid this problem by having a home delivery or returning home within a few hours after birth.

It helps to prepare your older child for the arrival of the baby. Accompanying you on routine doctor's appointments, listening to the baby's heartbeat, "helping" with preparations at home, and going with your husband to bring you and baby home from the hospital, help your child to feel a part of what is happening.

Sharing his mother with a strange little newcomer can be a "hard pill to swallow," especially for an only child, whether he's nursing or not. Many mothers find that nursing at this time offers the older child comfort and reassurance.

In her book, *Understanding Your Baby: A Course in Child Development 0-3 Years* (2), Dorothy Baldwin humorously illustrates how a child might feel towards a new sibling, but changes the characters to those of a husband and wife. The dialogue of the comic book-style cartoon goes like this:

Wife: I've got a surprise for you.

Husband: What then? Something nice for supper?

Wife: Listen. It's important. I've got another husband to come and live with us. Aren't we lucky?

Husband: What's-that-you-said?

Wife: Don't be cross. He'll be company for me while you're at work. And you can take him out in the evenings. Won't that be nice?

Husband: Who's cross? I'll kill him, that's all.

Wife: No you won't. You'll be nice to him and love him as much as I do. You are still my *first* husband. I still love you just as much. You don't have to be jealous. It's just that I want another husband.

A long separation when your new baby arrives can be confusing and upsetting to the child left at home. Sometimes

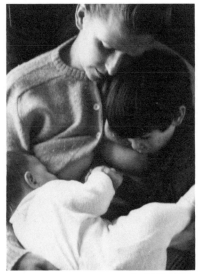

Betty nursing Joseph (left), and Daniel, who holds his brother's hand.

Sandra C. Wallace

it just can't be avoided, as when a mother has to have a cesarean delivery.

Betty's son Daniel was 3½ when his bother Joseph was born by cesarean section. Although Betty had tried to prepare Daniel with stories, conversations, and doll play, he reacted very strongly to the separation from his mother. He became rebellious and hostile towards his grandmother, who was caring for him during his mother's absence. When his mother returned home after a five-day hospital stay, at first Daniel rejected her. "For three months Daniel cried five or six times a day no matter what I did," says Betty. "Mostly I sat and nursed them both a great deal. This brought peace and quiet and love, and finally an acceptance of our new situation. Daniel began to pat the baby as they both nursed, then they began to play together at the breast." *

Fortunately, the arrival of a new baby is usually not so

---

* Ilg and Ames in *The Gesell Institute's Child Behavior* (3) state that at 3½ years old a child does go through this cycle of behavior normally. Nursing can be very helpful to mother and child at this time.

upsetting to the child at home. Jan says, "During our separation when I was in the hospital, Davey got along happily and hardly seemed to miss me." However, after Jan was home with Christie (the new baby) for a while, Davey nursed as often as he had six months earlier. Jan feels that nursing Davey helped them both adjust to the arrival of the new baby. She says:

> Nursing offered emotional comfort and stability to Davey. It helped keep Davey and me close, too. Like so many nursing mothers and babies, we'd had a good relationship. Nursing guaranteed that we still had frequent moments of special togetherness in spite of the demands of a new baby. For about nine months I was nursing two. Davey gradually weaned himself. It was not always easy nursing siblings, but most of the time I enjoyed it very much. To this day, Davey (3½) and Christie (21 months) have a close and loving relationship, and Davey is still happy when Christie nurses and is concerned if I don't go to her right away when she wants to nurse.

Change in Taste

Because breast milk reverts to colostrum, usually during the last stages of pregnancy, your newborn will still receive the benefits colostrum provides. (See Milk Supply in chapter 16, "Nursing While Pregnant.") However, your older child may not like its taste and may lose interest in nursing temporarily or completely. Also, colostrum can make an older child's stools very loose if he continues to nurse.

Nipple Tenderness

Nipple tenderness is common during pregnancy and is discussed in the Sore Nipples section of chapter 16, "Nursing While Pregnant." Many mothers report that they experience no nipple tenderness after birth. Keep in mind, though, that a newborn nurses differently and more frequently than a toddler. Some mothers who nursed a toddler while pregnant, and did no nipple preparation, reported extreme tenderness when nursing the newborn.

Engorgement

Nursing siblings may provide a bonus—most mothers experience little or no engorgement. Your breasts simply won't have the opportunity to become overly full!

The Early Weeks

During the early weeks of nursing a newborn and his older sibling, you may feel you are doing nothing but nursing. Many mothers find that their nursing toddlers suddenly want to nurse frequently.

This is the toddler's natural attempt to seek the reassurance that he is not being "shoved aside." He may be delighted at finding a suddenly ample milk supply. Once he realizes that he is secure in your love and that you accept him as he is, he will gradually nurse less. He may even completely wean, feeling that "nursing is for babies!"

Even a child who has already weaned may ask to nurse when he sees a new baby at his mother's breast. Many times he will nurse a little, giggle self-consciously, and slide off his mother's lap, secure in the knowledge that it's okay for him to be a "baby," too. However, some mothers find that instead of taking a little taste, then forgetting about it, the child resumes nursing on a regular basis, even though it has been some time since he last asked to nurse.

Again, the renewed interest is probably caused by many factors, not the least of which is the competition for your attention. If your toddler abandoned nursing during your pregnancy because of the changed taste of the milk or the diminished supply at that time, he may be thrilled with the new taste and abundance.

Carolyn became pregnant when her daughter, Laurie, was 15 months old and nursing three to four times a day. Since they both enjoyed these nursings, Carolyn decided to let Laurie continue nursing as long as she wished. "Besides," says Carolyn, "it was the perfect way to interest her in taking an afternoon nap that we both really needed." When Carolyn was eight months pregnant, Laurie began to lose interest in nursing, and stopped nursing completely shortly before her brother was born. The first time Laurie saw the baby nurse, she asked to nurse, too. Carolyn expected Laurie to take a taste, then climb down, but instead "she settled down and nursed for quite a while." Carolyn says, "I enjoyed it too, because I had missed her while I was in the hospital, and she felt good in my arms. Anyway, I felt it was more natural than pushing her out of the nest for the newcomer. Laurie went back to a three-times-a-day routine until she weaned completely six months later."

Suzanne had a similar experience with her little girl, Jennifer, who had weaned shortly before her sister was born. However, though Jennifer was again interested in nursing, she'd forgotten how to do it. Suzanne says, "I had to teach Jennifer how to suck. Her tongue was not covering her bottom teeth and she was hurting me, but after a little instruction to refresh her memory, she was off and sucking away."

On the other hand, Peggy nursed her third child until she went to deliver the baby. After she returned home a couple of days later, her toddler asked to nurse and then stated with irritation, "Milk's hot—I like mine from the refrigerator," and he never asked to nurse again.

To Each His Own?

Some mothers find that reserving a particular breast for each child works well for them. It can help the toddler accept the fact that the new baby is also nursing, if they have separate breasts. Other mothers are concerned that even this partial denial of the breast may be emotionally upsetting to the older child. And, since your babies may take different amounts of milk, you *may* look somewhat lopsided, with one breast bigger than the other.

One mother who *did* nurse each child from separate

breasts and was happy with it says, "In our situation (an only child having to accept a newcomer), I felt it eased the tension for Shannon to know that 'her breast was just hers.' Since the new baby was completely nursed on one side, I always held him, at nonnursing times, on the other side."

Perhaps one reason some mothers prefer to nurse their babies from separate breasts is because of their concern that infection may pass from one baby to the other. Since the nipples are self-cleansing, it is unlikely that this will happen. In her book, *The Family Book of Child Care* (4), Dr. Niles Newton writes:

> The idea of not cleaning nipples is deeply shocking to some people. They do not realize that the body itself controls germs on the nipple in two different ways. Sweat mixed with skin oil tends to kill germs. The largest sweat glands on the body are found on the nipple, and the skin oil secretions increase during pregnancy in preparation for breastfeeding. Secondly, breast milk is itself antiseptic when it first comes out of the breast. Experiments indicate that newly secreted breast milk is 100 times as potent as newly secreted cow's milk in killing germs.

Simultaneous or Individual Nursings?

Nursing siblings simultaneously is much easier than nursing newborn twins simultaneously because the older child is able to position himself at the breast.

During the early weeks you can let your older child settle in your lap, then lay the baby on top of him. Or, you can sit on a couch or sit propped up in bed with the baby in one arm and the older sibling sitting next to you. It is helpful to have extra pillows handy to support your arms if they get tired. You can nurse the two in the "football hold," as with twins. One mother says she found it very relaxing to sit cross-legged on the floor with one baby on each side. She says it wasn't hard to manage, either, because the older child could climb on and off mother's lap herself.

During her pregnancy, Betty showed her little boy, Al,

pictures of twins nursing together. She found this helped Al to understand that the new baby would need to nurse, too. She says:

> When I brought James home from the hospital, Al always nursed when he did. At first I held both of the boys as they nursed. Later, Al would sit at my side and nurse. Now they don't nurse together unless Al stops playing and stands next to me. They enjoy taking turns and being held. Al doesn't mind waiting as long as he knows his side is waiting. Al nurses on the right side at night and on the left side during the day.

Most mothers who have nursed siblings together treasure those moments. Rose, who nursed three-year-old Mary for a year after her brother Eric was born, says:

> Looking back on the time when I was nursing both Mary and Eric, I feel really glad I did it. I think that continuing to nurse Mary after Eric was born made the whole adjustment of sharing Mommy much easier for her. Nursing gave her comfort, solace, and reassurance as nothing else could have. Those times when I was nursing them simultaneously are special memories. They were particularly close moments. I'll never forget our first night together home from the hospital. I was propped up on pillows in bed, 12-hour-old Eric was asleep at one breast, and Mary was asleep at the other with her arm protectively around her new brother. A cherished moment indeed! I'd do it all again.

And she did. When Eric was not yet 2½, and nursing, baby Cliff arrived. Rose says:

> Because Eric was younger and less mature than Mary was when he was born, accepting a new baby was really hard for him. He was still so much a baby himself. If Eric hadn't been nursing at the time Cliff was born, I'm afraid we would have pushed him to "grow up" before he was ready to. With a new baby to care for, I probably would have expected Eric to be more independent and self-sufficient. But nursing Eric provided me with a constant

reminder: "Hey, Mom, I'm a baby, too. Just let me be me. I'll grow up soon enough." Once again I discovered that there is a special camaraderie that develops between siblings who are introduced at their mother's breast.

A mother who chooses to nurse the babies individually, rather than simultaneously, should be flexible when the older sibling asks to nurse at the same time as the baby. It is difficult for a small child to understand "waiting his turn," especially when a week or two previously he was allowed to nurse when he wished. He may see this as a rejection and build feelings of resentment.

Pearl found it easier for her to nurse her daughter Laurie and her baby, Doug, separately. She says, "Laurie never showed resentment at her brother's nursing. We chose her room for Doug's nursings, and thus Laurie could do as she pleased without any 'no-no's'. I often got down on the floor and played with her, or she drew her rocker up to mine and held her doll."

Nursing Older Siblings

Nursing a toddler and an older child can be as heartwarming as nursing an infant and a toddler. As the infant grows older he not only becomes more responsive to you, but to his sibling as well, and they will begin to play together at the breast. Claudia, nursing her two boys, ages three and two, says, "The boys . . . tease each other when nursing at the same time. The three of us piled up in the rocker or lying on the bed are quite a sight. My husband just laughs. We all enjoy the situation very much."

Lindsey says of nursing three-year-old Michael and one-year-old Rena, "Rena loves to share her milk with her big brother. It isn't always easy to nurse siblings, but when they fall asleep holding each other's hand and me, I feel good inside."

Night Nursings

Night nursings, when both toddler and baby awake at the same time, may present a problem. However, with some thoughtful planning, it does not have to be insurmountable.

As one mother says, "I decided to learn to sleep while nursing two just as I had when nursing one. The only way I have found to nurse two while sleeping is flat on my back with one on each side. It is hard for a tiny baby to nurse with mother in that position, but putting a bed pillow under him solved that nicely for me."

Other mothers are comfortable sleeping with the baby lying across the chest and the toddler beside them. Or you might try lying on your left side with your baby at your left breast, and your toddler lying over your right hip from behind to nurse from your right (top) breast.

After a while, it may be that only one of your babies wakes for nursing during the night, while the other one sleeps through. And it may not be the younger baby that wakes.

Having two children in bed with parents may be a rather crowded sleeping arrangement. For this reason, a king-sized bed may be worth the investment. Some couples find that an extra bed pushed up against the mother's side of their bed works just as well. Other couples have abandoned traditional sleeping arrangements and simply spread several mattresses on the floor for a single "sleeping room" for the entire family. Valerie says she had one baby at the head of her bed and one at the foot. She slept on top of the bed and alternated between the children at night. "This way they each had their own time with me. Sometimes it worked, sometimes both woke at the same time and I nursed them together."

Children sleeping with their parents is a controversial subject. It is a matter of personal taste and individual choice. Those who do choose to make the parental bed a *family* bed find that this need not detract from parental lovemaking.

For more on children sleeping in their parents' bed, see these listings in the Bibliography: Tine Thevenin's *The Family*

Bed: An Age-Old Concept in Child Rearing (5); *The Family Book of Child Care* by Niles Newton (6); *Touching: The Human Significance of the Skin* by Ashley Montagu (7); and *Mother Love: The Book of Natural Child Rearing* by Alice Bricklin (8).

Nursing in Public

Although it is possible to nurse a small baby discreetly in public, it is sometimes difficult to do with a toddler, much less a toddler and a baby at the same time. Distracting the older child for a time with toys or with interesting activities usually helps. If the child is old enough to understand, a simple explanation followed by "I'll nurse you as soon as we get home," or "Wait until we get to the car," may be enough to deter him. If this is not possible, try to find a secluded place where you can nurse him quietly.

When One or Both Babies Are Adopted

Some parents who wish to adopt a baby do so while their toddler is nursing enough to maintain the mother's milk supply. With milk already there, the adopted baby is encouraged to suck, and the additional stimulation increases the milk supply.

But Jessie had a different experience. Having been unsuccessful in trying to conceive her second child, she and her husband decided to apply for adoption. They received their son, Eric, when he was 2½ days old. Jessie nursed him using the Lact-Aid supplementer, donor breast milk and formula. Jessie says:

> Twenty days after we received Eric, I conceived our second daughter, Melinda. During my pregnancy I continued to nurse Eric with the Lact-Aid with formula. After arriving home from the hospital with Melinda, I nursed Eric twice with the Lact-Aid. Forty hours after the birth,

my milk came in. That morning I did not need the supplementer. At last, Eric had my milk, his birthright; he
was ten months old!

Some mothers have nursed siblings who were both
adopted. Karen and her husband adopted one baby who was
5½ months old, and then several months later adopted a 3½-
month-old baby. Karen had difficulty interesting them in
nursing and resorted to the Lact-Aid supplementer. Eventually,
though, both the babies nursed naturally, without the supplementer.

For more information on the Lact-Aid, see Special Feeders
and Feeding Techniques in chapter 2, "Nursing Techniques"
and *Supplementing at the Breast* in the Supplemental Food
section of chapter 15, "Inducing or Reestablishing Your Milk
Supply."

Taking Care of Yourself

The amount of time spent nursing a newborn and a toddler
need not be a strain on you. Drink plenty of fluids and try to be
especially conscientious about your diet. Vitamins may be
helpful in combating fatigue and that overtired feeling, but
rest is essential, too. See chapter 3, "Nutrition for Mother and
Baby."

Housework should be minimal. The dust and clutter will
be there tomorrow, but never again will your little ones need
you as they do now. Remind yourself that *people are more
important than things,* then turn your back on the unmade beds
and dirty dishes. Nursing encourages you to sit and relax at
various times during the day which is a definite advantage during the early weeks when you need the rest. It is satisfying to
realize nursing's importance to your whole family. You are
contributing to their health and growing characters. Your
husband benefits, too, from having a happy wife.

Ups and Downs

There will probably be times when you really don't feel

like nursing. Why feel guilty when it is a normal reaction to a sometimes trying situation? One mother, who nursed both a newborn and a two-year-old, says, "I got to the point where I didn't *want* to nurse my two-year-old and I felt guilty. I'd try to nurse her, but it would make me feel irritable. That made me feel terrible. I couldn't imagine not wanting to nurse."

If you feel this way, reassess your priorities. Remind yourself that you have the ability to satisfy many important emotional needs by nursing your baby. Perhaps a walk in the fresh air with your little one, or enjoying a warm bubble bath together will help relieve the tension and help you to regain your perspective.

Jan describes her mixed emotions:

> I often felt the positive emotions of love and happiness toward my children and myself, but at other times I felt that I was being used physically almost beyond my limit. Sometimes my husband's interest in sex seemed to me like just one more person who wanted to use me for something. . . . I don't know to what extent a new mother with two small children feels these things regardless of nursing experience. I never felt that I was nursing two because it was my duty, however. I always felt I was doing so by choice. I never regretted it, but I didn't always enjoy it.

Most mothers experience these mixed emotions while nursing siblings. Suzanne, while nursing her one-year-old and three-year-old, said: "At times I was irritated when my three-year-old still wanted to nurse, after my 'don't offer', 'don't refuse', 'distract' tests. I noticed that she rarely asked to nurse away from home, however. It was mostly when she was tired, frustrated, or hurt." Suzanne was able to have a sense of humor about the whole situation. She tells about asking her daughter, "What do you want for breakfast?" Jennifer answered the question with a twinkle in her eye, saying, "Milk . . . breast milk!"

Suzanne describes their nursing relationship:

Jennifer learned to accept rather gracefully that baby got first preference and she had to wait. In a way she was *too* easily put off. One particular morning Jennifer asked several times to breastfeed and I told her to wait for one seemingly necessary thing and then another. Finally, she said despairingly, as she went out the back door, "Call me when my breastfeed's ready!" Bless her heart . . . and I did call her, too. Often, after I had put her off and she had momentarily forgotten about it, I called her to me and told her that "I owe you a breastfeed, you want it now?" Usually, she gratefully crawled up for a few minutes.

In a speech presented at the 1972 state meeting of La Leche League of Oklahoma, Norma Jane Bumgarner summed it up beautifully when she said:

> No matter how virtuous a mother may feel about it, nursing two can be maddening and hectic at times. It can be particularly hard if a mother's family or friends cannot support her decision. Many mothers, though, have survived the special problems of nursing siblings, along with the fun of watching camaraderie develop between their little ones, especially when they are nursing together. These mothers feel good about their decision because, while fully meeting the needs of their new babies, they have not had to deny their older babies this focus of love and security they have relied upon since birth. (9)

Your Cheering Squad

As in all breastfeeding situations, a father's support and encouragement are important. When you nurse siblings, the father's role takes on added significance. Even the mother who has considerable nursing experience needs reassurance.

Some parents find it helpful for the father to take over the care of the older child in the evenings. This gives the mother a "breather," and the opportunity to give the new baby undivided attention, while the older child can enjoy special times with his father.

A husband can be more understanding if you share the

positive aspects of nursing two babies and not just the negative. Otherwise your husband may wonder why you are doing it. Tell him about the silly, fun things that happen as a result of nursing two. Point out how you've noticed that your older child is learning to lovingly accept his new sibling as he begins to realize that the baby's life will enrich his own, not impoverish it.

Harsh criticism from family and friends can really undermine your confidence. Let's face it—we all need to feel "accepted" by our peers, and if we are made to feel odd, it can be quite depressing. One way to handle this situation is with a straightforward discussion about what you feel is important and why. Once the people involved realize how strongly you believe in what you are doing, chances are they will respect your views.

You should try to surround yourself with those who share your enthusiasm towards breastfeeding and mothering. Attending La Leche League meetings can be a great morale booster. As one mother so aptly put it, "It's like getting my mothering batteries recharged."

Chapter 18

Nursing Twins

Breastfeeding twins is practical and possible. In fact it's much more efficient than having to fix and store double the usual number of bottles every day.

Many of us who have nursed twins feel breastfeeding promotes a special closeness with each twin individually, which otherwise might be much harder to achieve. Nursing time can be a time to relax—perhaps your only time to rest during the whole day! At night, you'll get more sleep, having no bottles to warm. The fact that breastfeeding is less expensive is a double advantage with twins. Breast milk is best for any baby and with complications such as allergies or premature births, breastfeeding could be absolutely imperative.

Preparation

Since more than half of twin births are premature, be sure to start your nipple preparation early if you have advance notice that twins are on the way. You'll be nursing twice as much as a mother with one baby, but this needn't be a problem if you're adequately prepared.

Milk Supply

Don't worry about your milk supply being adequate. Your breasts will produce according to the law of supply and demand, and there probably will be enough milk right from the start. Many mothers with slender builds and small breasts successfully nurse their twins.

When one or both babies go through a growth spurt, this increases the demand on your milk. Frequent nursing will build up your supply fast. Nurse them often, without regard for when they last nursed, and in a couple of days you'll have plenty of milk again. Remember your breasts are continually producing milk. If you just finished nursing 20 minutes ago and the same, or the other, twin now wants to nurse, you'll have another meal ready. You will have enough milk to completely supply all their needs until they're ready for solids (about six months) and to continue nursing them until they're ready to wean.

Supplemental bottles aren't really necessary; your babies won't need extra milk, water or juice. And since giving bottles can lead to more bottles and eventual weaning, it's wise to avoid them most of the time. But an occasional bottle is not disastrous, especially after the first six or eight weeks when your milk supply is well established. If you have allergies in your family, you'll want to use your own milk. Even if you're not concerned about allergies, it's still nice to use your own. That way you're sure your babies are getting the very best, and you won't need to worry about diminishing your milk supply.

In the Hospital

While you're in the hospital, try different positions for nursing (sitting up or lying down), to find the most relaxing for you. Try nursing both babies together, using pillows to support them. Remove a too-tight bra, take a hot shower to relieve engorgement and put anhydrous lanolin, Vaseline or A and D Ointment on your nipples to prevent soreness. Nurse your babies often for your own comfort as well as theirs.

The hospital staff may suggest bringing one baby at a feeding, alternating the baby they bring, so that it's "easier" on you. But it is better for your babies to nurse each feeding time, rather than receive a substitute. And the extra stimulation is better for you.

By nursing often in the first week, your nipples will be less tender and your breasts less engorged. Rooming-in makes un-limited nursing possible and is especially suited for twins. They frequently need to be nursed more often than the three- or four-hour interval that staff nurses are willing to cooperate with.

Simultaneous or Separate Nursings?

Dr. Spock once made a study of twins in which he found that the mothers who nursed both babies completely were the best organized, time-wise, and at an earlier date, than the mothers who partially nursed or bottlefed their babies. The mothers at the top of the list nursed their babies simul-taneously.

Most mothers of twins nurse simultaneously at some time. Although simultaneous nursing is a big time-saver, you may find you're more relaxed and comfortable nursing separately. And it's nice to give each child your undivided attention. Yet what do you do when both babies wake ravenously hungry at the same time? Whether you nurse separately or at the same time, the milk supply doesn't seem to be affected one way or the other. If you try simultaneous nursing one time and aren't able to manage it well, don't give up. Try it again at a later date when the babies aren't especially hungry. Have your husband help by bringing you the babies and getting you settled com-fortably with pillows.

A difference in birth weight or nursing patterns between your twins might affect whether simultaneous nursing at each feeding is reasonable. A five-pounder might want to nurse every two hours or more often, whereas a seven-pounder might soon settle into a three-hour feeding interval.

One mother who felt that simultaneous nursing did not work well for her twins explains:

> Michael nursed until his tummy was full and then slept for a long period, while Marita took less milk and slept for a shorter time. I fed whichever one happened to want it, but if they woke together a pacifier came in handy, to keep one quiet long enough for me to feed the other.

At nighttime, Michael could go six to eight hours without nursing. Usually when Marita woke, I fed her, then while my husband burped her I woke Michael and fed him. If they both woke together, my husband changed one while I fed the other and we each ended up with a baby to burp. Sounds rather involved, but we still managed to get enough sleep. (1)

If Simultaneous—How?

It's a lot easier to nurse twins together if you have help getting into position. You can sit in a rocking chair, on a couch, or on a bed. The arms of a chair are helpful and so is a footstool.

Use pillows to get each baby at a comfortable height for your breasts, and to support your arms. Get one baby started, then have someone help you position the other. Or, you can place the second baby on your legs or alongside you until you're ready for him.

Have fun trying out different positions for simultaneous nursing. Here are three to experiment with:

• You can nurse with each twin in a regular nursing position, across your body in front of you. One baby's body is against you; the other baby's body is against his twin. The babies' bodies are criss-crossed.

• You can nurse them with their bodies lying alongside yours, almost parallel.

• You can hold each in a "football hold" position, with his feet behind you. You definitely need help from pillows for this, otherwise your arms will tire.

I found a combination of the first and last methods the easiest; one baby at my right breast, her body across mine in usual nursing position, the second baby at my left breast, in a "football hold" position, with feet toward my back.

With the illustrations as a guide, see which position is best for you, or devise your own.

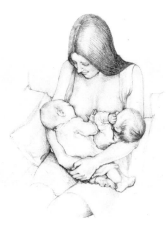

Nursing Positions

*Babies are criss-crossed, with sup-
port from mother's hands under
their buttocks. A pillow placed
under mother's right elbow helps
to support the lower baby, who is
the heavier of the two.*

*Babies are criss-crossed, but with-
out pillows under mother's arms.
Mother's hands are clasped for
support. Tiring, but useful in a
dressing room or ladies' lounge.*

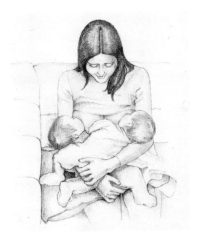

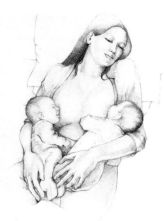

*Mother lies nearly flat on her back,
two pillows placed under her head.
Babies are in a "V," knees touching. Safe and comfortable position
for night feedings.*

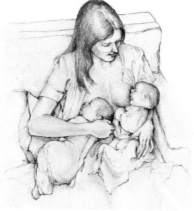

Babies facing same direction, with pillows supporting mother's elbows. A pillow on her lap may also be helpful.

Both babies in "football hold" position. Firm pillows are best, and the higher the pillows, the less the back strain. A footstool can add to comfort.

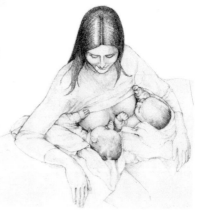

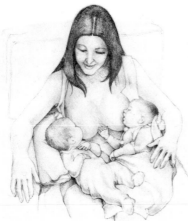

Babies lie parallel to mother's body. Pillows are placed behind mother's back and under each baby's head.

When you're by yourself and positioning tiny babies for simultaneous nursing, remember that they're not as fragile as we sometimes think. After placing one at your breast, using only your free hand to position the other baby won't hurt him.

By three months babies are easier to nurse simultaneously, because then they can hold their heads up and don't need as much help guiding the nipples towards their mouths.

When my twins were tiny babies and seemed to want a lot of nursing, we'd always settle down with pillows in the rocking chair after dinner. For the rest of the evening the babies would rock with me, and nurse and snooze at will, some of the time simultaneously, while I talked with my husband or three-year-old Suzy, watched television, and just enjoyed cuddling and nursing.

To Each His Own?

You can assign each of your babies his own breast or alternate between breasts.

Shawn consistently nursed the same baby on the same breast. "That way I was sure one wouldn't take all the milk and the other be left out. They each had their own supply so the stimulation was a demand schedule for each breast and each baby."

Some mothers nurse each baby from the same breast for one day, and switch breasts for alternate days. This has the advantage that each baby gets equal left and right visual stimulation and brain development while nursing.

Equal visual stimulation can also be accomplished by nursing each baby all the time from his "own breast," but alternating the position in which you hold him—sometimes across your body, sometimes in the "football hold."

I never worried about who had which breast, and it worked fine. When my twins nursed simultaneously, they each had one breast for the feeding. When they nursed separately, I offered both breasts to the nursing baby. She usually got filled up on one side, so at the next feeding I'd nurse from the fuller breast first (no matter who was nursing).

Scheduled or Demand Feedings?

Shawn's attempt at nursing her first baby lasted only one month, but she is now successfully nursing twins. "I figured out why I ran out of milk with my first baby," she says. "I had her on a bottle schedule, and the twins are on demand. That makes all the difference in a good start and proper stimulation. At nine months with the twins I still have plenty of milk."

Many mothers find demand feeding for each twin works out well. An exception might be if you're going out and want them both to nurse just before you leave. But aren't you nursing all day and night if you allow each twin to be fed on demand? Admittedly, it can seem that way, especially at first. But twins take up time no matter how they are fed. Four half-hour feedings in a four-hour span of time take the same amount of time whether they are following a prearranged schedule or are scattered at random throughout the four hours (assuming all nursings are separate nursings).

Jeanne nursed her twins strictly on demand, which averaged about 12 times in 24 hours. It was every 15 minutes at some times, every 4 hours at others. Some feedings were "snorts," some were 45 minutes, and others anywhere in between. Jeanne ignored the clock, feeling that withholding the breast because a certain amount of time had not passed would defeat the supply and demand phenomenon and tend to decrease the milk supply.

Can you still nurse each baby on demand at night, too? One mother who did says, "I kept the babies alongside our bed in a bassinet and buggy, and when one got hungry all I had to do was scoop the baby into bed, doze and nurse until the other one awakened, and then switch. This way the babies got the milk they wanted and I got the sleep I needed."

I had my own variation on demand nursing for nighttime. During the day I found it convenient to nurse each baby on demand, simultaneously if they were hungry at the same time. At night if they woke together, I nursed them simultaneously, but if one twin woke first I would nurse her, then awaken and

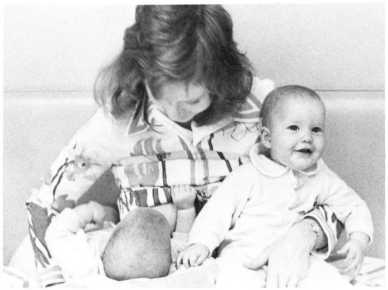

Sandra C. Wallace

With this arrangement, everyone's happy; one twin nurses while the other sits up to burp.

nurse her twin. This sort of "first come—both served" method could also be used during the day.

Burping

Some babies need burping while others don't. One mother of two sets of twins said that neither of the first set needed to burp, but both of the second set did.

When one baby is finished nursing, you can lay him face down across your lap and pat his back, while you continue to nurse the other. If they both need to burp, you can lay them across your lap, or lay one across your lap and "shoulder-burp" the other, using your free hand to pat one and then the other.

You can burp one baby sitting up, while continuing to nurse the other. Or, you can lay the baby on his tummy next to you on the bed and rub his back with your free hand. After burping, you can then bring him back with one hand for more nursing.

Solids

Your babies may want to start solids at different ages. One of ours became extra fussy at 4½ months, so we started solids. The other didn't start until 5½ months. Babies often have little interest in solids until they get a tooth, which can be around 9 months or later. A doctor may feel that the babies may get anemic on nothing but breast milk, but this is unlikely if the babies are thriving and weren't very premature.

When both your babies are eating solids, you can feed them together. Use one jar or bowl of food, one spoon, and alternate mouthfuls. Nurse them before the solids (if nursed *after* they'll not nurse as well and may wean too early). Or you can nurse one baby while you spoon feed the other with your free hand.

Teething

You may be glad you're nursing twins instead of a single baby if they get teeth at different times. If one baby drastically cuts down on his nursing (or quits for a few days) because of sore gums, you do have your other nursing baby to relieve your fullness.

On the other hand, if you happen to be nursing simultaneously when one baby decides to try out a new tooth, a sharp "No!" to him might just start both of them crying. Nurse them individually if you can for the next few days. Pretty soon the offender will learn not to bite while nursing.

Weight Gains

Although your twins will thrive on your breast milk, you may find a difference in their weight gains. This can be expected since each baby has his own rate of growth.

If one of your twins nurses more vigorously than the other, or more often, or for longer lengths of time, this may cause a noticeable difference in weight gains. Cindy says that in three months her boy had gained seven pounds while her girl had gained only four. The girl was healthy and thriving as was her brother, but he just nursed more often and longer than she did.

Weaning

Twins, like single babies in the same family, may wean at different ages. Sometimes one twin may continue to nurse despite an apparent readiness to wean, because the other twin is still interested in nursing. Mothers of twins usually hope the twins will want to wean a little later than single babies. The twin babies seem to need this prolonged closeness with mother, and as they get older, nursing may be the only time a twin has mother all to himself. Most mothers realize this and hesitate to wean arbitrarily. Most like the baby-led weaning idea.

If your twins are your first nursing babies, you may be surprised that nursing can continue for so long. You can of course encourage them to wean much sooner, but there is no age limit on nursing. Those of us who have nursed babies until they decided to wean themselves have found this a very satisfying way to end the nursing relationship.

Jeanne had an interesting experience with her twins and weaning. Weaned prior to a period of separation from Jeanne, they *unweaned* after the seven weeks during which they saw very little of her. Jeanne offered to nurse them, to ease their feelings of rejection. Her daughter nursed for short periods (three to five minutes), but her son nursed more heartily. A month after Jeanne was home continuously, he weaned again, while his sister continued token nursing a little longer.

Time to Yourself

If you feel you need some time for yourself or to be alone with your husband, a few hours out when the babies are settled into a schedule and take a 1½- to 2-hour nap may work best. Lunchtime can be a good choice. If your babies are taking their long nap from approximately 11:00 A.M. to 1:00 P.M., usually lunch is a little quicker and cheaper than dinner out.

It's best to avoid using bottles and missing feedings if possible. You'll be less likely to run the risk of getting overtired and getting too full, which could lead to a breast infection. Realistically, however, there just may be times when a bottle may seem practical. For example, if the twins have settled into different nursing schedules, and you're out shopping with one baby, you may not get back before a sleeping baby at home awakes and needs to nurse. It's good if you can have some extra breast milk in your freezer to tide him over. A bottle still might be avoided by giving the expressed milk by cup or spoon.

For the mother of twins, taking just one baby out with her may be enough of a refreshing novelty to provide a welcome respite from "double trouble." Another possibility is to take the babysitter with you, to entertain the babies between nursings.

Get Help!

Learn to accept graciously any offers of help. Spend all your available time in baby care and resting. Especially while your babies are young, you'll find that sleep, not milk supply, is your biggest problem. Sleep during feedings when you need to, having someone else bring the babies to you to nurse. Let others do housework, cooking, car-pooling, etc. Rearrange your priorities so that you are not exhausted all the time.

As one mother of twins put it, "The first year is tough. The first three months are 'impossible', but somehow you survive. Maybe your husband will take the babies out in the stroller for one hour while you take a nap. I was able to lie down whenever the babies napped after I decided dirty dishes and unmade beds could wait forever."

A high school girl to help out after school, a baby carrier (or two), a diaper service, a local market that delivers groceries—all these can allow you the time to pay attention to your husband and love your babies. It will be too late to enjoy them in the same way when they're older.

Traveling with Nursing Twins

Don't think you'll be stuck at home all the time with nursing twins. It's so much easier to go places with them than with bottlefed babies, because there's no need to carry along bottles and bottle equipment.

You can nurse your babies in the car if someone else is driving. One mother sat between her twins in the back seat. They were securely restrained in backward-facing infant car seats, while she wore a seat belt. When they wanted to nurse, she was able to lean over the hungry one.

For more about traveling with twins, see chapter 24, "Traveling with a Nursing Baby."

Helpful Hints with Twins

You'll appreciate all the time-saving hints you can get. Here are a few ideas that worked with my twins:

To save steps we had a bathinette in the bathroom at one end of our house; at the other end we put a pad on top of our dryer and used that as a second changing area.

We no longer worried about a bath a day. Once a week (or even less) is probably sufficient if you wash their faces and bottoms well daily.

Dad pitched in on the weekends and in the evenings; he would bathe one baby while I fed the other, cook and help with the laundry.

Our three-year-old, Suzy, was delighted to help in many ways. She brought diapers or tissues, helped bathe the babies and feed them solids, made her own bed, and helped to cook. While I nursed, I sometimes read to her, or sang songs with her, or watched her work a puzzle.

Here are some tips from other mothers of twins:

"You can save steps by wheeling the babies from room to room in a baby buggy, or put one in a stroller and carry one in your arms."

"You can rock one baby in a rocking chair and rock the buggy with the other foot."

"While the twins were small I found it very handy to use

an oblong laundry basket to carry them to the car. A car bed was just too bulky and heavy for me to handle."

"My 4½- and 2½-year-old children helped by setting and clearing the table, getting items I needed, and talking to the babies or singing to them."

"At night I kept the twins in one Port-a-Crib in my room until they were three months old. This was easier for me and they seemed to like the warmth of each other and always nestled together."

"I couldn't tell the twins apart at first, so for the first few weeks I kept their name bracelets on. I also had a chart so I could be sure each was getting sufficient milk. I would rotate the twins so the one that didn't get a lot at one feeding would get the fuller breast the next feeding." Here is an example of one of the charts:

Time	Twin	Breast	Comment	Twin	Breast	Comment
12:00 A.M.	Joni	L	vigorous	Kathi	R	vigorous
3:30 A.M.	Kathi	L	vigorous	Joni	R	pokey, sleepy
6:00 A.M.	Joni	L	vigorous	Kathi	R	vigorous
8:00 A.M.	Joni	L	vigorous	Kathi	R	vigorous
11:30 A.M.	Joni	L	pokey	Kathi	R	vigorous
2:00 P.M.	Kathi	L	vigorous	Joni	R	pokey
5:15 P.M.	Joni	L	vigorous	Kathi	R	pokey, sleepy
7:00 P.M.	Kathi	L	vigorous	Joni	R	vigorous
10:00 P.M.	Kathi	L	vigorous	Joni	R	vigorous
12:00 A.M.	Kathi	L	vigorous	Joni	R	vigorous

Complications

If you have complications, such as premature babies or a cesarean birth, ask for your babies as soon after delivery as possible. Even if you are not allowed to nurse them for several days, or even weeks, you can express your milk and request that the hospital give it to the babies. Once you return home you can build up your supply and continue with normal nursing.

Even when babies are healthy at birth, one may have to return to the hospital. To read how one nursing mother of twins managed, see the section, Hospitalized Child and

Another Nursing Baby in chapter 12, "When Baby Is Sick or Hospitalized."

Nursing Triplets

If your bundle of joy turns out to be three bundles, you can nurse them all. Here is what Shirley says about breastfeeding her three babies:

> The babies were born five weeks early by cesarean section. During the ten days in the hospital, I was only allowed one baby at a feeding, and they insisted on bottlefeeding the other two.
>
> Once we returned home I began nursing in earnest. At the end of two weeks, I only needed four to eight ounces of supplement a day. By the time my trio was two months old, they were totally breastfed.
>
> Around 6 months I started them on solids, and they were gradually weaned at 16, 17, and 18 months. (2)

Some mothers of triplets feed two at once, others feed them all individually. The frequency of nursings, not the length, is what counts. One mother found a king-size chair to be helpful, as she kept one baby at her side, one nursing, and the third lying across her lap. A chart can help keep track of the situation: note who was fed, the time of feeding, which breast, whether supplemented, and wet or messy diapers.

Discounting the Myths

Many people who haven't heard that you can nurse twins are very surprised, and some absolutely refuse to believe it. Don't let them discourage you, though. If someone hasn't nursed *one* baby successfully, it's hard for that person to imagine you can do it with twins.

Here are some reasons a mother of twins was given for why she couldn't nurse, along with her answers.

Objection	Reply
You'll eat like a horse.	I'd gained 40 lbs. while pregnant. By eating moderately and only when hungry, I've lost all 40 lbs. now that the babies are ready for solids (4½ months).
You'll be tired.	No more than nursing one, I find.
You'll have no time for the older children.	I use the nursing time for family time and have found no jealousy.

Not only friends and relatives, but sometimes doctors and nurses question whether it's possible to nurse twins. Listen well with one ear and let all the poor advice go out the other.

Your Cheering Squad

The more encouragement and help you have from those around you, the easier it will be for you to nurse your twins or triplets.

Mothers of twins and triplets say it is especially helpful to get in touch with a supportive pediatrician *before* the babies' birth, and to be in touch with a mother who has nursed twins or triplets. (You can contact one through La Leche League.)

There are also Mothers of Twins clubs, where you can meet with other mothers to discuss and share practical ideas on twin care. To find the one nearest you, contact your newspaper or write to the Twins Mothers National Organization, listed in Appendix: Organizations to Help the Nursing Mother.

Chapter 19

Nursing an Older Baby

He's a curly-headed cherub with a devilish glint in his eyes,
A noisy bundle of mischief, about pint-sized.
He bangs with his hammer, the favorite of his toys,
And people tell me, "He's all boy!"
But then in the night when he comes to me,
I'm suddenly aware of his vulnerability.
He seems so helpless, so innocent, so small,
It seems like just yesterday he was learning to crawl.
He snuggles up close, seeking my breast,
And even in sleep, nurses with zest.
Once more I am grateful for these moments we share,
And whisper softly, "Whenever you need me, I'll be there."

Eric, My Nursing Toddler
by Rose A. Sodergren

When does a baby cross the threshold and actually become an older nursing baby? As a mother, how can you recognize when baby enters this stage? Is it the cuddly four-month-old who is friendly with everyone but still needs mother for his food? Is it the eight-month-old who loves to squish his food through ten tiny fingers as he eats his solids, but still gets his milk from mother? Maybe it's the one-year-old crying in the night because that new tooth is hurting. Snuggling with mother and nursing is all the comfort he needs to fall asleep again. Or perhaps it is the lively fifteen-month-old toddler who needs comfort after a fall; or that rebellious eighteen-month-old who says, "No, No, No," but still wants the comfort and security of being allowed to nurse. (1)

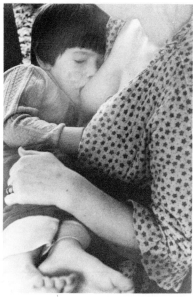

Nursing an older child provides him with emotional benefits, as well as being a rewarding experience for mother.

Sandra C. Wallace

No matter at what age your baby is labeled "older," it is true that as he begins eating other foods, he becomes less dependent upon nursing as a source of nourishment. Why, then, should you continue to nurse?

Though your little one may no longer need the nutritional benefits of breastfeeding, he may very well need the emotional benefits. As he explores that big world out there and is confronted with new and often frightening situations, he may need the warm reassurance that nursing offers.

There will probably be times when you'll find yourself wondering if he's going to nurse forever, but for the most part, nursing an older child is a deeply rewarding experience. The older your baby gets, the more responsive he becomes. He smiles and gurgles, and reaches up to give you love pats. As he learns to talk, he will delight you by responding verbally to nursing. It feels so satisfying when, after having a little "snack," your toddler looks at you with eyes full of love and says, "Mmm, that was good!"

Dependence-Independence

Probably the most common question about nursing toddlers is, "Can it make the child too dependent upon his mother?" This is a natural concern for mothers brought up in a society that expects infants to sleep through the night at six weeks, potty train by one year and completely wean shortly thereafter—a society that in general expects them to act like miniature adults instead of children.

It *is* true that the nursing baby is dependent on his mother for comfort. These are "the dependent years" that we hear so much about, and it makes sense for us to allow children to be dependent and to be there when they need us most. It is an important time in a child's life, for it is a time when they learn to trust others.

It seems contradictory to expect our little ones to magically become independent at some arbitrary age with no consideration for individual differences. Real independence isn't something you can force on a child. It's something he reaches out for, a little at a time, as he's ready. When a child is forced to become independent before he's ready, he's likely to react by becoming more dependent than ever before. He becomes confused and upset. He cannot begin to understand why suddenly he is expected to abandon all his baby ways which a week before were quite acceptable. In his confusion he understandably seeks out his main source of reassurance and security—mother. He wants to be with her constantly. He may cry if she merely goes to another room. The more "clinging" he becomes, the more determined are his parents that he is overly dependent and that he must "grow up." And so the vicious cycle continues.

In her book *Mother Love, The Book of Natural Child Rearing* (2), Alice Bricklin writes that a child's sense of trust and dependence on people is basically formed during the first few years. This is the basis for love as the baby comes to know and understand it. Without being able to rely on someone's comfort in response to cries (a child's only form of communication before learning to talk), the child's reactions to people's behavior can become mixed. This is because it is difficult for a child to understand why a parent will respond to some cries but not to others. The child becomes confused and in many cases apathetic.

However, if a child is accepted and loved just as he is, and allowed the freedom to outgrow each phase of babyhood, toddlerhood, and childhood at his own pace, he will grow into independence and emotional security as an older child and an adult.

For babies with special problems, such as those requiring many hospitalizations, nursing into toddlerhood gives them a security which is vitally important to them.

As Dr. Thomas Harris writes in his bestseller, *I'm O.K.— You're O.K.* (3), "If you baby a baby when he's a baby, you won't have to baby him the rest of his life."

Weaning

Weaning begins the day your baby takes his first mouthful of some food other than breast milk. As he begins to eat more and more other foods, he will probably nurse less and less, until he is nursing only to sleep, or during times of stress or illness, or after an accident. As your child grows and becomes secure in the knowledge that you'll be there whenever he needs you, he'll gradually decrease the amount of nursing. One day you'll realize it's been several days or weeks since he has asked to nurse. As his demands to be nursed decrease so will your milk supply. When he does wean, your breasts will have gradually adjusted, too. Natural, or baby-led, weaning is usually a gradual process that extends over a period of time. Just as baby gradually learns to walk, talk, and eat with a spoon, so will he wean from his mother's breast.

NOTE: This steady, gradual weaning process is not, however, the pattern with all toddlers. Certain children have sucking urges until four years old or longer that peak in frequency around 18 months. (4) Also, babies sometimes increase their nighttime nursings, if they get too absorbed in daytime activities to nurse during the day. Children with these sucking needs who are not breastfed find satisfaction with pacifiers, thumb sucking, or bottles.

In order to confidently accept the idea of natural weaning, try to look at it from your child's point of view. Once you do this it is easier to continue despite possible criticism from friends or relatives.

To help you understand how your child feels when he is being weaned, think how you would feel if you smoked and really enjoyed your cigarettes. Then one day you decided to quit. You've made the decision yourself; you're ready to give it up, you feel good about it and proud of your accomplishment. Imagine, though, how you would feel if someone you dearly loved (your spouse, for example) came up to you and said, "That's it, no more smoking," and took your cigarettes away. You'd be nervous and upset, for the person you love most has deprived you of something you enjoy. This might be how a child feels if all of a sudden his mother says to him, "You're two years old, you don't need to nurse anymore."

Early or abrupt weaning can be a deeply traumatic experience for a child. Pick up any psychology book and you're likely to find numerous case studies describing emotional disturbances in adulthood that were caused by how people were weaned. It doesn't seem wise to pick some arbitrary age and say this is the "right" time to wean your child when it has been proven over and over that each child will wean himself when he is ready.

There may be times when you might consider gently encouraging your child to wean, for example, if another child is on the way. (See chapter 16, "Nursing While Pregnant," and chapter 17, "Nursing Siblings.") But even then, weaning should be a gradual process. No child should be asked to quit "cold turkey."

If you believe your child may be nursing from boredom, try suggesting an alternative such as playing a game, reading a story, taking a walk, painting a picture, baking cookies, washing dishes (young children enjoy *anything* having to do with water), raking leaves, or going to the park. The possibilities are endless for activities in which you can *both* be involved.

You may find that many times your baby will happily accept such an alternative because asking to nurse was merely a bid for your attention anyway. Some mothers find that a conscious effort to spend more time doing things with a child decreases the number of times he asks to be nursed. However, there will be times when your child genuinely *needs* to nurse. Remember, he *will* give it up when he's ready to. Don't worry about nursing *too* long. It is virtually impossible to force an unwilling child to nurse.

Those who yield to societal pressure and wean their babies themselves often regret it later. One mother told me, "I nursed Liza for eight months and everybody approved when I weaned her. However, I sat and rocked her to sleep while she sucked her thumb every night until she was 2½."

Our twins were a little over two years old when they nursed for the last time. About a month after they had weaned, Karen asked to nurse again. I was willing, but she just sat with her mouth in position on my right breast, seeming not to know what to do. She was down from my lap in a few seconds. Then she pointed to my left breast and said, "Sharon's." "Do you want to nurse there?" I asked. "Uh huh." Karen climbed back on my lap, but again didn't suck when her mouth was in position. She got down, and said, "Sharon nurse." Sharon, busily playing nearby, voiced her own opinion of the proposal with an emphatic, "No!" They never asked to nurse again, which made me a little sad, for after they had weaned I looked back over the time they had nursed and realized what an interesting and wonderful adventure it had been.

Advantages of Nursing

Benefits to Baby

The road from infancy to childhood is not a smooth one. There are bumps, bruises, colds, the flu. Other stressful situations to cope with are moving, traveling long distances, and visiting relatives. Such situations bring with them feelings of unhappiness and insecurity which the nursing toddler has a direct and simple solution for—he indicates in his own way his desire to nurse. Within minutes the problem is solved.

As one mother put it, "What do you do with a fussy two-year-old in the middle of the night if you can't nurse him back to sleep in five minutes flat?"

For allergic children, the importance of prolonged nursing takes on added significance. Lada's little girl, Eleanor, was born totally allergic to almost all food except breast milk. If Eleanor had not been nursed, she would have been hospitalized and fed intravenously. Lada says:

> Our total medical bills for the first two years were well under $100—compared to those of friend who had a highly allergic child who was weaned at five months. That child could tolerate several foods. Between the ages of five months and two years, that family spent over $4,000 on doctors, hospitals, and medicines. For the highly allergic child, breastfeeding saves great sums of money as well as a great deal of trauma.

Some children are so allergic they need to be hospitalized even though they are breastfed. Continued breastfeeding is greatly beneficial to them. (See Dr. Kimball's statement in *Your Diet during Lactation,* in the section Preventive Measures, chapter 11, "Dealing with Allergies.") Janet describes her experience:

> My 23-month-old daughter, Jolayne, is still an enthusiastic nurser, although she is a severe asthmatic. During her many hospital stays, I stay with her "round-the-clock," frequently nursing her both for reassurance and for her prescribed need for constant intake of fluids. In fact, the doctors and I have a deal that as long as I frequently nurse her, she is not required to have the otherwise mandatory I.V. . . . She's allergic to all dairy products, and soy and beef protein, so thank heaven she still nurses.

Benefits to Mother

Many times nursing an older child is a godsend for mother as well as child. Frequently a mother who is nursing an older child is looked upon as a martyr because she is "giving so much of herself" to her child. Some people don't seem to consider all mother gets in return.

Suzanne, nursing her three-year-old daughter, Jennifer, said:

I am not nursing "a three-year-old." I am nursing Jennifer who has gradually grown into this relationship with me. So often new mothers are led to believe that they are going to suddenly wake up one morning and nurse an unwieldy child, but this just isn't so. The times I nurse Jenni are *intense* personal communications in which we take mutual pleasure.

Jeanne has boy-girl twins who weaned at age 2½. When they were 3, their 14-year-old sister was hospitalized for seven weeks for two major surgeries. Jeanne stayed with her after each surgery for several entire days, not seeing the twins at all. Jeanne says:

After the first days of separation, both babies appeared to be feeling rejected. I immediately offered the breast, and both graciously accepted this symbol of love-in-spite-of-separation. . . . My offering of love was important to them; but their acceptance of it gave me the strength I so desperately needed at such a traumatic time.

Everyone Benefits

Besides becoming more independent and self-confident, children who are nursed until they wean themselves seem to share another, perhaps more important quality: a loving acceptance of others.

Bette's little girl, Sarah, nursed until shortly before her sixth birthday. Bette says:

Sarah is a really great person—I don't know of anyone who hasn't commented that they really liked her and what a nice child she is. I feel she's the person she is largely because she was given love and attention when she needed it. She's rarely around me now, with school and friends. Sarah's kindergarten teacher commented that if the other children in her class were to know as much about people at the end of the year as Sarah did already, she would consider herself a successful teacher. She said Sarah was helpful without being condescending, kind, thoughtful, and imaginative. For the first time with my children I feel *I* had a lot to do with encouraging such positive attributes.

These qualities are particularly important to mothers like Tina who is partially blind (she has only 10 percent of her vision). Speaking of her two-year-old nursing son, Aaron, Tina says:

I used to wrestle with the problem of "you're spoiling your baby" . . . but now I'm happy because he's more independent than most children his age and more content. Some mothers seem to want their children to grow up so fast that they end up by missing out on basic security. This comes out later when they cling to mother, are very withdrawn, or extremely aggressive. A child's needs should be thought over. Give him his security and tender care now. Be with him while you can and he will leave you happily and you will let him go because you have shared all the moments you needed with him. You won't have to say, "Why didn't I spend more time with him?" If we give our children a bond of love and security as their foundation, then they will love us, too. I feel that our nursing relationship has made us so close that Aaron understands many things already. If I lose something, he always finds it for me. He learns not to hide important things because he doesn't want to hurt Mommy. He always waits patiently while I take the extra time I need to dress or take care of him.

Pam concludes by saying, "The joy I have found nursing

my boy as he has grown older, the love and cherished time together seems to grow with the months. . . . It's not spoiling a child to make a habit of showing love."

Biting

Many times, when biting occurs, it's towards the end of a feeding when baby isn't really interested in nursing anymore, and wants to play. If this happens, immediately tell your baby, "No" (gently the first time). If he bites again during the feeding, stop nursing and perhaps put him down for a few minutes. This will help him learn that he should not bite you.

At the next feeding, if he tries to bite again, say, "No," more firmly. Stop nursing when your baby begins to lose interest, to avoid a bite.

Brigid, the mother of an infant *born* with a fully grown tooth, says that after about two weeks, even her tiny baby had learned what a firm "No!" meant, and was nursing beautifully without any biting. (See If Baby Bites in chapter 4, "Breast and Nipple Problems.")

In addition to firm "No's" it's important to give positive reinforcement for correct behavior, too. By this I mean that if your baby nurses correctly, stroke him, tell him soothingly, "Yes, that's right, honey, that's the right way to nurse," or whatever words are natural for you. And learn *why* baby bites. Even though we can't allow it, baby is often giving us a very valid message through the only way he can communicate— biting. The message may be: stop talking on the phone or to your company and pay attention to me; stop chastising the older children while I'm nursing (they often act up then), and love me; I need a quiet room (sometimes a baby will put hands over his eyes or ears while nursing—you get the message); or I need eye-to-eye contact with you now, mother. As always when children misbehave, we have to show them firmly that we can't permit the misbehavior, and yet we must seek the causes for it and remedy them whenever possible.

It's also well to keep in mind that a baby nurses with his tongue over his bottom teeth, and he must pull his tongue in before biting. If your baby is becoming a biter you can watch carefully for this change in nursing rhythm and anticipate a bite.

To withdraw your nipple from your baby's mouth, don't pull him off the breast or you may get a sore nipple. Release the suction by slipping your finger into the corner of his mouth. Closing the baby's nostrils is also a quick, effective way to stop a bite.

Some babies have more of a tendency to bite when they are teething. This inclination usually declines after the tooth is in.

Your baby may enjoy chewing on hard, cold things while teething, but once a tooth is through he may prefer just the opposite to try out the new tooth. He may want something soft and squishy. Avoid a bite at this time by offering alternatives he can really sink his teeth into, such as a nice, thick, juicy piece of meat, or a slice of toast.

Nursing in Public

Nursing an older child in public may present a problem, especially when the child is old enough to verbally express his desire to nurse. Because of society's attitudes, it can be disconcerting, if not downright embarrassing, when suddenly, in the middle of the supermarket your little one exclaims, "Mama, I want to nurse!"

Many mothers find that using a special word for nursing helps to avoid this situation. Marsha, when nursing her son, Matt, started referring to his "snuzzling," a word coined from his nuzzling and her snuggling.

Other mothers use words like "num-nums" and "loves" to refer to nursing. That way when a child asks to nurse in public only his mother knows what he means and can respond accordingly.

If a child's need to be nursed is not urgent or if there's no privacy available, you may wish to wait until you're home or in the car. This is best handled by saying something like, "Okay, I'll nurse you as soon as we get home (or to the car or

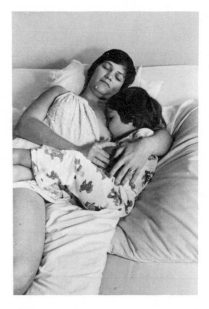

Night Nursings

A child goes to the natural source of comfort and security—his mother's breast.

whatever)." This is a positive answer and is often more readily accepted by the child than a flat, "No, I can't nurse you now." Anticipating your child's needs helps to avoid having to refuse to nurse. Try to anticipate your child's hunger or thirst by offering him something before he has to ask to nurse.

Night Nursings

It is common for young children to wake at night. They know nothing of the "rule" that says they're supposed to sleep through the night in their own beds in their own rooms. When a child wakes at night, he feels lonesome, perhaps anxious, maybe a little scared. Naturally he looks for his parents, especially his mother. Whether nursing or not, this is very normal. If he is nursing he will probably seek the comfort of his mother's breast and nurse until he feels secure again. You can put a pillow between your child and your husband to keep him from kicking his father while nursing.

Some mothers find that when a nursing child wakes at night, he is able to get out of his bed and come to his parents' bed on his own. Once there he can practically "help himself" to his warm snack of mother's milk with minimal interruption to their sleep.

The need to come into the parental bed may continue even after the child weans, but just as he weans from the breast, so will he eventually leave the comfort of his parents' bed.

Nursing Your Son

If your nursing child is a boy, you may notice that even as a small infant he has occasional erections while nursing. (Bottlefed boys have erections too, when they nurse on their bottles.)

NOTE: Erections are not so noticeable with a bulky diaper on an infant, but they are common at any age, for nonsexual emotional reasons (fear, tension, anger). (5)

Dealing with Conflicts

Your Own Feelings

As nursing continues past nine months, a year, two years, your relationship with your baby will probably change. Eventually he may only want to nurse when he is hurt or frightened or tired. Nursing becomes even more personal than with a younger baby.

Even though you enjoy nursing most of the time and think it's wonderful that your baby is getting this superior nutrition and the other benefits of breastfeeding, there may be times when you become impatient or wonder if you really want to continue. Perhaps your husband or someone else has made a remark that has raised doubts in your mind. Second thoughts and self-doubts emerge occasionally, no matter what project we undertake. Self-evaluation and reassessment of our priorities are a normal part of life and in no way belong exclusively to the mother nursing an older child. As with any worthwhile endeavor, our "off" moments while nursing usually are overshadowed by all the good ones.

427

Here is what one mother, Lynne, experienced:

I was so glad to be able to offer nursing when the world was too frustrating to Jason, or when he was overtired. Jason was all mine at those special times. When he went through "difficult" cycles of behavior, nursing kept me not only tuned in but also loving him.

When Jason was three, nursing was mostly at night or at home. This happened so naturally. He just plain wasn't interested in nursing when there were other things to see and do.

I did periodically experience feelings of not wanting to nurse an older child. These feelings were scary for me. I didn't understand, and I felt guilty. I loved Jason so much. They first appeared when Jason was around 2½. I'm sure they were related to outside pressure. But also I began to feel that it was nature's way. These times of wondering whether or not I was doing the right thing in nursing Jason never lasted long. Jason's need for nursing and being close to Mommy always came across *loud* and clear.

People's Attitudes

Nursing an older child may sometimes be annoying or inconvenient, just as mothering in general can be, but the biggest disadvantage many times lies, not in the nursing relationship itself, but in others' attitudes towards it. Friends and relatives may consider you some sort of "oddball." Others, even doctors, may think that you nurse for sexual gratification. They seem to completely overlook the needs of the child. There seems to be added concern if the nursing child is a boy. This may stem in part from our society's attitude that breasts are primarily sex objects, and also from the fact that boys have occasional erections while nursing.

Even though in some countries children are nursed until they are five or six years old, it just isn't "the thing to do" here in the United States. You may try to explain to people why you are nursing, that your child still needs this, that the two of you just enjoy it, that it is best for you. However, as one mother said:

> I could explain, but I was limited by people's ability to really *understand* what I was saying. They just didn't seem to hear. This is something mothers nursing an older child have to contend with. You do a lot of growing as far as your values go when you learn to look at nursing, and weaning, from the point of view of a child's needs. There were times when the outside pressure made me wonder if I was really doing the right thing, after all. I guess it's normal for you to wonder, when you're in the minority.

Ours is practically the only culture in the world that encourages premature weaning from the breast. It is acceptable for a child to have a bottle, suck his thumb, or have a security blanket until he is three or older, but unacceptable for a child to receive this comfort and security at his mother's breast. Is it really emotionally healthy for a child to seek solace from objects rather than another human being?

Nursing an older child is not unnatural, as some may imply, but it may be *uncultural.* Still, how can you cope with others' attitudes? What do you say when Aunt Betty discovers that four-year-old Johnny is "still" nursing?

Rose offers this solution:

> I found that people's reaction of shock and dismay was because they'd simply never come in contact with it before. By explaining that instead of a thumb, bottle, or blanket, Mary had me, they were able to understand a little better. I also added that I was glad Mary could get this security and comfort from me, a person, rather than an inanimate object that couldn't love back. This type of explanation was usually quite well received. Sometimes I would also point out how important gradual weaning is, and that many emotional problems are caused by how and when a child is weaned; I simply refused to take the responsibility that "now" was the right time for my child because I knew she'd wean when she was ready.

Fathers

Sometimes fathers who accept breastfeeding as normal and natural for infants may not be so accepting as the baby grows older. Some fathers urge their wives to wean before mother and baby are ready.

Your husband may be concerned, perhaps even without fully realizing it, that mother might remain the focus of the child's attention, when *he* wants to have his share. He may want your attention more, too. He may be worried that he'll be "tied down" indefinitely with a child who continues to nurse, or be concerned about night nursings interfering with sex.

What can you do about these concerns? First of all, remember that each family is different; each family must work out its own solutions when conflicting views are present. These thoughts from other mothers may give you ideas for your own situation.

Communication. Communication is a must to understanding each other and coping with problems. When feelings are repressed, they tend to get out of proportion. Explain yourself fully. Never take it for granted that your mate understands what you are saying. Be specific, not general. If your husband wants you to wean, urge him to talk about *why* he thinks you should do so. Listen to him. Accept his feelings. Tell him why *you* want to continue, why it is good for *his* baby. Your husband needs to know your feelings in order to understand them. Much of the trouble can be avoided or greatly minimized by talking about mixed feelings and the reasons behind them while baby is very young. Reading and discussing such books as *Touching* (6) and *The Family Bed* (7) can help you grow together in your views about the nursing toddler.

While baby is still little, encourage your husband to play an active role in his life. He may not feel a need then to compete with you for your child's attention as the child grows older. It's a good idea for father and baby to have special times alone with each other, right from birth, even if only for five or ten minutes a day.

If the baby gets upset being away from you, don't push it; it will only make it worse to force the issue. Your husband can take the baby in the bathtub with him, perhaps while you are in the room, too, so baby doesn't panic. Or, how about going to the park? You can sit on the bench while father pushes baby on the swing. *You* suggest things to do, since you're familiar with your baby's favorite games and toys. Do this while baby is fresh, not tired or cranky. Always start out with a rested, happy baby, and take it slowly.

Your husband's competition for *your* attention can be alleviated if you make special efforts to do nice things for him, too. For example:

• Spend at least five minutes a day sharing the good things. Pick a time of day that is quiet, maybe morning before you get out of bed or over a cup of coffee, or at bedtime as you snuggle close together.

• Surprise him—love notes left in obvious places or in his lunch box.

• Write down your feelings. Sometimes that's the only way you can say them. Also write him a love letter and send it in the mail.

• Find out what he feels are the essential tasks. If you take care of them, he won't be so ready to notice other things left undone.

• Plan a candlelight supper of his favorite foods.

• Keep in touch. Go up to him and rub his back or ruffle his hair or pat his hand. Sit next to him and hold his hand while you are nursing the baby.

• Share with him the happy, funny things that happen as a result of nursing an older baby.

• No one likes to be taken for granted. Tell him how much he means to you, how you count on him for his love and support. Tell him you think he's a terrific husband and father.

Being Tied Down.   Being tied down with a baby, whether breastfed or not, is largely how you look at it. My husband and I found it was a lot easier just to pick up and go on an outing than it would have been if we'd had to take bottles and warming equipment along. It was so easy to nurse in the car or plane whenever a baby got hungry.

A conflict may arise if a baby has a need to be with mother *all* the time. He is miserable if she leaves him with a babysitter or with father. He needs to be nursed to sleep. He wakes up several times during the night wanting the reassurance of nursing and mother's presence. As baby gets older, this could become increasingly irritating to a father who wants his wife to leave the baby with a sitter while they go out for an evening. What can you do about this?

It helps to recognize that whether breastfed or bottlefed, some babies are more dependent in the first year or two. They need the presence of mother to develop the emotional security that carries them through life. While you are in the middle of this intense dependence, it seems endless, but it really isn't.

During this period of intense dependence, you can try keeping a record of baby's sleeping habits for a week or so. Maybe you'll discover a particular pattern that you can work around. For example, if baby sleeps a couple of hours at night before waking to nurse, you and your husband could go to a nearby restaurant for a late dinner. If baby should awake before you get home, the sitter can call the restaurant and you can be home in a matter of minutes.

Perhaps you and your husband would enjoy going to an occasional movie. Simply take your nursing baby along, dressed in pajamas ready for bed. Nurse him to sleep in the darkness of the theater while you and your husband enjoy the show. Other times, you may be able to take your baby with you for a social evening or even a weekend away. Perhaps you can take a babysitter along with you who will entertain or watch your nursing baby between feedings. Of course, there may be times when your husband can go out without you, as in the case of job-related social activities.

One couple discovered this ingenious idea: every once in a while mother, father and baby would spend the weekend at a motel. No one had to cook, make beds, or clean house. It was a change of environment for all of them. They ate and slept whenever the mood struck. All came back home refreshed!

And finally, here is what one mother and her husband decided:

> After discussing "being tied down," we decided it really doesn't matter all that much about having an evening out. It's just easier to wait a bit. There'll still be a whole lot of life left after the baby is older, is ready to accept our temporary absence, and is secure in the knowledge that we will return.

Baby in Parents' Bed.   Some babies continue to wake during the night. Some nurse for many months or years. Others start sleeping through the night when they are a few months old but may still have occasional wakeful nights (perhaps because of an immunization, a bad dream, or teething) and need the comfort of nursing.

As your baby grows into toddlerhood night nursings in bed might be viewed with some resentment. However, they can be taken as an interesting challenge, especially in regard to lovemaking.

Look for a way in which each one's needs can be met. A child's need to be with parents is not restricted to *nursing* babies. Many children who are *bottlefed* also wake frequently and want company. Sleeping together can be viewed as an opportunity to extend the amount of time you share your parental love with your child.

As for lovemaking, one mother wrote, "If the baby sleeps with you and sometimes wakens, try making love in another part of the house. Many sex manuals suggest this as a way of putting some variety and zing into your sex life anyway. Or how about outside under the stars when it's warm? Once in a while, call your husband and proposition him to come home at lunchtime. Meet him in a nightie and forget lunch."

One mother wrote me:

> Our baby frequently wakes up about 10:00 P.M. I'm still up at that time, so I nurse and rock him awhile until he goes back to sleep. He usually sleeps a few hours before coming into our bed, so we have ample time for lovemaking. There are times when our lovemaking is interrupted. At these times it's no big deal. I bring the baby into our bed and nurse him back to sleep while my husband and I continue to snuggle and caress each other to keep in the mood. Frankly, these interruptions often make it that much better in the end for us. Anticipation can heighten arousal! Occasionally we go to bed ourselves when we put the baby down around 8:00 P.M.

Another mother said she and her husband resolved the conflict about bringing the baby into their bed when he woke crying in the night by having baby sleep alongside father. Both the baby and his father liked this. Baby loved the protection of sleeping under his father's arm, and Dad did not feel left out any more. Once or twice a night, when baby was thirsty, he would climb over to his mother to nurse, but then climb back to his father for cuddling.

Mary White, one of the founding mothers of La Leche League, tells how she and her husband have come to manage their own "sleepless smalls":

> With the last several children I have simply let them stay with me until they are asleep and then moved them into their own beds. Frequently this meant two, three, or four hours uninterrupted time before they woke up and cried to be picked up and nursed again. So I again tucked them in between us, nursed them back to sleep, and then, if I

was still awake, moved them back to their own beds.

Sometimes this didn't work, as the minute head touched bedsheet they woke up again. In that case, I decided that the only thing to do was to get into the restless baby's bed rather than bring the baby to our bed. Now, this is really easier than it sounds, because I found that babies do very well in a regular size bed from the time they are two or so. Surprisingly, they rarely fall out. Before that age, I simply spread out enough blankets on the floor to be comfortable and lay down there with the baby. Then when he dropped off to sleep, I was the one who did the moving and he wasn't disturbed at all. This way, you can see that we really didn't have a child in bed with us all night at all.

Maybe we're just lucky, but the fact is that as we've become "old hands" at parenting and more relaxed and cheerful about responding promptly to the babies' needs, we've rarely been upset for long by a wakeful child. From the time a little one is three or so she or he sleeps happily with an older sister or brother. (8)

Breasts. Some mothers find that their breasts are more sensitive while they are nursing, and they don't want them handled too much. On the other hand, you may find that your breasts are *less* sensitive to touch and thus need more stimulation by your husband. Tell him, so he will understand why you are reacting the way you do.

One mother said, "When our first baby was little, my husband did not like the taste of breast milk, so he did not fondle my breasts much. Actually, it wasn't so much a matter of disliking the taste as it was his feeling that that was for baby, not for him, and if he 'nursed' he'd be depriving his child of her breast milk. Also, he thought that after nursing the baby all day, I wouldn't like it if he 'nursed.' We talked about it, and once his true feelings were out in the open, it was easier for him to overcome his inhibitions. Now he loves it!"

Some men get upset when they see an older nursing baby play with the nipple of the breast that is not being nursed at the time. But this is a normal occurrence and many older nurslings do this.

To sum up, open, honest communication between husband and wife is essential, especially when conflicts occur. Each family must find its own particular solutions. Leave room for failure. Your first solution may not quite work, so try again. A willingness to make some adjustments goes a long way. Breastfeeding won't last forever, and your child will be a more secure and happy person because both his parents met his needs when he most needed them.

Comments from
Satisfied Customers and Admirers

Ranking high on the list of treasured childhood memories are the comments that the children themselves make about nursing. They are funny, candid, and often wise beyond their years.

Toddler: Mommy, can I N-U-R-S-E?

Mother: Why are you spelling it?

Toddler: So no one else will know.

Five-year-old Greg asked his mother one day, "How come Stephen (18 months old) isn't still nursing and he's so little yet?" His mother says, "Wouldn't it be nice if the rest of society felt the same way?"

Mary says that when she asked her son if he wanted a "drinkie" he changed it to a "winkie." As an older nursing baby, it was always acceptable when he asked for a "winkie" when out in public.

A toddler explained to other children who fell or were unhappy for some reason, "Mommy will nurse you and you will feel better." Sometimes the toddler even said, "I will nurse you and you will feel better."

One little boy, when asked if he remembered when he used to "have a breast," said very seriously, "No, I don't suck on your breast anymore, I am a little kid, not a baby. Your breasts are just loving things." His mother concludes, "I thought that if all he can remember about nursing is that it was loving, then those two years were really special."

Bette tells of something her daughter Sarah said "which made all those night nursings seem worth it. When she was four, she placed her doll's crib right next to her bed. She explained that 'if my baby needs me in the night I'll be right there.'" Bette adds, "Right then I felt she would probably be a better mother to her first child than I was to mine."

When asked to help her mother with a list of advantages of breastfeeding, five-year-old Laurie thought for a moment, then offered, "Because it makes the baby happy." "Why else do you think babies should be nursed?" asked the mother. "Because it makes the mother happy," was the prompt reply.

Lori wrote: "One day last week was particularly frustrating for our 18-month-old nursing toddler. Her four-year-old brother repeatedly took her toys and teased her, saying, 'They are mine, Jennifer, they are all *mine!*' Later that evening, she crawled into my lap, patted my breast, and with a look of triumph, grinned and whispered, 'Mine.'"

Perhaps the most poignant comment comes from a child who himself was bottlefed. Tricia tells this story:

> While we were visiting relatives, I slipped into a quiet room, away from household noise and older children's hubbub to nurse two-month-old Brian. As he and I relaxed together, the door opened softly to admit Danny, my four-year-old nephew. Danny had never seen a baby feeding at the breast; he was both fascinated and puzzled.
>
> "What's the baby doing?" he asked.
>
> "He's nursing," I answered. "This is how he gets his food."
>
> "What's that?" was the next question, a finger pointed at my breast.
>
> "That's part of me," I said. "I have milk there for the baby."
>
> For a moment Danny was quiet, busily sorting out that information. Then the light dawned.
>
> "Oh," he said, drawing on his four-year-old knowledge of anatomy. "I understand now. You feed him from your heart."

And finally, here is how one satisfied mother describes it:

Nursing a toddler is not always fun,
It seems that nothing else ever gets done.
Nursing an infant is peaceful and sweet,
But nursing a toddler with mud on his feet?
With peanut butter mouth and a handful of cheese,
He pushes you down and climbs on your knees,
He positions himself 'till he's comfy and steady,
Then tugs on your blouse so you know that he's ready.
You look down and smile and you give him a drink,
Knowing those dishes are piled in the sink,
Knowing the clutter is still on the floor,
Hoping that nobody comes to the door.
Oh heck, you lean down and you give him a kiss.
What can you do that's more important than this?

Nursing a Toddler
by Maryann Malecki

Your Cheering Squad

Because of the criticism nursing an older child may draw from friends, relatives, or even doctors, the nursing mother in this situation needs a special kind of support and encouragement. Your husband's support is very valuable. Contact with others in the same situation can do much to reassure you that you're not the "freak" others may seem to think you are. Such contact is made possible through attending La Leche League meetings. Some La Leche League groups have couples' nights or fathers' nights. Consult the list of recommended readings in the Bibliography for books that can offer reassurance and insight.

The husband's role is summed up beautifully by an experienced father of two breastfed children. He says:

Nursing is a relationship between two people. It's more than a mere biological function. The husband must see this and accept it as good for both wife and child or he will unconsciously become a barrier to the relationship. To his wife it is a unique experience of her womanhood and an opportunity to give of her substance to one she loves. To the child breastfeeding not only gives the best healthful food but also submerges the child in warmth and security. This complete personal acceptance, as so many mothers attest, seems to develop emotional security and independence of character in the breastfed child. If the husband really believes this, the sacrifices he makes are pretty easy. An untidy house, children in bed with parents, unsympathetic doctors and relatives—these barriers are overcome together. If people are important to the couple, the "price" paid is nothing compared with the personal dividends.

Chapter 20

Nursing Strikes and One-Sided Nursing

Reasons for Nursing Strikes

Living through a nursing strike can be a frustrating experience for the whole family. Hopefully, you can find out what is wrong, and find a quick solution. But sometimes it's not that easy. You want to nurse your baby. You know he is hungry. You want to comfort him. Yet, he cries, perhaps takes a few sucks, screams, spits out the nipple, bites, turns away, or shoves you away with his hands. Faced with this behavior, you may feel rejected, frustrated and impatient. As one mother said, "You reach a point for a little while where you just can't cope."

Nursing strikes do indeed require a great deal of patience and understanding. It helps to keep in mind that it's not you, it's the child. Keep attuned to your baby's moods and actions; they can help you figure out what is going on.

The reasons babies go on nursing strikes are as varied as babies themselves. It can happen at any age. Sometimes the same baby may have more than one nursing strike, perhaps for different reasons. Nursing strikes may last a few days, a week or sometimes longer.

If you can discover the reason your baby goes on a nursing strike you may be able to do something about it. At least your understanding of the problem will help you through this difficult time.

Teething Pain

When a baby is teething, his gums are very sensitive.

Some babies increase their nursing at this time, turning to nursing for comfort. Other babies turn away from nursing temporarily because it simply hurts to suck. When you settle down to nurse, your baby may bite, stiffen or fuss. Medication for his gums may help. Nursing in a different position may change the pressure to a different part of his gums. Try nursing lying down, or using the "football hold." (See illustration in section Simultaneous or Separate Nursings?, chapter 18, "Nursing Twins.") If he's old enough to drink water or juice from a cup he can get some liquids that way.

Herpes: Sores in Baby's Mouth

Sores in baby's mouth also make it painful for him to nurse. Joni's 18-month-old son, Jason, a frequent and contented nurser, suddenly stopped for no apparent reason. For an entire day he refused all nourishment and wouldn't take water. The reason he couldn't stand anything in his mouth became apparent when the doctor diagnosed the open sores on his gums, tongue and throat as herpes. This is similar to cold sores, but much more extensive and painful. Joni describes how she handled the situation:

> The doctor said there was no medication to ease the discomfort so we could only wait it out and force fluids. Dehydration was a very real possibility and then hospitalization would be necessary. We fed him with a teaspoon every chance we got and found he would only accept small quantities of tea after trying milk, water, and yogurt.
>
> The next day Jason could handle a little broth but still could not nurse although he tried desperately to hold the nipple in his mouth. We went through all the motions of our normal nursing pattern such as rocking, singing songs and a great deal of body contact. They did seem to comfort him a great deal during the three days that he did not nurse. When he resumed it was only for a short time, but each day he nursed longer and soon we were back nursing much the same as before the herpes.

Congestion in Nose and Throat

Sometimes a baby will go on a nursing strike when he gets a stuffed-up nose. He can't breathe comfortably while he is nursing and stops to inhale through his mouth. This can happen along with teething, if he gets a cold, or with another illness. If your baby has a problem with congestion, oral decongestants or infant-strength nose drops before a nursing may help, but your doctor must determine if the baby is old enough. A humidifier in the room helps the baby tolerate the congestion. Breast milk is less likely than cow's milk to aggravate the congestion.

Baby Feels Rejected

If a baby feels rejected, unwanted, or as if he has done something wrong, this may prompt him to stop nursing.

Regina says her son Michael suddenly stopped nursing at 5½ months. She then realized that her two older children had started using nursing time as "Mommy can't stop us now!" time, and she had been retaliating by shouting. Michael was probably frightened, thinking she was shouting at *him*. She solved the problem by giving the older children something interesting to do while she nursed Michael in the quiet of his room. When she gradually reintroduced him to the noisy "outside" world, she used soft singing as her only contribution to the sound effects. (1)

When a baby starts to get teeth, it's a natural thing for him to try biting while he is nursing. Your flinching, or sharp "No!" could puzzle the baby, until he figures out why you are reacting this way. Your unhappiness with him, coupled with his discomfort from teething, may make him decide not to nurse anymore. You can try just touching a finger to his mouth, as a gentle reminder to stop biting. (See also Biting, chapter 19, "Nursing an Older Baby.")

When Eric was six months old, Rose was busy with the hectic process of moving. Without realizing it, she would sit down to nurse Eric with the attitude, "Okay, kid, let's get this over with, so I can get back to work." Eric sensed this, and even though he was ravenously hungry, he absolutely refused to nurse unless she lay down with him and gave him the total, relaxed attention he deserved. As soon as she realized what the problem was, the situation improved immediately.

Easily Distracted Baby

Some very sensitive babies, when they are a few weeks or a few months old, begin to be distracted by their surroundings while nursing. A nursing strike may be a baby's way of expressing his displeasure with what's going on.

What can you do in such a situation? Maybe you can figure out what is going on in your baby's mind. If distractions upset him so much, avoid them as much as possible. Before beginning to nurse, take toddlers to the toilet, prepare a plate of finger foods, provide story books, take the telephone off the hook and have tissues and something to drink within reach. You might find your baby will nurse contentedly if he is alone with you in a quiet room, apart from all activity. You might have to do this for several weeks, when you want to calm your baby to nurse. (2)

Mother's Let-Down

As a baby gets older a mother's let-down may get slower, and the baby may be impatient to get the milk, which could lead to a refusal to nurse. The less baby nurses, the slower the let-down. Expressing a little milk before nursing might help shorten the time it takes for the let-down to occur, once the baby is at the breast.

A let-down that is too strong for the baby to handle can also trigger a nursing strike. When John was three weeks old, he began to refuse to nurse. This went on for four weeks, during which he gained no weight. His mother, Darcy, found she could rock him to sleep with a pacifier in his mouth, then nurse him in his sleep for a long time. She did this for many months until he was able to relax enough to nurse while awake. In cases like Darcy's, where the let-down may be too strong, expressing some milk and waiting to nurse until after the let-down and initial surge of milk may be helpful. See Over-abundant Milk Supply, chapter 7, "Newborn and Infant Problems."

Preference for Bottle

The way a baby sucks to get milk from a bottle differs from his sucking when breastfeeding. The milk almost drips out from a bottle, but with breastfeeding, your baby has to draw out the milk (this promotes better mouth and jaw formation). If they are offered an occasional bottle some babies become confused or are lazy nursers, and choose bottles rather than nursing.

How many bottles can you offer, without running this risk? It's hard to say. It depends on the individual baby, but it's best to use bottles only when needed. In *The Family Book of Child Care* (3), Niles Newton says, "If you give a bottle to your new baby twice a week, simply accept the fact that it will probably mean your baby will be totally bottlefed by the time he is three or four months old. It just works out this way most of the time. The bottlefeeding deprives the breast of some stimulation and teaches the baby to suck less hard. Psychologically, that feeling of 'you belong to me and I belong to you and there are no substitutes' disappears. One bottle usually leads to another."

If your baby is turning away from breastfeeding, and prefers a bottle, what can you do? Before offering a bottle, first offer to nurse him. Expressing a little milk before nursing will help get your milk flowing and the taste of it may encourage your baby to start nursing. Something sweet, like honey, on your nipple may help, too. (Just add a dab—don't overdo it.) If he is too fussy to try nursing when he is very hungry, try a little later in the feeding, and try nursing him in his sleep. It's best if the milk in the bottle can be your own milk, instead of sweetened formula. If you can offer him other milk from a spoon or cup, he'll have a greater need to turn to you to fulfill his sucking needs. You might also try slightly diluting milk you give in a bottle. See *Reducing Supplement* in the Supplemental Food section, chapter 15, "Inducing or Reestablishing Your Milk Supply."

Vastly Dwindling Milk Supply

If your milk supply decreases greatly, your baby may scream with frustration as he tries to nurse. You might have a poor let-down because his screaming upsets you and because you simply don't have much milk. This can start a cycle which can end in a baby's turning against nursing.

There are several reasons for a dwindling milk supply. Some mothers get involved in a lot of things. As they become very busy, they find it's easy to have someone give their babies a bottle. If the babies fuss a bit when they do sit down to nurse, the mothers may become discouraged and give them bottles.

A mother who is under a lot of stress and doesn't find it easy to relax may find that her let-down reflex is not working well.

The "Pill" can decrease supply. Hormonal changes during pregnancy sometimes cause a decrease in the milk supply or a change in the taste of the milk. Decongestants like Contac and other cold or hay fever remedies have also been known to cause decreased supply.

A baby who is used to a fast flow and good supply in the early days of nursing may begin to suck lazily as he grows older, and his ineffectual sucking may mean he doesn't get enough milk even though he may spend long periods at the breast. This may cause your supply to drop.

Early introduction of solids can also cut into the milk supply, with some babies. With a tummy full of food, a baby is not as likely to be interested in nursing. The less he nurses, the less your breasts will be stimulated to produce milk. Most breastfed babies don't need solids for about six months.

The remedy for a decreased milk supply depends on the

baby and the reason for the decreased supply. Some babies go on a nursing strike and can never again be coaxed into nursing. If you've been especially busy, try cutting down on your activities, for a few days at least. Some mothers cut out solids. Others do away with bottles and are there to nurse the baby any time he wants. Watch your baby's diapers (six to eight wet diapers a day are enough), particularly if he is a young baby; if he seems too dry, you can give him water from a clean cup, syringe, or spoon. See chapter 2, "Nursing Techniques," for a discussion of How to Insure a Good Milk Supply.

Milk's Taste

The taste of the milk may change because of menstruation or the onset of it, pregnancy, or the use of an oral contraceptive or other drugs. Smell and taste are closely related. If you are wearing a new perfume or have used perfumed cream or soap, the milk or nipple may seem to have a different taste. Once a foreign substance is removed there should be an improvement.

Separation from Mother

If you and your baby are separated for a few days, perhaps because one of you is hospitalized, or because you are away from him on a trip, the close nursing bond may be broken. If one of you is hospitalized, try to continue nursing during the hospitalization. One mother I know went away on a ten-day trip when her baby was five months old. When she returned her baby refused to nurse; he would only take a bottle. You can't always tell what your baby's reaction will be. Depending on his personality, he may feel rejected and reject you, too.

Is It a Nursing
Strike or Weaning?

How do you distinguish between a nursing strike and the baby signaling weaning? It may not be obvious, especially if the baby is several months old and there is no apparent reason for him to be on a nursing strike. If for several days you have been trying to find a cause and have been encouraging him to nurse, but he still refuses, it may be that he wants to wean. You may not be prepared for this if you were expecting weaning to occur much later. It can be disappointing at first, but your baby still wants and needs *you*, even though he no longer wants to breastfeed. If you are still unsure about whether it's a nursing strike, offer now and then to nurse him. Should he decide he wants to resume, you will be able to build up your supply again by frequent nursings.

The Baby Won't Nurse: Checklist

Whether your baby refuses to nurse at one feeding or more, or from one breast or both, here is a list of ideas you might check for finding the problem and possible solutions.

Physical Search

Before stripping the baby, see if his clothes fit comfortably. Then look for rashes. Are hair, lint, or threads in places where they cause discomfort? Check his hair, eyes, fingernails, toenails, genitals. Note the color of his skin on fingers, toes, ears, trunk, limbs, face. Is his belly stiff or bloated? What's in his mouth when you look with a flashlight? While pushing his tongue down with a spoon, check the color of his throat; a fiery red means it's sore, pink means it isn't. Suspect an earache if he pulls at his ear or cries when swallowing. If you have access to an otoscope, look at the ear yourself; white skin is normal, pink or red signals an infection. Rub a finger over his gums; any lumps or sharp edges almost through the skin mean baby's teething. He may either pull away from your finger or lean closer so you can continue to rub. If he merely sucks your finger, he's not teething. Fever, loose bowel movements, drooling and crankiness may also accompany the new teeth. Finally, note any differences in body temperature, crying and behavior.

Emotional Search

All babies respond to feelings rather than words, regardless of how they are fed. What were your feelings about the baby or about breastfeeding before the baby refused to nurse? Might he be responding to some mixed emotions? Are you particularly tense because of a domestic situation? Financial problem? Pain, apprehension, tiredness or frustration? Could these feelings be influencing baby's behavior?

Some Ideas That Have Worked for Others

(Many of these ideas have already been described throughout the book, but are repeated here for quick reference.)

Drink a relaxing beverage.

Touch your nipple or rub baby's gums with ice just before the feeding.

Wear a plastic breast shield between feedings (for inverted nipples).

Dab honey on your nipple or in his mouth.

Stand up to put him to breast, and sway or walk.

Use the "football hold."

Nurse in a different position when in bed.

Go in a darkened room; outside; be with others; away from others.

Put him to breast while he's asleep.

Stop shouting at other children while nursing.

Move away from loud and distracting noises.

Put on some soft music.

Stop using a new perfume.

Nurse him nude, skin to skin.

Stop taking medication, birth control pills.

Avoid foods with monosodium glutamate (possible allergy).

Express milk until you get a let-down, then start nursing.

Express, feed some milk with a spoon, then put baby to breast.

Trickle extra milk in baby's mouth while nursing.

Use breast pump or hand expression to increase supply.

Hot weather? Put dampened diaper over your arm where his head rests, or lie down with your nipple in his mouth, but bodies not touching.

Stop using supplements or offering other liquids in cups.

The solutions for refusal to nurse are varied. Some babies begin to nurse again as suddenly as they stopped. You may never discover why the baby went on a nursing strike, which is fine if you can help him back to the breast anyway. When a baby does not nurse and does not gain weight over a week or more, there is cause for concern. In this case, medical attention is needed as well as breastfeeding information.

One-Sided Nursing

For various reasons, mothers and nursing babies sometimes prefer nursing from just one breast. The preference may be only temporary or it may continue until the baby weans. Some mothers are satisfied with one-sided nursing; others try to encourage the baby to return to nursing from both breasts.

By Baby's Choice

Some babies seem to prefer one breast because it is closer to mother's heartbeat. Others favor a breast because they get more milk more easily from it, due to a physiological difference in the breasts. A breast infection can change the taste of the milk in one breast, causing a baby to turn to the other. An earache or teething discomfort may also account for his choice of a favored side.

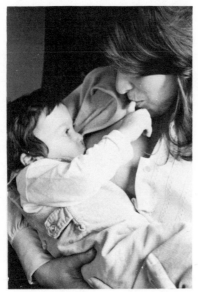

Georgia, nursing Brett.

When Brett was 1 month old, Georgia had a breast infection in her left breast, which developed into an abscess. The doctor advised her not to nurse from that side, so Brett nursed satisfactorily from the right breast only, for more than 2 years.

Sandra C. Wallace

By Mother's Choice

Some mothers find nursing more comfortable on one side than on the other. Elissa, who nursed all of her children on one breast, says, "I just preferred the left side. I soon stopped forcing myself to use the right side and my milk became more copious in my left breast. I still had some milk in my right one and always knew I could use it fully with a little effort, but my babies all seemed satisfied with just one breast."

If you feel more comfortable holding your baby on one side, but don't want to encourage one-sided nursing, you may need to make a conscious effort not to favor that side. Due to a childhood accident, Sheri's left arm was weak and sometimes ached. When she held her baby she had a natural tendency to use her right arm. Perhaps sensing tension, her baby became reluctant to nurse from the left side. After Sheri used pillows to support her left arm during nursing, her baby began nursing from either side.

Let-Down and Milk Supply

If one breast produces more milk or has a faster let-down than the other, the baby may prefer the breast from which he can obtain the milk more readily, or the one from which the flow is slower.

You may be able to build up the supply in a breast by offering it first at each feeding for several days, although a very hungry baby may be too impatient to suck from that breast first. Try stimulating the milk supply by expressing from that breast between feedings or by using a breast pump. You might also encourage your baby to nurse from the more slowly flowing side by feeding him extra breast milk with an eyedropper or a Lact-Aid supplementer as he is nursing. (4)

A plugged duct might inhibit the flow of milk and cause a slow let-down. See Plugged Ducts section in chapter 4, "Breast and Nipple Problems," for what to do about this.

Differences in Nipples

Some mothers whose nipples are different sizes find their babies prefer the smaller nipple, while other mothers say their babies prefer the larger one. The favorite nipple may be the one where the let-down is faster. If one nipple is inverted, the baby may have difficulty latching onto that breast.

Jody's babies did not accept both breasts equally until they were about six weeks old. She noticed that with the breast they avoided, the milk shot *up* from the nipple as well as forward. To encourage her babies to nurse from that breast, when they were hungriest she nursed them on the breast they were avoiding. She nursed them in their sleep and sometimes gently awakened them to let them know where they were nursing!

Nursing Positions

Try nursing in different positions. Sit in different chairs, lie down, stand, and change holds to place the pressure on different areas of the nipple. When sitting down, you can hold your baby in the usual position at his favorite breast, then switch him to the other breast almost without changing his position. If you are nursing him from the right breast, with his feet pointing to your left, you can move your body and move him to your left breast while his feet remain pointed in the same direction. He then ends up in the "football hold."

If you nurse your baby in bed at night, always nursing him in the same position and from the same breast, he may begin to prefer that position and breast during the daytime as well. Sleep on the opposite side of the bed some of the time so that your baby will still be facing you, but lying on a different side. Also, you can nurse your baby in bed from both breasts while he stays in the same position. After finishing with the first breast, simply turn your body to offer him the second breast.

Nursing in different positions and alternating sides is necessary for bilateral eye muscle development. If your baby is nursing from one breast and in the same position over a long period of time, make sure to hold him on the other side when not nursing, to ensure the eye muscles an equal chance of developing normally.

Is There Enough Milk from One Breast Only?

Many mothers who do nurse their babies from one breast only encounter no supply problem even when they have a good-sized, vigorous nurser. As one mother says, "A woman naturally seems to have an ability to supply twins, so nursing one baby on one side fits within this ability."

Other mothers find they have to gradually work up to a sufficient amount. This may depend on the baby's age, nursing patterns, and the situation.

Excess Milk

Will unused milk in one breast leave you uncomfortably engorged? Many mothers find no problem with this, especially if their babies gradually begin to prefer one side. However, there is no harm to you if you have excess milk in one breast. Express some milk whenever your breast becomes uncomfortably full. You can use a breast pump, or express by hand. You may only need to do this occasionally. Most mothers find that the unused side eventually dries up completely.

One-Sided Nursing's Effect on Your Appearance

Mothers vary in the amount of the "unbalanced effect" they get from one-sided nursing, and their reactions to this vary, too. A mother who found a difference said, "Most clothes didn't matter, but I couldn't wear anything clingy. To solve that problem I went to a store that fits women who have had a breast removed and ordered a false breast. This false breast was the most natural looking one I could find. Made of soft, flesh-colored rubber, it had a nipple on it, and was filled with a gel. It was covered with a washable (removable) bralike material, and it felt almost like a real breast and looked very real when inside a bra. I didn't wear it every day, only with clingy clothes."

Mastectomy

The question of whether it's safe for a mother to nurse after having had a mastectomy has no clear-cut answer. There is no conclusive evidence to indicate whether breastfeeding afterwards is or is not harmful to a mother's health. Due to this unproven status and lack of specific guidelines, you are advised to consult several surgeons before making a decision.

Does nursing reactivate a cancer? Medical authorities are divided on this issue. Certain doctors advise against nursing, feeling that the hormones involved with lactation are of the type that will stimulate residual malignant cells to grow. Others contend that nursing will not necessarily trigger a recurrence of cancer. Dr. Michael J. Brennan of the Michigan Cancer Foundation says, "I do not think that nursing aggra-

453

vates a tumor or even breast cancer. If eradicative surgery has succeeded and removed all the cancer from a woman, there is no reason for her to act any differently from then on, than she would have had she never had a cancer."

Even doctors who agree that *nursing* is not harmful differ on the risk posed by *pregnancy*. Certain authorities see pregnancy as more likely than nursing to increase the estrogen level which could stimulate malignant cells.

There is general agreement that a woman who has had a mastectomy doesn't endanger her *baby* by breastfeeding. The idea that cancer is a virus and could be passed through a mother's milk is discounted, and it is widely accepted that a tendency to cancer is passed on genetically, instead. Dr. Laman A. Gray, of Louisville, Kentucky, says: "The ability to breastfeed depends on the amount of milk available. If the woman has sufficient milk to nourish her child, I can see no danger to the baby." (5)

When deciding whether to nurse, you should take into consideration how long ago your mastectomy was performed. A previous operation probably will not interfere with your ability to breastfeed. If yours was a recent operation, exhaustion, pain, chemotherapy or radiation therapy could adversely affect your physical condition. It is possible to nurse following an operation and mothers have done it, but it may be a strain. Trying different positions may lessen the discomfort of a sore back and muscles. Nurse lying down, or if sitting up, have someone else hold the baby or use pillows to prop him up.

As for whether you will have enough milk to nurse from one side only, it is possible, as the previous examples of one-sided nursing have shown. Mothers have been able to fully breastfeed their babies following removal of one breast. Besides undergoing a mastectomy, one woman also had a lump removed from her remaining breast when she was five months pregnant. After consulting several doctors and weighing their advice, she decided to nurse. She was able to maintain a good milk supply and never needed to supplement. (6)

Chapter 21

Nursing during
Stressful Times

*God, grant me serenity to accept the things I cannot
change; Courage to change the things I can; and Wisdom
to know the difference.*

> Dr. Reinhold Niebuhr
> Professor of Applied Christianity
> Union Theological Seminary

Dealing with Stress

What qualifies as an upsetting situation, and in particular,
upsetting to a nursing mother? Problems may be mild or
severe: the baby is fussy, friends may disapprove of nursing,
the car has a flat tire, a family member becomes ill, a death
occurs. A situation that is very upsetting to one person may
not affect another person to the same degree. No matter what
triggers the upset, stress is the result of any pressure that taxes
your resources.

There is a popular myth that in order to be able to breastfeed, you must be in good physical and emotional health, have
a healthy, full-term baby, have two properly shaped and placed
breasts and nipples, maintain a bright outlook on life, and stay
relaxed.

The myth continues: you should not lose sleep, eat poorly,
get sick, get divorced, bear criticism, go to graduate school, go
bankrupt, become pregnant, do physical labor, meet professional obligations, be exposed to death or dying. What
fantasy! Women in Nazi concentration camps nursed their

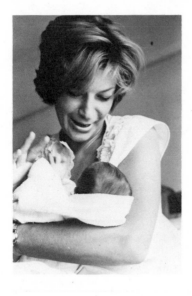

Women in varied situations have coped with emotional and physical upsets, while still maintaining the breastfeeding relationship. A tranquil, sedentary life is by no means a must for successfully nursing your baby.

babies under atrocious conditions. Margaret Court, a professional tennis player, nursed and played in tennis tournaments. Natalie Wood nursed while she maintained her career as an actress, taking her nursing babies on the set with her. These are just some prominent examples of women whose lifestyles discount the myth.

Family Communication

When one member of a family is upset, the entire family is affected. No matter how hard you try, you cannot prevent others from sensing your anxiety, since unspoken messages come across loud and clear. Being honest with yourself and telling your family what you want and how you feel can help ease relations. When you let your family know how you want them to help you, they learn how to express themselves.

A family's mutual support is invaluable in handling stressful situations. A family which works together to solve a problem functions at a higher level than before.

One mother, Sonia, wrote about her need for comforting and acceptance. Her baby had a very poor sucking reflex for several months. It took patience, understanding and a lot of extra effort to continue breastfeeding in the face of such remarks as "Your baby is allergic to your milk," and "You're upsetting yourself so much, that's why your milk's not letting down." Sonia says:

> My husband was very good, but he just didn't realize the amount of time the two children took. My most desperate need was to talk with someone, someone who could know just what I was going through and could understand and comfort me. Neither my husband nor our parents could accept that ours was a very sick baby, and the demands on me far outweighed what I could tolerate. I was very lucky to have a good friend who was also a La Leche League leader and who had a willing ear.

Anxiety and Fatigue

Both anxiety and fatigue can distort your view of what is really happening and hamper your ability to handle a situation. Exhausted? Get some rest. Overwhelmed? Get some help. Can't eat? Concoct nutritious drinks yourself or stock up on fruit or vegetable juices. Losing your milk? Nurse the baby more often. Simple solutions exist, but may be difficult to find when you're upset. If at times you think you're a failure as a mother, you share a feeling common to almost every mother who has ever lived.

Events Unrelated to Nursing

When your baby seems fussy and hungry, do you have doubts about your milk supply? Of course, the baby may be teething, ready for solids, catching a cold, or reflecting your fatigue. But if this is not the case, ask yourself what has happened recently that might have caused you some concern. Something unrelated to breastfeeding may be bothering you. For example, one mother was concerned because she had forgotten to put stamps on her birth announcements and they had all just been returned. At the next feeding when she tried to nurse, there was no milk (or so it seemed). Her supply was back to normal though, at later feedings.

Does this mean you must always avoid stressful situations? Must your milk supply have special attention? Do you feel "different" because you're lactating? Without doubt, your milk supply is influenced by pain, fatigue, anxiety and fear. (1) However, this influence need not be adverse or long lasting. With information, desire, and support you can cope with almost any obstacle. (2)

Lada describes how she combined nursing with an active lifestyle:

> I've spent over eight years nursing babies, in sickness and in health, emotionally tranquil, or emotionally distraught. The baby always got fed. Nursing has not prevented me from leading an active life. When my fourth baby was three months old, I went to work full time. Then I entered law school which was one giant trauma, with the pressures of studying and exams. I found that my emotional state seldom affected my milk supply. The only time my milk wouldn't let down was just before I played in the finals of a city tennis tournament. I couldn't salivate or lactate, I was so nervous. I have also suffered an emotional trauma sufficient to cause amnesia, but my milk supply was uninterrupted. No one stays healthy, calm, and relaxed for eight years; nursing doesn't have to depend on a stress-free environment.

How do you weather the storms while nursing? It helps to keep in mind:

- Milk can be obtained directly by the baby, or by breast pump even if you are not relaxed.

- Nursing stimulates production of the hormone prolactin, which helps you relax.

- Drinking plenty of liquids is vital to secreting milk.

● For emergencies, keeping some extra breast milk in your freezer is good insurance.

● If you have started to wean, reconsider. Once you regain composure you'll be able to provide plenty of milk for your baby.

Reactions to Upsets

What does being emotionally upset mean to you? What happens? A group of fifty nursing mothers completed the following sentence: "When I am emotionally upset, I feel _____ (a feeling) and then I _____ (a behavior)." (3) Responses to this sentence were varied and revealed the uniqueness of reaction to stress as well as similarities. Following are examples:

When I am emotionally upset,

I feel	frustrated	and then I	cry
	anxious		go in circles
	tense		fuss a lot
	frightened		can't sleep
	angry		spank the kids
	depressed		eat
	pessimistic		argue
	worthless		wish I were dead
	sensitive		get my feelings hurt
	burdened		lose my appetite

It's interesting that no two of the respondents answered with the same paired words.

A way to share feelings and information with your husband is for each of you to complete a sentence such as: "When my spouse gets upset, I feel _____ (a feeling) and then I _____ (a behavior)." Perceptions of each other may differ from what you anticipated. Checking out these differences and validating your anticipations is part of communicating effectively. Breastfeeding can be an easy function when your marriage grows along with your baby.

Despite open channels of communication, situations may arise that elicit a different response from each of you. Imagine that you are a nursing mother and your husband has invited some business friends over for the evening. As usual, you nurse your baby discreetly. Nobody seems to notice until later, when the baby burps up a little milk. Someone remarks she didn't notice your giving him a bottle; you reply that he is breastfed.

When the guests have gone, your husband surprises you with a request. He wants you to nurse the baby in the privacy of the bedroom from now on, as he heard a negative comment from his colleague. Would you . . .

do as he asks?

refuse him?

compromise?

avoid entertaining?

have him take his friends elsewhere?

bribe, plead, threaten, accuse?

tell him how you feel?

Talking about and accepting each other's feelings can help you to discover more about each other. It is okay to "see it differently" and still feel good about yourself and the other person.

Effect of Hormones on Emotions, Milk Supply, Conception

Your emotions and your milk supply are influenced by the hormones prolactin and oxytocin. Prolactin is reputed to be one of the most expensive substances produced by the body, and it cannot be synthesized. It is involved in the development of your breasts and in stimulating milk production. It is also believed to stimulate and maintain a strong mothering instinct in pregnant and lactating women. Oxytocin is involved in the release of milk and in causing your uterus to contract, which stops the flow of blood after childbirth. These two hormones together have a tranquilizing effect that you may notice through a rush of peaceful, warm, or euphoric feelings when your baby nurses.

Prolactin is also involved in ovulation. When you nurse your baby, the sucking stimulation produces prolactin, which normally inhibits ovulation for several months. However, if you are upset for a few days and your let-down is affected or you nurse less frequently, there is a greater chance that you may become pregnant. The contraceptive effect of breastfeeding cannot be counted upon. If you do not want to become pregnant, use some other form of contraception (but not an oral contraceptive).

Expressing Milk

For some mothers, expressing (or pumping) milk even when they're completely relaxed seems a difficult task to accomplish. Is it any wonder then that they find it practically impossible to express milk when they are feeling tense? Even mothers who normally find it easy to express sometimes have difficulty when under stress. Your attitude can help.

Ginnie points out how important attitude is:

On the day of my daughter's operation, I tried to express milk for her and only got one ounce, total, from both breasts. I panicked and thought I was losing my milk. I became very depressed and called my La Leche League leader. She assured me I had not lost my milk and gave me encouragement. I tried to rest and drank plenty of fluids (wine and tea). Sure enough, the next time I expressed milk, my supply was more than adequate.

Another mother found she didn't have any milk buildup when her six-week-old daughter was hospitalized and was unable to nurse for two days. She says:

I had been very tense and worried about my baby, and my body just seemed to shut down production. I tried to express some milk to leave for the nurses to use while I made a quick trip home, but couldn't get more than a few drops. I didn't worry at all about having enough for my baby when she could resume nursing, and after a few nursings she got an adequate amount of milk. I was confident in my body's ability to let the supply meet the demand (no demand, no milk), so I didn't worry myself unnecessarily about trying to keep up full production when it wasn't needed.

Some Stressful Situations

There is no cookbook recipe for problem solving. Although approaches to solving problems are often suggested in this chapter (and throughout the book), they are merely meant to be springboards for your own solutions.

The following situations include descriptions of how some mothers have handled their stressful experiences and may provide reassurance and ideas about handling your own.

The Blues

The third day following childbirth is the traditional day for "the blues" to set in. Childbirth is considered to be one of the greatest challenges in a woman's life, and 10 to 40 percent of new mothers experience a depression from one day to two weeks postpartum.

The impersonal setting of a hospital plus separation from your husband may be enough to trigger a case of "the blues." But even with husband-coached childbirth, in a family-centered facility, you still may become depressed. Changes are taking place physically, emotionally and socially. Your parents may not be available to cheer you up. Your husband is experiencing the strange new status of fatherhood, and he, too, has anxious moments. Perhaps you have doubts about facing the very personal and private implications of becoming a mother. Did you know that some adoptive mothers experience the same "blue" feelings? (4)

The mixed emotions often seem to erupt on the third day, and the distress usually passes quickly. Whatever the cause, both you and your baby *will* survive, your milk *will* come in, your baby *will* get the nourishment and nurturing he needs. (5)

Early Separation

Early separation of mother and baby due to birth complications or other problems often has lasting effects on a mother's emotions.

Mothering feelings may need to be developed later if nature's instincts have been interfered with. One mother relates, "My baby and I were separated for a month after birth. I cared for her and went through all the motions of loving her, but I didn't feel that way. In fact, she was a stranger to me for the first five months before I began to feel genuinely motherly towards her."

Breastfeeding is one of the best ways to develop the closeness and mothering feelings that were disrupted by an early separation.

Thoughtless Remarks

Prejudiced or thoughtless remarks can add to the anxiety of an already upset mother. When you are feeling comfortable with yourself and your baby, the remarks are soon forgotten. When you feel insecure, remarks can hurt and build resentment. You can protect yourself in two ways:

- Be aware that the remark is a statement about the speaker's feelings or experience, not about you.

- Be aware that the remark could be a distorted perception rather than the truth.

People who need to increase their own feelings of worth

may do so at your expense by criticizing your actions. If you think that a person is prejudiced or thoughtless, and you feel defensive, angry or at a loss to reply courteously, these suggestions may be helpful:

- Give the speaker at least ten seconds to reformulate his comment. In other words, say nothing for ten seconds.

- A prejudiced person is not ready to hear your facts. There's no need for you to defend yourself, unless you choose to do so.

Other people may simply want information, in which case you give them facts. It is best to keep in mind, however, that the same statement, from different people, can mean different things. When someone says, "How long are you going to nurse the baby?" he may mean, "In my opinion that child should have been weaned months ago," or, simply, "You're the first of my friends who has nursed a baby. I'd like to know more about it." It's gratifying to tell people what you've learned, if information is what they are seeking. Even when a person doesn't agree with you, you can "agree to disagree," each respecting the other's right to his own opinion.

Deciding whether a remark is hostile or a matter of natural curiosity is difficult. If you give people the benefit of a doubt, tune in to their underlying needs, offer understanding and sympathy, and supply information if they seem to be asking for it, you may be surprised how few thoughtless remarks you do encounter.

The following is a collection of common remarks made to nursing mothers, what the meaning may be to the person making the comment, and examples of responses. This sample of possible answers can help you find your own satisfactory way of dealing with similar situations. Remember, *how* you reply can be just as important as *what* you say.

Remarks You May Encounter, Their Possible Meanings and Sample Responses

Remark	Meaning	Response
"How do you know your milk is rich enough?"	I feel unsuccessful at breastfeeding. Your success points out my failure. When you are doubtful, I'm more confident.	"Nature made it that way." "I only produce the richest kind!" "By the looks of my baby, I'd say he's doing pretty well!"
"Didn't you just nurse him?"	I'm not this attentive to my baby. I feel threatened by your commitment, your ability to think for yourself.	"We love to cuddle." "He evidently forgot!" "That's the nicest part; we're not tied to any schedule."
"Aren't you awfully tied down?"	I am fearful of intimacy, responsibility, commitment. I'd feel tied down if I were you.	"I'm indispensable and like it that way." "I sure appreciate your concern, but no, I'm not." "A nursing baby is so portable, it's really the opposite of being tied down."

Remarks You May Encounter, Their Possible Meanings and Sample Responses

Remark	Meaning	Response
From your mother: "I couldn't nurse, so don't be surprised if you can't, either."	I listened to poor advice. You are a good mother, therefore I must have been a bad mother. I didn't want to nurse and can't face that now.	"I feel fortunate I can do it, with the help of lots of information and support that you might not have had." "You've been such a wonderful mother, that's what's important." "Confidence is half the battle, and I'm certainly giving it my all!"
"If you nurse longer than three months, six months, nine months, a year, you'll become flat-chested or big-breasted."	Breasts are sex objects to me; if they changed, I'd lose some sexual identity and feel less feminine.	"That's not really a big concern of mine." "The change isn't that drastic." "Actually, it's pregnancy that causes the change in breasts."
"What if you get sick, baby gets sick, your milk doesn't agree with him?"	Will I be stuck with the baby's care if you get sick? I'd feel insecure if I were you.	"I'm enjoying my baby too much to spend time worrying about things like that." "I can see that you're worried, but he's doing fine." "One of the reasons I'm nursing is because babies are healthier on breast milk."

466

"You don't nurse him every time he cries, do you?"	I let mine cry. Is that wrong? I'm scared by commitment; it sounds inconvenient, burdensome.	"Sure, it's his way of telling me what he wants." "Not always; sometimes he just wants comforting." "Do you have some other ideas? This works well for us."
"If you weren't nursing him, I could help you more."	I feel left out. I feel jealous. I need some attention from you, too.	"But you've been so much help already! We could never have made it without you." "You'd probably like to hold him more. How about giving him his bath next time?"
"Don't be a martyr. You don't have to breastfeed to be a good mother."	I feel helpless, guilty, resentful, insecure.	"You know, you really are right. There are lots of wonderful mothers who bottle-feed." "Who's a martyr? I really enjoy breastfeeding."
"He'll never let you go; you're making him overly dependent."	I feel rejected when the baby refuses to come to me. I disagree with your ideas on child rearing.	"I understand that you see it that way, but we each have our own way of doing things." "Our closeness now will make him secure enough so that he can be independent."

Remarks You May Encounter, Their Possible Meanings and Sample Responses

Remark	Meaning	Response
"How long are you going to nurse that baby?"	I'm uncomfortable with baby-led weaning. I need your attention. I can't understand that sort of closeness.	"You're wondering when he'll wean? I'm curious about that, too." "That's up to him and how long he seems to need it." "I'm not worried, we're in no hurry to stop."
From your husband: "When can we get back to a more familiar schedule, go out more?"	I feel neglected, left out. I miss our old relationship. Help me adjust to fatherhood.	Make love at the earliest possible time and talk it over afterwards. Tell him how necessary he is to you and the baby and how you feel about him. Work out new ways to be together.
"You nursed only 17 months? I nursed for 3 years!"	I need for you to know that I can do it better, because I feel inferior in some ways. I need praise.	"You sound really happy about your nursing experience. I'm glad." "Your child certainly was lucky!" "Isn't it interesting how *individual* babies are?"

The Baby Won't Nurse

One of the more frustrating situations is when the baby refuses to nurse, which is called a "nursing strike." These are not unusual and are generally limited in time. His seeming "rejection" of your breast is his way of letting you know that something is wrong. His behavior may prompt you to become anxious or tense, and you may feel guilty and helpless. For suggestions on how to handle the situation, see chapter 20, "Nursing Strikes and One-Sided Nursing."

Night Nursing

A common source of stress to parents is the baby who needs less sleep through the night. One mother laments, "After many months of getting up with the baby several times every night, I am reaching the end of my rope. I just can't take it anymore. I'm irritable, grouchy, and miserable to live with, and I admit resenting the intrusion on my sleep." Frustration leads to upsets, especially when the individual differences in babies' sleep patterns are not understood.

Another mother whose baby does not yet sleep through the night feels differently: "I am lucky that I'm healthy and strong enough to meet the needs of my baby whenever he needs me. That's just part of being a mother."

Obviously, attitude has a lot to do with how you are affected by having an older baby who nurses at night. Many mothers have their babies sleep with them and find night nursing easy because they can doze during feedings. Some mothers have found that a twin bed rolled next to mother's is good to lie on while nursing baby back to sleep.

Night nursings are also discussed in chapter 19, "Nursing an Older Baby."

The Baby Who Doesn't Gain

A distressing situation for the entire family is the baby who nurses but does not gain enough weight. There are several labels to describe this: "low weight gain baby," "failure to thrive," "starvation diarrhea." *

The more critical situations involve babies who have symptoms other than low weight gain. Some of these are fretfulness, sleepiness, poor skin tone, poor muscle tone, stiff body, dehydration, fever, vomiting, diarrhea, green frothy stools. An emaciated baby who nurses three times a day and sleeps the remainder is in fact starving.

Frequent nursing but little weight gain may indicate a problem. It may be a case where the baby is not utilizing the milk or you are not producing and secreting enough.

Norma Jane's baby was a "low weight gain" baby, and the problem seemed to be a combination of poor sucking and inadequate milk supply. Norma Jane describes her attempts at improving her baby's weight gain:

> When the baby was two weeks old and had lost a full pound since birth, I became frantic. Friends supplied extra breast milk for a short time and were very supportive.
>
> I could express an ounce or two of my milk after Vincent's feedings, which indicated that he just wasn't sucking well and wasn't getting what milk was there. I started limiting our nursing sessions to about 20 minutes (because of his poor sucking, he would have nursed all day and not gotten enough milk). After the 20 minutes of breastfeeding, I would express what was left and give it to Vincent by spoon or with a Dixie cup. This way my breasts were completely emptied, stimulating them to produce more, and Vincent got more milk.
>
> We went on a two-hour schedule and once I got this system going, after four weeks, I stopped using any milk but my own. We struggled along with a minimum of wet diapers and a three-ounce weekly gain. Slowly, over the first six or seven weeks, his sucking improved and I

---

* According to La Leche League medical advisor Dr. Mark Thoman, lengthwise growth is the most important barometer of adequate nutrition. Weight often catches up later. In breastfeeding, calories often go into length, not weight.

stopped hand expressing. He was healthy, happy, developing normally, growing in length and in head circumference. Had any of these been different, we might not have let him stay so skinny. He obviously could have used more calories.

The pediatrician found a physician to evaluate my health status and try to find a way to improve my milk supply. We tried various possibilities, all to no avail. Then we decided to treat my high blood pressure. After it was brought to normal with medication, my baby's rate of gain became normal and stayed at this level. There were no bells or sirens to say that there was more milk. The baby's pattern of frequent nursing didn't change; I had no physical sensation of more milk; the only obvious change was on the scales.

Many mothers of low weight gain babies are not as fortunate as Norma Jane. They may switch to bottlefeeding unnecessarily, and then feel disappointment or guilt about the change. However, A. H. Maslow has found that mothers put this "guilt" to good use; they give their babies more mothering attention and their babies become quite secure. (6)

For further discussion of slow-gaining and fast-gaining babies, see chapter 7, "Newborn and Infant Problems."

Birth Defect Compounded by Stress Situation

Many times mothers who have babies with birth defects must also deal with other factors, such as many trips to the hospital, and several other children in the family to care for. In addition, some mothers have to deal with people or situations that may tend to interfere with nursing.

One mother who had three children under six years of age when her baby was born with a cleft palate, said that she had a difficult time attending to the needs of all the children. She found that the baby needed long and frequent nursings: an hour nursing, an hour being held. The baby slept at night, but hardly at all during the day. Then a further complication arose. The mother describes her experience:

I was managing to cope with my baby's condition.
Then a problem in the family threw me off track. A close
friend who was divorcing her husband became involved
with my brother and the whole situation left me emotionally drained. My milk supply, which had been precarious
to start with, dwindled to nothing despite frequent nursing. The baby became dehydrated quickly, and I had to
offer her supplementary formula until I could pull myself
together. It was another 2½ months before my milk supply
was built up enough so that we could do without supplements. Now I understand that the difficulty I was having
in nursing my baby was not just because of the cleft palate.
At the time I couldn't figure out why techniques which
worked for other babies with cleft palates did not work
well for us. But ours was a case of stress situation nursing.

Death

Death deals such a traumatic blow, it cannot be absorbed
all at once. It's important to know that grief is not just a
hollow agony, it is a healing process. Gradually, you work
through stages in your grief. Initially, you feel mental shock,
which can be very frightening. You may feel as if you are in
another world, unable to concentrate, physically numb and
emotionally drained. Denial is not uncommon during this
stage; your mind is not ready to accept the loss.

After the initial shock begins to fade, the recovery stage
begins. It is gradual and often frustrating. It is difficult to
concentrate on even simple tasks like making a meal. This
can be so frightening that you think you're losing your mind.
This, too, is a normal fear. But day by day, normal routines
become easier.

The final stage of grief is acceptance. It is one thing to
recover and survive the crisis. It is quite another to recover
and accept the loss. It takes a lot of soul-searching to come to
terms with a tragedy and put it in perspective. It seems impossible for a while that life will ever be normal and happy
again.

How is nursing affected by a death? Many mothers have found that nursing after the death of a member of the family is a great comfort to them, their babies, and ultimately the family. Your baby may sense your unhappiness and be fussier. Comforting him helps to take your mind off the pain of the moment. If you try to express milk to leave in a bottle when you go to the funeral, you may find you are unable to get a let-down. Later, when things have settled down a bit, you'll be able to nurse more easily. Even if there seems to be no let-down, nursing for comfort is important.

Often it is easier for parents to deal with a child's death from a physical ailment than from an accident. Kerry had a very difficult time emotionally when her older son accidentally drowned. Her baby, Chris, was two months old and nursing at the time. Kerry told me:

> Chris was with me at the wake and the funeral, and I found great comfort in holding him. The next two years I went through a period of great depression. My guilt made me cry and cry. What could I have done to prevent it? Was I a bad mother? I knew I had to learn to calm down. At least I had to do it for Chris's sake. His nursing was my only brightness in a grim two years. I believe nursing after a death can be a mental lifesaver. It keeps you in tune with the now, not with the past.

I asked Kerry's husband, Ron, to share his thoughts. He said:

> I think nursing was more of a help at the time than anything else. When Kerry was nursing she was relaxed and able to think more clearly. The nursing was more frequent than it had been, but then they both needed that. How did I feel about this increased time in nursing? It takes time away from a husband, but it's important for him to be understanding. A woman needs to feel that she is a mother, and that she is capable of doing something constructive. Nursing is a time when she and the baby are consoling each other. The best attitude to have is to be

understanding, loving, encouraging. Above all, do not put the blame on anyone. This will bring the family back together and closer than before.

For other mothers who have lost a child, Kerry advises seeking professional help in order to cope with the tendency to punish yourself with guilt. Reaching out to other people such as clergy, friends, and your family can provide the support you need. Reading about how other mothers have survived the loss of a child can also be helpful.

For other discussions on death, see also chapter 6, "Nursing a Premature Baby"; chapter 12, "When Baby Is Sick or Hospitalized"; chapter 13, "When Mother Is Sick or Hospitalized"; and chapter 25, "When You Go It Alone."

Self-Help Guide

Understanding the Problem

What are the facts of your situation?

What other information is necessary?

Has this happened before?

What worked then? Might it work now?

What are your pleasant feelings?

What are the feelings that you'd rather not have?

Are you able to tolerate frustration?

Are you aware of how you feel?

Finding Help

Are you actively seeking assistance from another significant person (husband, parent, friend, minister, counselor)?

What are your strengths?

What resources and supports are available to supplement your own strengths?

How can you find resources in your community?

Coping

How can the problem be separated into manageable bits and pieces?

What can you do to get through this situation a little bit at a time?

How are your strengths helping you to do well in other areas?

What is the best possible outcome; the ideal result?

What will happen in your family if the best possible outcome occurs?

What is the worst possible outcome; the most disastrous result?

What will happen in your family if the worst possible outcome occurs?

Resolving

"I will resolve to be calmer."

"I will recognize and accept my feelings."

"I will learn to accept the inevitable."

"I will explore what can be changed."

"I will try to be flexible and will adapt when it is necessary."

"I will keep my self-respect and develop my self-confidence."

"I will work toward removing barriers between myself and others."

Chapter 22

Mothers with Special Physical Problems

"I know how important it is for a young woman who has a physical problem to know that she is capable of fulfilling her biological roles of reproduction and lactation," says Diane Linda Miller, author and counselor on diabetes, pregnancy, and breastfeeding. Her own experience as a breastfeeding diabetic, and the experiences of many other mothers as described in this chapter, show that breastfeeding *can,* and in some cases *should* be done, for the benefit of both mother and baby.

In some of the situations discussed here, special procedures are necessary, with close supervision by a physician. The examples that are described are offered simply as *examples.* Often there are wide variations in the causes, symptoms, severity and treatment of a problem. Each situation is unique and generalizations should not be made. For example, the effects on a baby of medication taken by his mother vary with his age and weight. Also, if the baby is receiving other foods besides breast milk, the influence of the drug could be modified. A mother may be in such a weakened condition, for example, that she needs to take a drug which contraindicates breastfeeding, but which is necessary for her survival. In this case, there are options to explore, such as resumption of nursing when the mother's health allows or when the baby is older.

Diabetes

This is one of the most common serious metabolic disorders. A diabetic cannot manufacture an adequate amount of insulin (one of the agents needed for the conversion of sugars and starches to energy), which results in an abnormally high blood sugar level. Many diabetic mothers who nurse are juvenile diabetics, meaning that their disease began in childhood or adolescence. They must have daily injections of insulin and follow a prescribed diet.

It is important to have optimal medical care before, during, and after pregnancy. If you receive excellent care during pregnancy, it is possible to deliver a normal, full-term baby without any complications. And with your diabetes under control, breastfeeding can have many advantages for you and your baby.

Most diabetic mothers find that diabetes presents no problems for nursing, either for themselves or their babies. In fact, many mothers do better in controlling diabetes while nursing. Dr. Carolyn Rawlins, an obstetrician on La Leche League International's Professional Advisory Board, points out that diabetics must be watched more closely for breast infections, but generally, diabetic mothers who are on insulin do very well. (1)

Dr. Robert Jackson, a La Leche League International Professional Advisory Board member, whose primary interest is diabetes in children, says that there is considerable evidence that infants of diabetic mothers tend to be obese at birth, and obesity in childhood often extends into adult life. This is significant because obesity often precedes development of diabetes. It is especially beneficial for the baby of a diabetic mother to be breastfed, since breastfed infants develop fewer fat cells than formula-fed infants, reducing the likelihood of their becoming obese, and in turn, diabetic.

Babies of diabetic mothers often have problems with blood sugar levels immediately after birth. During pregnancy, the high blood sugar passes through the placenta to the baby, and in response, the baby produces a large amount of insulin to control it in his system. After birth, the high blood sugar from mother is cut off but the baby still produces an overabundance of insulin, which drives his blood sugar way down, and can cause hypoglycemia.

Your baby's blood sugar will be checked frequently during the first few days, and usually stabilizes in a day or two. Sometimes supplements of sugar water or formula (or breast milk if available) are given to prevent low blood sugar. However, the fewer oral supplements that are given, the more the baby nurses and the faster your milk supply will be established. It is very important to have a supportive pediatrician who will try hard to avoid supplements. When your own milk comes in, any oral and intravenous supplements will probably be discontinued.

A diabetic mother's milk is not adversely affected by her condition. The sugar content of her milk is no higher than that of a nondiabetic. While it is true that trace amounts of insulin are transferred into breast milk, an infant's digestive enzymes inactivate the hormone. (2) (3)

Diabetes does present a unique set of circumstances. Yet, according to Diane Linda Miller, who has helped many diabetic nursing mothers:

> After a high-risk pregnancy and delivery, nursing helps normalize your situation. High-risk care, as is the case with a diabetic mother, is often quite impersonal and often entails mother-infant separation. Breastfeeding involves frequent skin-to-skin contact which is essential in bonding the mother and infant. And this bonding is essential to the infant's emotional development. Breastfeeding helps to establish the diabetic mother's confidence in her body's ability to nourish her child.

Besides emotional benefits, there is evidence that the complex hormonal balance of nursing lessens diabetic symptoms. Many diabetic nursing mothers find they require less insulin.

While nursing, mothers with mild diabetes which can be controlled by diet alone simply need to maintain a high-quality diet, modify meal plans, and increase caloric intake.

The diabetic controlled by oral hypoglycemic agents can usually breastfeed. Although traces of drugs will be transferred to the baby through the milk, there has been no indication that normal doses of hypoglycemics are transferred in any amounts significant enough to harm a baby with normal glucose levels.

You may have to be more careful than other nursing mothers to avoid sore nipples, plugged ducts, and breast infections, and to treat them promptly if they develop. Infection, digestive upset, and emotional upset are variables which can disturb your diet-insulin-exercise balance during lactation. They require adjustment of insulin in order to keep blood glucose at a normal level.

A sudden loss of interest by the baby in nursing can lower your milk supply and make sugar control difficult. Some mothers can compensate for sugar in the urine by simply eating less; if this does not afford adequate control, you may need to take supplementary insulin under the direction of your doctor. When weaning occurs, it is best if this can be a gradual process, involving equally gradual changes in diet and insulin.

Diane Linda Miller was diagnosed as a brittle diabetic when she was 13 years old (brittle diabetes is a form which is particularly difficult to control). She was told she could never have children, and when she *did* have a child, she was told she could never breastfeed successfully. Despite this advice, Diane is now the mother of two healthy children who were both breastfed. She relates her nursing experience:

> In the beginning, I had problems nursing my daughter, Eden, because of my ignorance in handling my diabetes during lactation. I went into insulin shock several times, because milk production requires a great deal of sugar. Once my insulin dosage was decreased and my diet increased, I had no more problems. Before pregnancy, my normal routine was a minimum of 80 units of insulin with a minimum of 1,500 calories daily. During pregnancy, I took 150 to 200 units of insulin daily with 1,500 calories. When Eden was completely breastfed, I took 40 units daily and ate 3,000 calories.
>
> While I was working closely with my internist and pediatrician to balance my diet and insulin, I sometimes

had to give Eden formula. After two months, she was completely breastfed and she continued nursing until she weaned herself at 22 months.

When my son was born, I had my experience with Eden on which to base my dosage and diet. My insulin was immediately decreased to 40 units, and I was in complete control five days after delivery. (4)

Regular mealtimes and frequent snacks are a must if you are a nursing diabetic mother. If your blood sugar gets too low and triggers an insulin reaction, the let-down reflex may be inhibited either at the beginning or during nursing. Regular meals are vital to maintain a constant blood sugar level. It's important to have meals made ahead and other food easily available, so that one free hand can keep the diabetes in line while the other keeps the baby happy.

Babies of diabetic mothers often have problems after birth. With medical supervision, most of the time these problems are overcome. However, Leslie, who expressed her milk for her premature baby until he died at two weeks of age says:

A diabetic mother who is nursing and loses her baby will most likely need to be very careful about stopping lactation. Breast infections could crop up very easily unless she pumps her milk or hand expresses it. It is very hard to hand express milk after your child's death, though. I used Syntocinon on the occasions when I couldn't get a let-down. I chose not to have "dry-up" medication; I felt the prolactin would help smooth things out, and I think it did.

Nursing when you have diabetes can certainly be a challenge. For helpful information, see readings listed in the Bibliography and consult Appendix: Organizations to Help the Nursing Mother.

Hypoglycemia

Hypoglycemia involves lower than normal blood sugar and it is often an early stage of diabetes. Nursing has a

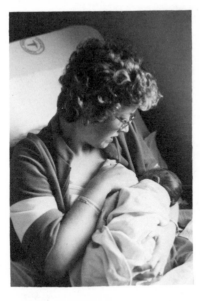

Andrew's first nursing with his diabetic mother, Michele.

Michele's doctors were not enthusiastic when she said she wanted to breastfeed. She was not allowed to nurse for 6 days following Andrew's birth. Breast milk and nursing were especially important for her son, who had a condition which made swallowing and retaining liquids and foods difficult. Bottle-feeding would have aggravated his problem, and he would not have thrived as he did while nursing.

variable effect, helping to stabilize the blood sugar in some cases.

One mother who suffered from weakness, tiredness, anxiety, and depression was diagnosed as hypoglycemic. A year before her child was born, she began carefully controlling her diet and her physical condition improved. Her intention was to nurse the new baby for a few months, regardless of how she, herself, felt, and to reevaluate the situation after that. By knowing which foods affected her adversely, she was able to keep a stable blood sugar level and successfully breastfed until her baby weaned 2½ years later. She said that because of her improved health, she felt better emotionally and this further helped her condition.

Thyroid Disorder

The thyroid gland controls the rate of all the body's metabolic processes. An underactive gland is fairly common, usually slow in causing symptoms, and is sometimes confused with other conditions with similar vague symptoms. An overactive gland results in a more dramatic illness, Graves disease.

If you have a thyroid problem, you need to be under the close supervision of a doctor who is supportive of your desire to breastfeed and can also monitor you, and perhaps your baby as well. Mothers with thyroid disorders can nurse their babies, except in severe cases.

Hypothyroidism (Underactive Thyroid)

Many mothers who take medication for an underactive thyroid have continued to nurse. According to Dr. Ernest Solomon, a La Leche League Professional Advisory Board member, "Thyroid can be taken while nursing because it only replaces what the mother is lacking." As with any medication you are taking, especially for long-term use, it is a good idea that you inform your baby's pediatrician of it.

A mother taking thyroid medication may be warned that it will pass through her breast milk to the baby, who will come to depend on the medication and not develop his own thyroid gland. *This is not true.* Dr. R. M. Blizzard, Pediatric Endocrinologist at Johns Hopkins Hospital, points out several experiments that have been done on the relation of this medication to breastfeeding. In these studies, infants were given thyroid medication for six months and when it was withdrawn, the infant's thyroid gland functioned on its own and normally. To quote Dr. Blizzard: "I would like to state that there is no reason to suspect that thyroid ingestion by lactating women in any way contraindicates breastfeeding." (5)

Thyroid deficiency can be a problem without a mother realizing it. Dr. Gregory White, one of La Leche League's Professional Advisory Board members, mentions that mothers who feel especially tired might consider having a thyroid test. He says:

> Frequently, new mothers complain of fatigue, poor appetite and depression, and generally just don't "feel well." Unfortunately, this is often erroneously blamed on breastfeeding. Once the possibility of anemia is ruled out she should have a simple thyroid test. If the level is shown

to be abnormal, then it is a simple matter to prescribe a thyroid supplement (which is harmless to the nursing infant). Mothers often report that they feel much better, are sleeping better, and even that their milk supply has improved. (6)

If your doctor starts you on thyroid medication while you are nursing, it is wise for him to begin with a low dosage, then gradually increase the amount. A mother who started on too high a dosage found her milk supply increased profusely at first, and she had trouble with plugged ducts.

Too much thyroid, too suddenly, may also make you a little "edgy." Jayne, who suffered from a nonfunctioning thyroid, says:

> When my daughter Angela was about three months old she went on a nursing strike that lasted on and off for five weeks. It began to become apparent to me that there was a connection between how much thyroid I was taking and her "strikes." It turned out that our doctor had prescribed twice as much thyroid as I actually needed in his zeal to get me back to normal. My nervousness at being so "hopped up" on thyroid *may* have caused Angela to react by not wanting to nurse. When my thyroid dosage was brought down to normal everything was great again.

Hyperthyroidism (Overactive Thyroid)

An overactive thyroid gland is a serious health problem. It puts a marked strain on the heart, nervous system, and muscles. A mother attempting to breastfeed will have difficulty keeping up with the extra nutritional and physical demands of lactation.

Treatment of hyperthyroidism may be urgent if the condition is severe. Treatment may involve antithyroid drugs, surgery, or radiation. Antithyroid drugs are controversial in terms of their effect on the nursing infant. According to *The Medical Letter on Drugs and Therapeutics*, Propylthiouracil

(PTU), a thyroid depressant, reaches a higher concentration in milk than in the mother's blood, possibly inhibiting the activity of the infant's thyroid gland. (7) In some instances, mothers treated with antithyroid drugs have nursed their babies successfully, with no ill effects on the baby. However, most medical consultants discourage such attempts as too risky. They feel that the drugs seem to cause hypothyroidism or slow weight gain in some infants. At best, the baby who's nursing must be monitored carefully by his doctor.

Surgery removes enough of the thyroid gland so that what is left cannot produce enough thyroid hormone to be overactive. Such surgery, followed by replacement therapy with thyroid extract, would allow nursing to continue if a mother's condition permitted.

Radiation would definitely preclude nursing, but it is seldom used as treatment any more. See *Diagnostic Tests* in the section on Drugs and the Nursing Mother, chapter 13, "When Mother Is Sick or Hospitalized."

Pregnancy

If you become pregnant and already have thyroid problems or are on a maintenance program, Dr. Richard Guttler, Assistant Clinical Professor of Medicine at the University of Southern California Medical School, suggests you have your thyroid checked once the pregnancy is positively established and also after delivery. With different pregnancies, you may require raising or lowering of your thyroid hormone prescription.

If you are nursing while pregnant, this will probably not increase your need for thyroid hormone therapy or other thyroid medication.

Epilepsy

Epilepsy is a disorder of the central nervous system. The cause is not known, but scientists have related it to defects in the brain, brain injury before, during, or after birth, poor nutrition, childhood fevers, some infectious diseases, brain tumors, and even some poisons. There is no cure, but at least half of epileptics achieve complete control of their seizures with medication; most of the remainder achieve partial control.

An epileptic mother taking medication may be concerned about whether the drug will affect her nursing baby. An article in *La Leche League News* discussing drugs for epilepsy offers the following comments:

> We have been getting inquiries about the drugs taken by the epileptic mother who wants to nurse her baby. We know, from the references in the literature as well as from the personal experiences of mothers themselves, and doctors who have seen them through the breastfeeding experience, that the drugs usually prescribed for this, namely Dilantin, Mysoline, Phenobarbital, and other barbiturates, are safe for use by the mother of a nursing baby. We know personally several mothers who have had more than one child and have nursed them successfully, all the while on their medications, with no problems due to these drugs.
>
> There is one good general rule regarding drugs and the nursing mother. Drugs *which have been found to be safe for use during pregnancy* are probably at least as safe or safer for use during the nursing period, as regards their effects on the baby. The reason for this is that drugs are more likely to pass directly to the child before birth through the placental barrier, than they would be to get to him through your milk, and then through his digestive system. *There are a few exceptions, of course, and this should be as carefully checked out as the drugs you might be taking while pregnant.* (8)

Lourdes has had two serious epileptic seizures in her life; the first when she was 14, the second when she was 21 and had a 2-year-old son. She had bottlefed this baby, and because he had allergy problems, she wanted to breastfeed the second, in hopes of avoiding the same problem. She wondered if her medication, Dilantin, would interfere with nursing, but after delivery, her doctor told her there was no danger and that she could go ahead and nurse. The dangerous time was during pregnancy when the baby was receiving the medication through her blood, but since he obviously didn't have any problems after birth, there was no reason not to nurse him. At 6 months, the neurologist tested the baby's blood and some milk from each breast; there were no traces of Dilantin to be found.

Maura's epilepsy, unlike Lourdes', has caused Maura *many*—sometimes eight, ten, or more—psychomotor seizures (complex partial seizures) per day and an occasional grand mal episode (generalized convulsion). Despite this, she has nursed all three of her boys. She says:

> I began having seizures at age 12, and I've never been completely controlled. During the 14 months my oldest boy was nursing, I took, at one time or another and in various combinations, some common anticonvulsants and other drugs used in seizure control. For example, at one point my medication consisted of Celontin, Mysoline, and Diamox. None of the drugs seemed to have any ill effects on my nursing baby.
>
> Some people are worried about the medication going into the milk and making the baby sleepy. I consulted many doctors with this question and all agreed that if any medication is secreted, it is in very minute amounts and shouldn't harm the baby. They told me to go ahead and nurse. I watched for drowsiness in my babies and the neurologist also checked for this, but they remained very active and alert.
>
> Breastfeeding has been a salvation for me, especially on days when I knew there was very little I could do for my child. At least I was giving the very best of myself in extremely important areas—food, warmth, affection, touch, and caring. I could never have gathered the strength or had the energy to give bottles.

Maura offers some practical pointers for epileptic mothers nursing babies:

- Have a playpen or Port-a-Crib on each level of the house. When a seizure is imminent, place the baby inside. Use gates across doorways and stairs so if you have a seizure, baby will be safe.

• Nurse baby in a *big* easy chair if possible. In the event of a generalized seizure, without warning, you will tend to remain stationary and baby will be safe.

• If you use a rocker, pad the arms. Fold a Turkish towel thickly and wrap it around each arm, pinning it securely. This provides a soft pillow for baby's head to rest upon in the event of a seizure, as well as being a comfortable rest for your arm. Extra pillows and cushions can also save you from bruises.

• At night, sleep with baby in bed with you. When I nursed the first child, I was always tired and dragged out, due to too many seizures, not enough sleep. With the second child, I just took him to bed. I used guard rails and pillows on the bed, and when no one was around, rested on the floor on a quilt.

• On outings with a nursing baby, it's a good idea to have a sticker taped to the buggy saying, "My mother has epilepsy" and containing information such as baby's name, your husband's work phone, and the name of a friend who can be reached to take care of the baby for a short time.

Blindness

A woman who is blind may be told that she cannot expect to have babies, but Kristin, a totally blind mother who has three breastfed children, certainly disagrees with that opinion:

When I became pregnant, I realized that one of my biggest problems was not knowing how to take care of a baby. My husband and I took childbirth classes, I attended La Leche League meetings, and we read aloud from several baby care books. (There are many such books in Braille now, plus tapes and talking books.) Once the baby was born, a Visiting Nurse helped me with the bathing and care.

I looked for basic techniques that would help me— such as Braille thermometers and scales, and an infa-feeder for older babies who have started solids. There is a way to keep socks together—the little hose clips or plastic disks which will go through the washer and dryer. There is a way to find a toddler—using bells on his shoes or a squirt of perfume on his back. A baby carrier is absolutely essential. There are ways to "babyproof" a house. For example, a lamp can be screwed down to a table so it can't tip over, and a lock can be put on the medicine cabinet.

There was no question in my mind that I would breastfeed; it was the best thing I could do for my baby and for myself. For a blind mother, breastfeeding is obviously very convenient. There are no trips to the store to buy formula, no trying to pour the formula into the bottle. It's easier when you're traveling and visiting people. You don't have as much to carry and you don't have to depend on others to warm a bottle for you, when you're in an unfamiliar home. Even with an older baby, breastfeeding still gives you time for touching and closeness.

While breastfeeding, a blind mother can tell when the baby smiles, by feeling the facial muscles move and fill out against her hand or breast. If a mother is aware of these changes, she can respond to the baby by smiling back and talking to him.

I found that breastfeeding gave a terrific lift to my self-image. As a blind woman growing up in our society, I noticed that people seemed to respond to my blindness rather than to other aspects of my being a woman. Consequently I feared that I might appear less attractive than others. The experience of bearing and breastfeeding my children has reinstated feelings of beauty and self-worth that I have carried with me into other life situations.

Another mother, Abby, who has been legally blind (partially sighted) all her life because of an inherited condition, says:

The fact that I was a handicapped person who wanted to have a baby was not easily accepted by many friends or by my husband's family. I felt a strong need to find people who would not communicate their doubts about how I was going to manage. A friend recommended a doctor who did both prenatal and postpartum care, and also saw babies. This meant I wouldn't have to start all over with someone else when the baby was born. He was completely supportive and encouraging.

The hospital was less helpful. They did what they could to help me nurse, but were extremely doubtful that I could care for a baby without help. One nurse insisted on putting my breast in the baby's mouth herself. Another, knowing full well I was breastfeeding successfully, gave my husband a lecture on how to bathe a baby and give formula when he came to take me home. It made me feel incompetent although I *knew* I could nurse and take care of him.*

Mothering ability should really be seen as the ability to have an enjoyable and satisfying relationship with a child. Any task that a mother can't do can be delegated without making her less of a mother. The exceptions, such as feeding an infant, are strikingly easier for a nursing mother than for one who bottlefeeds. I can't imagine ever living through the tasks of locating a can opener at night or finding a moving mouth with a demitasse spoon. A nursing mother has no cleanup problem at all for the first six months or so. Then it is easier to clean up bread or cheese crumbs than it is to find puréed spinach on the walls and ceilings. I would certainly long-term breastfeed another baby. Breastfeeding has immense psychological importance for a blind woman. Seeing my baby grow on my own breast milk, and knowing that I truly did not need any help gave me much needed confidence as a mother and allowed me to identify with womankind in a way I never did before.

For the benefit of blind mothers, most of La Leche League's information sheets and books (including *The Womanly Art of Breastfeeding*) are available on tape and in Braille. For an up-to-date list of all the publications available,

---

* A brief discussion of hospitalization for blind mother appears in Special Situations for Mother, chapter 14, "Working Together."

write to the International office, listed in Appendix: Organizations to Help the Nursing Mother, and ask for reprint no. 502.
This Special Publications list also includes La Leche League-
approved material available from Recordings for the Blind,
Library of Congress, and elsewhere. Also, blind mothers should
check with the regional library in their states for other resources
available to them.

Deafness

One evening I attended an unusual meeting. I was one of
only four people present who had normal hearing. The others
there were all young women who had complete or partial hearing loss and who came to learn about babies and breastfeeding. The other three people present who could hear, besides
myself, were two La Leche League leaders, and an interpreter.
As a leader spoke, the interpreter conveyed the information
through sign language to the mothers, and in a similar way
assisted the leader in answering their questions.

Bonney, a deaf mother who has been with the group the
longest, shared these thoughts about her endeavors to successfully nurse her babies:

> After my son was born, I was very confused by the advice
> from the nurses at the hospital about formula and nursing.
> The nurses outlined a rigid schedule, and told me I should
> give him formula after each nursing session. My son was
> fussy, cried a lot and had a poor weight gain. I wasn't
> happy giving him formula and became very upset think-
> ing that I didn't have enough milk.
>
> One day my husband's friend at work told him about
> a La Leche League group and suggested that I contact
> them. His wife had also had problems with breastfeeding.
> Sure enough, the La Leche League leader was helpful in
> answering my questions, and she invited me to the next
> meeting. My problems began to clear up; I learned how
> to increase my milk supply, my son gained weight, and I
> was able to nurse him completely.

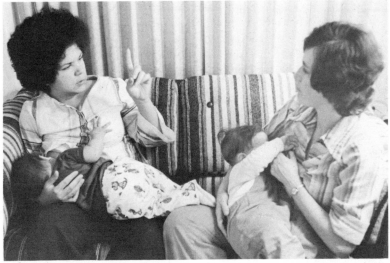

Sandra C. Wallace

Gloria (left) and Bonney (right) with their nursing babies at a special La Leche League meeting for hearing-impaired mothers.

Bonney's story is unique because usually deaf mothers will not contact a hearing person for help. Bonney was so enthusiastic about the help she received from attending La Leche League meetings that she urged other nursing friends who had hearing problems to attend. After several meetings, it was decided to hold special meetings for the hearing-impaired mothers, at which an interpreter would translate the words of the leader into sign language. The first meeting was held in February, 1976, in Arcadia, California. Hearing-impaired mothers now come to the monthly meetings from many cities in the Los Angeles area.

Stephanie Merritt, one of the leaders of the hearing-impaired group, says:

> Breastfeeding knowledge and guidance are greatly needed by these mothers. The hazards of ignorance and misinformation which hamper many mothers in their attempts to

breastfeed are even greater for the hearing-impaired mother. The breastfeeding relationship is especially important because it fosters a closeness and love-bond that may help offset the isolation the mother and baby feel as the baby grows and verbal communication begins to take on more importance.

Another La Leche League group of deaf mothers is located in Denver, Colorado. The leader of this group, Joyce Meshko, has a good understanding of the deaf since her parents are deaf-mutes. Knowing sign language, she is able to communicate directly with the mothers in her group, without an interpreter.

Muscular Dystrophy

Muscular dystrophy can attack people of all ages. Usually, the older the patient is when the disease begins, the more slowly it progresses. The ailment in adults sometimes continues for 20 to 30 years or more. But some become helpless within a few months. (9)

Dorie suffers from Kugelberg-Welander's pseudodystrophy, which is similar to muscular dystrophy. Both diseases result in muscle weakness. In Dorie's case, she has had this condition since she was a small child. She explains how her physical affliction didn't prevent her from nursing:

> My husband and I had wanted a baby very, very much. When my daughter, Lynn, was born I knew that I didn't have the strength to carry or lift her—so how could I be the kind of mother I wanted to be? My only solution was to nurse her.
>
> Even though I couldn't pick her up (I could only lift three pounds), I could still lean over the crib and nurse her. When I wanted to hold her to nurse, someone was always with me who could lift her up and hand her to me. My husband made a special chair, like the frame of a backrest, that we put on the bed so I could sit back and nurse her comfortably. I also nursed lying down on the bed.

Eight years later, Dorie gave birth to a ten-pound boy whom she nursed for 2½ years. Her story points out that even though certain disorders can make mothers helpless to a degree, it is still possible for them to provide their infants with the advantages of breastfeeding.

Your Cheering Squad

Maura, the epileptic mother who has many psychomotor seizures daily, is nevertheless a very active person, camping, canning and freezing vegetables which she raises herself, crocheting, carving wood and doing rough carpentry. She is a gourmet cook and an assistant Cub Scout leader. She says:

I think that my ability to be the active, happy person I am today is the result of my greatly improved self-image. Normal pregnancies, beautiful births, and long nursing periods were some of the strongest positive aspects of my life. The loving support given to me by my husband and children, and the real, honest caring by my physician, plus better management of my epilepsy have allowed me to develop a very positive attitude about myself.

Communication with the doctor is very important. Respect your doctor's judgment but make sure he understands how strongly you feel about nursing. Mothers under the care of a specialist may find the pediatrician can be helpful even if the specialist isn't.

The encouragement of friends can do a lot to boost your sometimes sagging spirits. You may encounter some people who cast doubts on what you are doing. Don't allow their comments to discourage you; listen instead to those who support your nursing, and feel secure in the knowledge that you are doing the best for your baby.

Chapter 23

Nursing and Working

Is it possible for you to be a working mother and also breastfeed your baby? The answer is not simple. It involves several considerations, one of which is—do I *need* to go to work? As one mother candidly put it, "A lot of us work and nurse our babies, but it's never easy on baby or on Mom."

Mary Ann Cahill, in "Breastfeeding and Working" (1), mentions that one of the strongest reasons for breastfeeding when working is the fact that nursing is associated only with mother. Anyone can give a bottle. But baby at the breast is reserved for mother.

If you work away from home, the comfort and security that nursing brings during the times you are together will be especially important. You may return home tired with a million chores to do. But you cannot "prop" a breast. You must sit down and relax, and hold and cuddle your baby as you nurse him. Breastfeeding improves the quality of the time you spend with your baby.

In this chapter you will read about various ways mothers have managed to work while caring for a breastfed baby. It *can* be done. Certainly no mother should feel that if she has to work, she cannot nurse her baby.

Freedom of Choice

Working, even while your baby is young, can be an enticing prospect. But so can the full-time job of being a mother. A working woman contributes to society by making use of her talents. A woman also makes a valuable contribution to society by helping to shape emotionally healthy, secure, loving individuals.

The truly liberated woman is one who is able to shape her life regardless of what society dictates. For some, this means staying at home and raising children, while for others this means entering the working world. Women have a right to choose and enjoy either option, motherhood or career—or both.

Standard of Living, Standard of Loving

If you work, will it be to meet a definite financial need? Or will it be to raise your family's standard of living? By deferring work, you would be able to devote more time and energy to your baby and family . . . you could raise your standard of *loving* instead.

Considering expenses, have you figured out what your net income will be if you work? The cost of your sitter, transportation, clothing, meals out, perhaps cleaning help, an occasional shampoo and set will all come out of your pay. The amount remaining can be surprisingly small. Also, consider the cost of formula and baby food if your baby is not completely breastfed. A six months' supply can equal the price of a major appliance such as a refrigerator or washing machine! There may also be the expense of extra doctor visits, since formula-fed infants tend to have more illness which can be compounded by allergies.

Some mothers choose to contact a social agency for financial help rather than return to work. Aid to Dependent Children, food stamps, and other programs are possible alternatives to working. Many states allow extra funds for lactating mothers.

It's certainly not all sweetness and light to stay home with your baby. There are dirty diapers and clutter, dirty clothes and dishes, hurt fingers and hurt feelings. These exist whether you work or not. But there's also so much that's precious that you might miss if you're not home. While my babies were nursing, I held a part-time summer job, much of which I could do at home. That allowed me to share in very special moments, when my little ones took their first steps and asked their first questions.

Timing Your Return to Work

It would be ideal if each mother could stay home while her children are very young. A mother's presence is important to her baby, beyond being the source of milk.

Separation can be hard on a young child. Dr. Niles Newton, a noted psychologist, says, "Beginning around age three, the child's understanding of time and the security of the greater world begin to have more meaning to him. Now he can begin to accept such explanations as 'mother will return by bedtime.'" (2)

If you cannot stay home during your baby's early years, the longer you can manage to wait before starting to work, the better. Many businesses allow maternity leaves, and your company may consider extending its usual maternity leave while you are nursing. Or, your employer may allow you to start working shorter hours, gradually working up to a full shift. See if part of the job can be done at home, or perhaps two mothers can split the same job.

Karyn has successfully combined nursing with her embassy job as vice-consul. She says:

> While working, you need certain skills, such as expressing milk easily and maintaining a good milk supply in relation to the baby's needs. Perhaps these come easier to an experienced mother—but they can be taught even to a first-timer. I would strongly recommend that a first-time mother make a special effort to be with her baby for as many months as possible while she is becoming accustomed to nursing.

Babysitting

If you decide to work, how can you see that your baby is adequately cared for?

An entirely satisfactory babysitting arrangement is often hard to obtain. The physical care may be sufficient, but if given routinely and without much warmth or interest, your baby's complete needs aren't being met. A mother often has difficulty finding someone whom she can trust to love and mother her baby.

A series of babysitters can be disastrous. A child needs one face, one way of handling, in order to have maximum emotional and physical development.

In a child care center, babies are exposed to many faces. Some seem to take this in stride; others don't. If you're considering using a child care center, find out first if the teachers have nursed their own babies. And remember, a teacher may say she favors nursing, but actually may resent caring for a nursing baby if she did not nurse her own. Day care centers are usually better suited for the three- to four-year-old. The staffing and care aren't geared towards the individual needs of babies under three years.

One mother leaves her baby in a nonprofit Child Development Center, started by the American Association of University Women. The teachers there have breastfed their own children and are very supportive of nursing. Another mother found a church day nursery to be a good setting for her young baby.

A sitter or a teacher in a child care center who is lukewarm about breastfeeding may become interested if you take her to La Leche League meetings or discuss breastfeeding information with her. If she's not at least supportive in a positive way, try to find someone else. Her feelings about breastfeeding may influence her feelings for the baby and in turn affect how she cares for him.

Regardless of your babysitting arrangement, it's a good idea to allow enough time to nurse your baby as the very last thing you do before you leave him. If the sitter comes to your house and you're dressed, sit down and nurse your baby before leaving. If you take your baby to a sitter, nurse him at her house, before you leave. When you return, the very first thing you should do is nurse your baby. Even if he is not hungry, and only sucks for a couple of minutes, hold him, let him feel reassured knowing you're there.

Emotional Aspects

Nursing can fill an emotional need when mothers find it a financial necessity to work. Suzette, a single mother, says, "I felt guilty at having to be away from my baby, but the fact that I, through nursing, was providing something that no one else could, created a valuable bond that will always last. The psychological benefits we received could never be measured."

Some mothers who start to work and are separated from their babies find their emotions to be quite different from what they expected. Instead of enjoying a gay, stimulating atmosphere, they're miserable. One mother spent her first day at work almost on the verge of tears. Weeks later she found she still couldn't concentrate fully on her work, distracted by worries about her baby and having separation anxieties of her own. Her daughter reacted to the separation by looking forlorn all day, and losing interest in eating. This mother decided the best thing to do was to quit her job and devote her time to her baby.

Long-Term or Temporary?

A successful nursing-working arrangement can continue as long as necessary. Be glad you are making the effort to at least partially provide your baby with the closeness, reassurance, and physical benefits of nursing at this time.

Some babies are not as adaptable as others to having a working mother. One mother had an irregular schedule and it did not work. Some babies may refuse bottles. One baby who had been sucking her thumb stopped soon after her mother quit work and was home enough to let her nurse as often as she wished.

But for however long you combine nursing and working, you are giving your baby something no one else can give him. He needs all the warmth, closeness and love you can give him in the time you two are together and you just might find the nursing experience even more beautiful and meaningful as you continue it.

Milk Supply

Will your milk supply be affected if you go to work? Many working and nursing mothers find that it's not. You can continue nursing even during your working hours, or you can express milk at home or at work.

Hopefully, you can wait until your baby is at least three months old before returning to work. Your milk supply will be well established, and physically you are likely to be in better shape than if you return sooner.

If you're overly tired, your milk supply can be affected. A mother can feel very self-sufficient as she becomes accustomed to handling two jobs—that of mother and working woman. She may take on more and more, trying to do everything she did before the baby was born. This, together with irregular nursing, can result in a plugged milk duct or breast infection. A diminished amount of milk is an indicator of body stress, and signals that you need to get more rest. Simple things like nursing lying down, taking naps on weekends, and eating nutritious food can keep your energy level from dropping too low.

Handling Two Roles

The grass is not always greener. . . . A job can be boring, or add pressures and mounting responsibilities. Even if you're working at home, you're really facing at least four projects that you are responsible for: your baby, your work, housekeeping and milk production. Handling all of these well re-

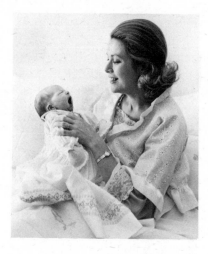

H. S. H. Princess Grace of Monaco nursed her 3 children. Here she is shown with H. S. H. Princess Stéphanie.

"I have many duties and obligations of State, but my family comes first. I would have liked to have breastfed my children for a much longer period than I did. But, at the beginning, when they first needed me and I, them, State had to wait upon mother." (3)

quires a considerable amount of mental and physical stamina.

Your chances of successfully combining nursing and working will be greatly enhanced if your efforts are supported by your husband and doctor. You can favorably influence your employer by pointing out that breastfed babies are healthier;

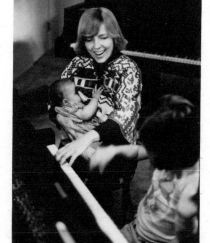

Anne Chapman Tullar

Working at Home

"I have found that my students have all reacted almost nonchalantly to the addition of my nursing baby to their piano lessons."
Mary Ann

that means less time lost from the job staying home to care for a sick baby.

Nursing mothers in many occupations have successfully met their dual responsibilities. I have corresponded with mothers who are saleswomen, bookkeepers, teachers, nurses, actresses, secretaries, scientists, lawyers, and professional tennis players. Others are part-time and full-time students. Some have flexible schedules, some have jobs requiring occasional long absences from their babies. They all agree that problems can be overcome.

There are several possible ways for you to combine nursing and working. One or more of the suggestions that follow may be workable for you.

Complete Breastfeeding

Working at Home

The best working situation, from your baby's point of view, is if you can work at home, setting your own hours, meanwhile nursing and caring for him as he needs you. Some mothers teach classes at home, do contract typing, sew or make alterations, iron, bake special cakes, sell various products, take care of other children, or develop special skills in handicrafts or sewing. Others are artists, writers and photographers.

Mother and Baby Go to Work

If you are determined not to leave your breastfed baby, you may be able to solve the problem by taking your baby to work. It is by no means easy or always convenient, but it can be done under some circumstances. Certain jobs are more conducive than others to having an older and more active child along. Working in a nursery care center or preschool are two such examples.

Meline co-manages a health food store, accompanied by her 20-month-old son. She firmly believes that it is possible

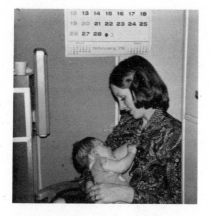

Lynn works part-time in a gift shop, accompanied by her 3½-month-old son. She nurses Ian in a private office where she also has a porta-bassinet for his naps. The gift wrapping table in the office doubles as Ian's diaper-changing table. In between naps, Ian is perched in his Infanseat in the store window. A young baby like Ian can go to work with his mother and "stay put" as no older baby could be expected to do.

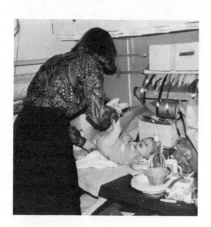

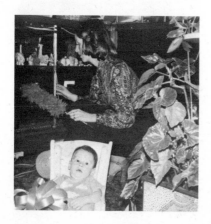

502

to work competently and efficiently in a small business, with a nursing baby along. As long as another person is present, she sees no reason why the working situation shouldn't run smoothly. Meline says, "A woman in this situation might be willing to take a reduction in the usual salary for the convenience of taking her baby along. I have no babysitting fees, and I'm able to breastfeed and be close to my baby while I'm working."

In the store, Meline places nonbreakable items on the lower shelves and keeps lots of toys behind the counters. In between selling, unpacking orders and dealing with customers, she manages to spend time with her son, and he is never bored. The advantage of this arrangement is that it allows her son unrestricted access to her, something that's very important for a child at this age.

Mother Goes to Work
While Baby Stays at Home

Working while your nursing baby stays at home with a sitter can still allow you to completely breastfeed. However, an agreement that satisfies his need for food won't entirely satisfy his need for your closeness and mothering. Expect him to require more of your time when you are at home. His need for mothering is likely to be unpredictable. There are cycles when children are more independent, and others when they have a greater need for your emotional support.

You might start with a part-time job, requiring you to be away from him only a few hours at a time. Keep in mind that a few hours each day will be easier on the nursing routine than two or three full working days, even though the total hours per week may be the same. You may want to leave an emergency bottle, which can contain your own milk, in case your baby gets hungry early one day.

If you need to work longer hours as your baby grows older, you'll find that when you start solids he'll be able to go longer between feedings. Then, when he's able to drink several ounces of juice from a cup (about seven to ten months), he may be satisfied with that all day, with no need for midday nursing or bottles. Nursing in the morning and evening when you are available may be sufficient.

If you want to nurse your baby during the hours that you are working, you may be able to do so, occasionally or on a regular basis. Shari began her teaching job when her baby was 10½ months old. She nursed Trevin at 8:00 A.M., 11:00 A.M., 3:00 P.M., and any time later in the afternoon, evening, and night.

If you're lucky enough to have a flexible work schedule, you can adapt it to your baby's needs. One mother who is a social worker goes home between cases to nurse her baby and then returns to work. This mother evidently has both a flexible work schedule and a flexible baby, one who is satisfied with only nursing when his mother appears. Not all babies are so adaptable.

Employers are sometimes adaptable, though. Perhaps you can combine your morning coffee break with your lunch hour, to allow a longer time to return home and leisurely nurse your baby.

Sitter Near Work

If you want to continue nursing your baby during working hours, but work too far from home to make it possible, you might do what Lada did. Her baby, Eleanor, was born allergic to almost all food except breast milk, so nursing was essential.

When Eleanor was three months old, Lada went back to work full time. She called the county welfare department for a list of licensed child care homes and found one two blocks from work. Lada nursed her baby on coffee breaks and at lunch, and found that Eleanor was often satisfied in five or ten minutes. Although many babies do need longer than that at a nursing, this may be a workable solution for you.

If you don't take time to nurse according to your baby's needs during the day, remember that he gets 60 to 90 percent of the milk in a breast in the first seven to ten minutes. He receives adequate nourishment, but this does not satisfy all of his sucking needs. Once you're home, he will probably want to nurse more, to fill his oral needs and to make up for the cuddling he has missed during your absence.

Baby Brought to Mother

Angie had to return to work when her second baby was three months old, to help cover some large medical expenses. The baby was very ill and could tolerate nothing but breast milk. Angie had no choice but to nurse him, since he refused to take a bottle, even if it contained breast milk. By having a sitter bring the baby to her, she was able to breastfeed him at work.

If you feel this arrangement would be good for you, talk to your employer. Tell him how important this is, how you may not have as much milk as you'd like to have if you're away from your baby all day. There's always a restroom, or lounge, or even the parking lot and the car, where you can nurse your baby.

An advantage to having your baby brought to you, rather than your going to him, is that it saves you travel time. It may be the only way you can be with your baby during the day. There are things to consider, though: your baby may have to go out in cold, rainy weather; he may have to be awakened from naps; and you'll need to find a sitter willing to make the trip.

Partial Bottlefeeding

Leaving Your Own Milk

If you are not able to nurse your baby during the day and he must receive his milk from a bottle, he can still enjoy the benefits of breast milk.

A couple of weeks before returning to work, practice expressing your milk, by hand or with a breast pump. Freeze the milk you express, and you'll start work with a good supply for your baby.

When you're on a working schedule, a good time to express milk is early in the morning. You're rested, it's quiet, and you have an abundant supply. Trying to express when you're in a hurry may create so much tension that the milk just won't let down. You can express on one side while nursing your baby on the other.

You can also express milk while you are at work. Nel returned to work as a research biologist while her baby, Iris, was still totally breastfeeding. Every morning, she collected four ounces of milk while nursing Iris. At noon she collected eight ounces, with the help of an oxytocin spray. When she came home from work, she collected another four ounces while nursing. This gave her two bottles for the next day. On weekends she saved a few more ounces if she had fallen behind during the week. She usually stayed four bottles ahead. To save milk while nursing, Nel held Iris on one arm with a small jar or bottle in that hand. Then, with her other hand, she expressed milk, which she refrigerated immediately to inhibit bacteria growth. By the time Iris was six months old, she was eating twice a day and Nel no longer had to express the eight ounces at noon.

When you're expressing milk at work, you can express from one breast at a time, every few minutes alternating the breast from which you're expressing, or you can express from both breasts at the same time.

Kendra developed an extremely efficient, easy method of rapid hand expression when she returned to work as an executive secretary. She found that a brisk walk around the block before expressing aided her let-down reflex. Then, in the privacy of a vacant locked room, she expressed from both breasts at the same time, into two bottles. Kendra had first tried a manual pump. But she discovered that in 15 minutes with hand expression she could express as much milk as it had taken her 40 minutes to obtain with the manual pump.

Kendra's son drank 18 to 20 ounces of milk the day after she expressed it. On Friday she froze the milk to be used on Monday. She kept two or three extra bottles in the baby-sitter's freezer in case she didn't express as much one day. On weekends she didn't express at all, but just enjoyed unlimited nursing with her baby.

Do people comment about it if you mention you express milk at work? One mother, Karyn, says:

> I never made a big point of what I was doing, nor did I try to hide it. If I wanted, I could have carried the bottle in my purse; perhaps keeping it in a paper bag in the refrigerator. But I never bothered to be devious.
>
> Once or twice someone got up courage to ask me what it was I had in the bottle, and I would just smile and answer that it was breast milk that I was expressing for my baby at home. By and large they were very nonchalant about it. People tend to be casual about routines unless you yourself seem to be terribly embarrassed, and then they notice what you are doing. I never had any problem with it at all.

Nursing and working mothers have found many ways to express and nurse at work. "Breastfeeding and Working" (4) mentions expressing in the ladies' restroom or in a fitting room in a retail store. Any sterile container can be used to hold your milk. The serving can be tailored to fit baby's need. If he is hungry, the sitter can warm a packet or two of milk (by holding them under hot running water) and take the edge off his hunger without spoiling his appetite for a nursing session once mother returns.

Many businesses, offices, and factories have a refrigerator somewhere on the premises where you can store the milk. Lunchroom managers may also be willing to relinquish a little refrigerator space. If there is no refrigeration available, you can use a Thermos. While still at home, sterilize the Thermos with boiling water. Then let it cool and fill it with crushed ice. At work, pour the ice out and express into the Thermos. Be sure the milk stays cold until you get home.

Leaving Regular Milk or Formula

Expressing milk may not be necessary if your baby is able

to drink regular milk from a bottle. If you are going to leave bottles of formula during your absence, be sure that your own supply is well established before you start substituting formula. Also, nurse frequently during the time you are home with your baby.

For some mothers, the question of milk supply can be critical. They need to nurse at regular intervals during the day in order to maintain an adequate supply.

For other mothers, once the milk supply is well established, they can then substitute formula or regular milk for one or more feedings a day. The milk supply adjusts to the smaller amount needed, and they still nurse all they want on weekends and evenings.

Irene worked part-time as a lawyer two days a week from the time her baby, Susan, was two months old. The baby-sitter gave Susan bottles while Irene was at work. Irene tried to work on nonconsecutive days so that her breasts did not get too full. She also cut down a bit on her fluid intake on the days she was at work.

A teacher with a full-time-plus job says she was never able to master manual expression. The sitter, who believed in breast-feeding, seldom gave more than two eight-ounce bottles of formula to the baby during the day. If the baby was hungry near the time for his mother to return, the sitter hugged and rocked him a lot and gave him a small amount of formula so that he was still eager to nurse when his mother came home. This mother says:

> During those first four or five months at work, I had some very wet moments around noon and midafternoon when the let-down reflex occurred. I would cross my arms and squeeze, but that was not always adequate. I really just put up with a damp front. My co-workers and students knew I was nursing my baby and breast milk never stained anything either washable or dry cleanable.*

---

* It is uncommon to have a problem with leaking for four or five months. A mother's breasts usually adjust in three or four weeks.

If your baby is quite young, he may be perfectly willing to sleep longer during the day and nurse in the evening, at night, and the early morning. The more nursings you skip during the day, the more he is likely to want to nurse when you are home. A baby who was sleeping through the night may want nightly nursings once you start working. Night feedings needn't be much of a problem, though. You can just bring your baby to bed with you and go back to sleep while he nurses. As long as the baby is kept warm you don't even need to change him for these night feedings.

Bottle Problems

Each baby reacts differently to bottlefeeding, so if your working arrangement requires use of bottles, be prepared for anything from enthusiasm to outright rejection.

Some babies may refuse a bottle from their mothers, but willingly take it from other people. They probably equate mother with nursing, and aren't willing to settle for a bottle in her arms. To accustom baby to the bottle, you may have to ask your husband to give one for a couple of weeks at one or two daily feedings, before you start work.

On the other hand, some babies prefer a bottle to nursing, once they discover how easily the milk flows from the regular bottle nipples. It might be worthwhile to get nipples with small holes so your baby has to work harder to get the milk from the bottle. The Nuk nipple is physiologically designed to help the baby suck in a manner as similar as possible to breastfeeding, which is better for your baby's jaw development. Also, to prevent "lazy sucking," a spoon, eyedropper or spouted cup can be used instead of a bottle for some of the feedings. However, no substitute can replace you.

Attending School

If you are a nursing mother attending school, you are in a position similar to the working mother, and have the same options available to you. You may be able to nurse your baby between classes, or express milk to leave with a sitter. You may even be able to take your tiny baby with you to class! Try it, perhaps checking first with the instructor. If your baby has been fussy, always seeming to need you while you're in class, you might find that he'll be much more content when he's with you. Nurse him well before class, and if possible put him in a cloth carrier that can be used in front or back. With a cardigan sweater or stole on over baby and carrier, you're available for inconspicuous nursing. He may surprise you and sleep right through your class. Should he want to nurse, nurse him on the breast opposite your writing hand, so you can still take notes.

Separation for a Few Days

If your job takes you away from home for several days, perhaps you can take your nursing baby with you. It's so much easier to travel with a nursing baby than with one who is bottlefed.

If you feel your baby absolutely cannot accompany you, the separation does not have to cause abrupt and permanent weaning. While you are gone, you can use plastic breast shields to catch any milk that drips. (Discard the milk, of course.) You can also express milk several times a day to relieve fullness and to keep up your supply. When you return, your baby may want to make up for lost time by nursing extra long and more often.

There is a risk involved in not taking your baby with you when you are away from home for several days. He may accept your absence and happily resume nursing when you return. Or, he may be very unhappy and confused. Sometimes babies who are separated from their mothers seem to reject them for a few days when they return, regardless of whether they are breastfed or not. Be prepared for this, and patiently keep offering to nurse him.

Enlisting Father's Aid

A supportive husband, ready and willing to help with shopping, cooking, and housework can make a difference in simplifying the life of a working nursing mother.

It's especially nice if the two of you can pick up your baby from the child care center or babysitter after work, allowing you to nurse the baby while your husband drives.

If your husband's hours allow him to take care of the baby while you are working, take advantage of the situation. He will be able to supply the emotional as well as physical needs of your child, better than any hired sitter.

Helpful Hints

Shortcuts are very important for a working mother, so that more of her time at home can be devoted to her baby and family. Make the most of your moments with your baby. Look at him and talk to him while nursing. Caress him and play with him while diapering and bathing him. Read to him, or look at picture books with him. If the amount of time you spend with your baby is limited by your working arrangement, it's up to you to make every minute count when you're with him.

Chapter 24

Traveling with a Nursing Baby

Though it's nice to be home with your baby, it's certainly not a necessity all the time. Many mothers have found that when baby is nursing rather than bottlefeeding, it's far easier to take off on the spur of the moment, go shopping, run errands, visit the doctor, travel on a vacation, and even move from one town to another.

Traveling with a nursing baby means less paraphernalia to carry along. This is quite an advantage when you're already toting a diaper bag, shopping bags, suitcases, or a camera. There is no worry about how much milk to take, refrigerating or warming it, or whether there is a restaurant or store open. Breast milk that is spit up doesn't stain or have an unpleasant smell, so there is less changing to do than with a formula-fed baby. Nursing can also calm the hunger pangs of an older child while waiting for food to be served in a restaurant.

Nursing can be very handy if you're traveling and an emergency arises. Mothers have been stranded far from any source of baby food or formula. Because they were breast-feeding, their babies were well fed. If a trip takes longer than you planned, you know there is always safe and nutritious food for the baby.

A family who moved from California to New York with six-week-old twins found they had to wait three weeks before the moving van arrived with their furniture. They were in an empty house without any appliances during that time. As the mother says, "Where would I have been if I'd had to worry about sterile bottles and nipples, to say nothing of trying to keep formula from spoiling?"

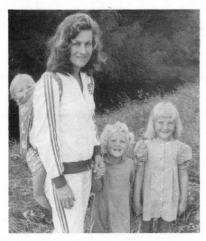

Alison, a top New Zealand distance runner, with daughters Shannon Lia (14 months), Karla (3 years), and Toni (5 years).

"I am convinced that breastfeeding is possible in almost any situation. I run because I want to and I breastfeed because I want to. My manager no longer asks if I'm taking my baby along. He just asks, 'Do you want me to book a cot at the hotel?'"

Alison

Some of the following travel ideas, although intended for longer pleasure trips, can also be useful for errands and visits to the doctor.

Traveling with Infants

Many parents have found that the best time to travel with a baby is during the first few months when he hasn't begun solids, doesn't crawl yet, and sleeps a lot. All he needs is mother. This section describes a variety of situations in which young nursing babies have traveled with their mothers.

While your baby is young can be a perfect time to take him on a camping trip. Kit tells how she shared the pleasure of the outdoors with her baby:

My husband and I decided to try backpacking with Laura when she was ten weeks old. On the trail I carried her in front in a baby sling, with my gear and her things in my pack. I had brought the foam mattress from the bassinet for Laura to sleep on, and the corner of the tent and our packs formed the sides of her bed. In between hiking, fishing and swimming I always found a nice shady place to feed her and keep her happy. It was wonderful to be able to include her in our enjoyment. And we *were* able

513

to enjoy the trip because we weren't burdened with the extra weight and extra preparations of bottles and formula. (1)

Baby carriers can be useful when sightseeing, as well as when backpacking with baby. Mary Jeanne used a carrier for her five-month-old nursing baby, Herbert, during a trip to the World's Fair. Mary Jeanne explains:

With the Happy Baby Carrier, the baby can be carried in front or in back. I used the front-carry style as this permitted me to sit down for a show or a rest and to take the baby out for nursing without removing the carrier. Also, with the baby in front I could see what he was doing, talk to him, wipe his mouth when necessary, and keep his face out of the sun.

We planned our activities around things we thought our four-year-old daughter would enjoy, making no special plans to accommodate the baby. And the only equipment I had to bring was a change of disposable diapers. Herbert didn't sleep as much during the day as he ordinarily did, and was perfectly willing to nurse no matter where we were. (2)

One thing to beware of, when staying with relatives or friends, is that you do not skip a lot of feedings. If Grandma keeps encouraging you to go off and visit your friends, it's all too easy for your milk supply to dwindle if she gives formula or baby food during your absence. Baths, walks, and diaper changing are fine for Grandma, but it's best if only you do the feeding. As an occasional alternative, you might leave your expressed milk for Grandma to give baby from a bottle. If your milk supply does diminish, remember, you can rebuild it.

Traveling with Toddlers

For toddlers, nursing provides food when the baby may

otherwise be distracted or reluctant to eat in a strange place. It is also a source of emotional comfort in unfamiliar surroundings. It not only helps the child relax when traveling, but the mother as well.

Many babies love to nurse in the car, and it's almost as popular as the rocking chair. Some mothers just lean over to the baby to nurse while he remains fastened in the car seat or seat belt. You may instead prefer to nurse before starting a trip, then stop for a nursing break when baby gets hungry.

Nursing discreetly while traveling can be more of a challenge with an older baby who may want to help himself, and may play while nursing. Clothes chosen with discreet nursing in mind are especially good to wear when traveling with a toddler. Having a special word for nursing may also make requests less obvious to those around you. See Clothing for Discreet Nursing in chapter 2, "Nursing Techniques," and Nursing in Public, chapter 19, "Nursing an Older Baby."

Before she became pregnant, Nel thought the last thing in the world she wanted to do was nurse a baby among strangers. Then one weekend she and her husband went on a trip with a couple who had a nursing baby. Nel says:

> I was really impressed with the convenience of traveling with a breastfed baby. All my friend needed were a few changes of clothes. She nursed the baby in the car between places and everyone was happy. Our own trip to England a year and a half later with our nine-month-old daughter gave me a chance to try nursing while traveling. One advantage to having her along was that the diaper changes, nursing, and feeding slowed us down somewhat and we did not get as tired as we had on our honeymoon, when we rushed to see everything.
>
> My ideas about nursing among strangers have obviously changed. I found myself nursing her on the train out of London which was full of men (after starting to feed her when there were just the three of us in the car). She was happy, full and content, which made me feel good, too.

Traveling with Twins

Running errands around town or traveling across the country *can* be accomplished when you have twin babies. It's easiest, of course, if father is along to help. When traveling by car you can sit between the babies and simply nurse them when they are hungry.

I had a twin stroller which was especially useful when my twins were small, for taking them to the doctor's by myself. For going shopping in the grocery store, I had one twin in a baby carrier and one in an infant seat in the front of the shopping cart.

Breastfeeding is doubly convenient when traveling alone with twins. I remember taking three-year-old Suzy to story hour at the library. Walking along the street and into the library, I'd hold Suzy with one hand, have one baby in an infant seat and the other in a baby carrier. Not having to be bothered with bottles was wonderful.

My husband and I planned a weekend trip, leaving our seven-month-old twins behind with a sitter. We left on Saturday, just after the morning nursing. While I was gone, Karen drank breast milk from a bottle. Sharon, who refused a bottle, was given lots of milk in her baby food. I used Netsy milk cups to catch leaking milk during the day, emptying them in a bathroom every two or three hours. I also expressed once in the hotel room. When we returned late Sunday, I made up for my absence with a long, leisurely nursing session.

How do you transport twin babies in a car? Probably the safest way is by using individual car seats. A quick, easy, inexpensive method when the twins are tiny is to put a blanket-lined box on the floor in each half of the back seat area.

A Port-a-Crib will fit in the back seat of a car or in the rear area of a station wagon. A piece of wood covered with foam rubber, then vinyl, can divide it into two areas so that the babies do not bump each other when the car stops suddenly. The Port-a-Crib bumper pad provides protection around the outside of the crib.

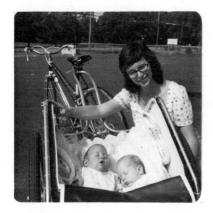

Marti with 3½-month-old twins, Stewart and Brian.

Marti, her husband, and twin sons participated in a 300-mile bicycle tour. The boys slept in the trailer, hitched behind their father's bicycle. Every few hours the group would stop so the boys could nurse. The trailer, called a "Bugger," is manufactured by Cannondale. Made of rip-stop nylon laced to a tubular metal frame, it rides on 2 wheels and is attached to the bicycle seat post. The entire front zips open, and a plastic insert is available which seats 2 children.

For more information, contact:
Cannondale
35 Pulaski Street
Stamford, CT 06902

You can also use a regular crib mattress in the back seat of the car. Support it by packing the wells with articles you won't need while traveling, up to the level of the seat. Put pillows at each end to cover the windows and door knobs to prevent injury. There are undoubtedly many other safe ways of transporting babies. Ask other parents what they do.

Moving

The situation may arise where a family with a baby must move. The move is, of course, simplified when you're breastfeeding. Many times items get lost or misplaced, and for children who are attached to something, the loss can be upsetting. A breastfed baby, though, is attached to mother and as long as baby and mother are together the move is more relaxed. With nursing, there is nothing to lose.

Babies are sometimes weaned prior to a move because someone suggests that the move will then be easier on mother.

However, keep in mind that moving is a lot of work under any circumstance. Mothers become exhausted; babies tend to pick up on this and demand more attention. A baby who has been accustomed to the comfort of nursing and is then denied it can be inconsolable. Sometimes a baby, sensing the tension involved in preparing for a move, refuses to nurse until mother relaxes with him. If you plan on fairly frequent nursings during the packing and unpacking stages of your move, your baby will be assured that all is well (despite the unusual activity and surroundings) and you will get the needed rest.

One family was able to easily handle a move of 800 miles with four-month-old twins. They fixed a safe bed for the babies in the car, which mother drove while father followed in a truck. For feedings, they would pull over in a service area or rest stop and the mother would nurse in the car. She made a point of drinking plenty of fluids at these times. They took it easy, making as many stops as were needed, and were not unduly tired when they finally arrived at their new home.

Once you arrive, be prepared for your baby to refuse foods for a few days and want only to nurse and be carried a lot, until he feels at ease in his new home. Just keep his favorite foods handy so that when he is ready, they are available.

It may take a while for you to get to know people in your new community. Getting to know other nursing mothers is a nice way to start and if you have questions or a problem related to breastfeeding, your new friends may be able to help. Find out if there is a La Leche League group near you. Look in the phone book or write to the International office. Your doctor, a Red Cross instructor, or a childbirth instructor might also be able to help you locate other nursing mothers.

Local Travel

Traveling around town, shopping, visiting, running errands, doctor's visits, driving the older children to lessons or meetings—all work out nicely with a breastfed baby. All you

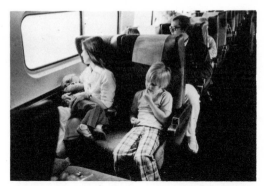

Train Travel

Discreet nursing allows a mother to enjoy the scenery without having to worry about warming bottles of formula.

Sandra C. Wallace

need is a baby carrier, a few diapers, and yourself. If you're running many errands, some types of baby carriers can be worn while driving, with baby in the car seat. Each time you get out, just pop baby back into the carrier. (See Time and Energy Savers, in chapter 2, "Nursing Techniques.")

While shopping on hot days you don't need to be concerned about baby's milk spoiling. It is always at the proper temperature. Trips to the park or beach are easier to handle with a breastfed baby, because there's less paraphernalia to carry. And baby is much more content on these day-long treks when mother and food are always nearby.

Breastfeeding can also uncomplicate visits to the doctor. Long waits pass more pleasantly if you nurse your baby during that time. It's a relief not to have to worry about how many bottles to take along, in case visits turn out to be longer than you expected.

If you are not yet comfortable about nursing around strangers, practice in front of a mirror to assure yourself you are covered sufficiently. This gives you confidence that you can nurse in public. Nursing in front of your husband for his critique can be helpful to you and reassuring to him that you can be discreet. Other nursing mothers who have traveled can be a wonderful source of ideas, too. As one mother said, "A crying baby who is waiting for formula to heat excites more attention than a peacefully nursing baby."

Traveling by Plane

When traveling by air with a breastfed baby, it's good to nurse during takeoff and landing or any other time when the air pressure changes. Baby naturally swallows then, to "pop" his ears. Besides, the noise of the jet engines can be frightening, and nursing is a good way to comfort him.

Here are some ideas on simplifying air travel, from a La Leche League publication:

• Select a time of day when air travel is lighter. Flight attendants are able to offer more attention if the flight is not full. The unused seats allow baby more room for naps, play and diapering.

• Request bulkhead seating (first row of seats in each part of the cabin which has a wall or wide space, not a row of seats, in front of it). The extra space is handy for a bassinet or play area.

• Whether you have two seats or a row of seats at your disposal, you'll find it more comfortable if arm rests are removed. If there are no extra seats, an airline pillow can be placed over the space where the arm rest was, between mother and father, for a third seat.

• Many airlines have in-flight bassinets which can be reserved at seat selection time. These cannot be used at takeoff or landing. At those times, you must hold your baby for safety.

• The 747 is the only large plane which has a fold-down changing table in one of its bathrooms. A sign on the door indicates this extra feature.

• In an on-board diaper bag, pack more diapers than you think will be needed and include one change of clothes. A wet washcloth in a plastic bag is valuable for post-meal wipe-ups. Also include nutritious snacks and a few toys suitable for a confined space.

- At mealtime, the flight attendant can serve one parent while the other tends to the baby. Extra seats between you often make this unnecessary as baby can be easily maneuvered and cared for as both parents eat. (3)

A nursing mother who has traveled a great deal and who is also a former flight attendant, wrote:

For very long trips abroad it is a temptation to make the trip all at once. By limiting travel to more brief segments, with layovers, you allow for gradual adjustment. Coping with a time change, such as from New York to London, can be an exhausting ordeal. Nursing is a real plus since you can sleep and nurse at the same time. The problem is that baby tends to stay on the *old* time and mother usually misses quite a lot of sleep because of this. So, stay extra well nourished and try to get help with the little ones so you can take some naps.

Food for Traveling

Children's eating patterns may change while traveling. Infants often seem to nurse more than usual, because nursing means security. Probably mother has more time, having fewer everyday pressures, and notices her baby's needs more quickly. Older babies who are eating solids often nurse more when traveling, for a sense of security in new surroundings or as a pleasant diversion if they're bored.

Traveling with toddlers and children presents a challenge to maintain a normal diet. Restaurants generally don't serve fresh fruits and vegetables, and much of the food is fried or very spicy. While staying in hotels, food bought at grocery stores can provide an alternative to restaurant fare. Yogurt and fruits, for example, are good choices. Grocery stores near hotels often serve individual portions.

Portable baby food grinders can be taken anywhere and

provide instant baby food. When selecting from restaurant menus, choose foods that are wholesome and nutritious to grind for your baby. To avoid any allergic reactions, stay away from "mixed" foods, like stews, because you will have no idea what ingredients were used in preparing them. Avoid changes in diet as much as possible while traveling because of unknown reactions your baby may have.

In a restaurant, nursing at a counter can be difficult with a toddler, but it can be done. When seated at a table, a chair that faces the fewest other tables offers more privacy.

Always having things on hand for between-meal snacks can help fill hungry tummies when there is no place to stop and eat. Cheeses wrapped in foil, fruits, raw vegetables, and nuts are easy to pack and can be bought at supermarkets wherever you are. A small jar of peanut butter and crackers is another good choice. It's fun for everyone to have his own container (plastic bag, or can with lid) containing a mixture of "goodies." One mother fixes a concoction of chopped fruits and unsalted nuts to tide over her carful of healthy appetites.

Individual lunches which contain plenty of protein and travel well can include a cold chop, hard-boiled egg, apple and dried fruits. Some foods can stay at room temperature; others can be kept fresh in an ice bucket or insulated bag with ice. Take along a large Thermos of cold water; it quenches thirst as no soda pop can do. Homemade lemonade is a good choice, too.

Long periods of driving, when everyone becomes tired, too hungry, and too cramped, are especially hard on children. Interrupt lengthy travel with breaks of 15 to 30 minutes in the fresh air to stretch and exercise.

Additional Tips

Here are some further ideas other mothers have found helpful when traveling with children:

- It is convenient to have a child's car harness which fits snugly, allows him to stand or sit on pillows and see out the window, but keeps him from being thrown around.

• If a child tends to be carsick, keep the seats as clear as possible. Watch for signs of yawning, coughing, sudden silence. Carry a plastic bowl with lid, old diaper, and air freshener. For the older baby, munching dry crackers can be used as an antidote.

• Keep a bag in the car containing a complete change of clothing to fit any child, insect repellent, soothing lotion, Band-aids, tissues, bag for trash, prepackaged moist towelettes, towel, books, pencils and paper. Surprises can be included, to be shared when you have "passed six red cars" or "come to the next town."

Chapter 25

When You Go It Alone

The single-parent family has special needs, and you, at the head of it, may feel overwhelmed by the responsibilities involved in meeting those needs. Being the planner, doer, and then evaluator is frequently coupled with too little time, not enough sleep, feeling overwhelmed, and occasional loneliness. Physically and emotionally, breastfeeding may ease the stresses of single parenting and provide a comfortable means of coping with your family's needs as well as your own.

If You Are Widowed

Some mothers who are widowed while they are still nursing find no change in the baby's nursing pattern. Other mothers find that the child nurses considerably more, or temporarily loses interest in nursing.

When Carla became a widow, her baby, Patrick, was eight months old. The other children were ten, eight, and four years old. Carla shares the following:

> During those first months after Gary died, I lost weight from not eating, and from being tired and upset. My milk supply was really down for a couple of weeks. Patrick was less interested in nursing, would nurse only a short time, and then still be hungry. Since he was getting solids, I didn't worry about his getting enough milk, just about his getting comfort. This drop in my milk supply was temporary, and it came back as I became more stable.
>
> For me, the main advantages of nursing were emotional. My feeling of helplessness was lessened because I

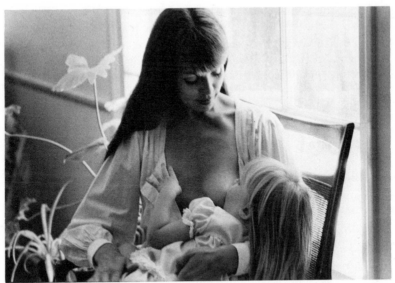

Sandra C. Wallace

The intimacy and loving involved with breastfeeding your baby can help ease you through emotionally troubled times.

was nursing; my baby was getting cuddling and attention, and *I* was doing it, not somebody else. The children needed me, and that meant I had less time for self-pity. Caring for them put some structure into my life.

About a month after Gary died, I thought Patrick was weaning. He'd had juice at the sitter's and he became used to the bottle. He just fooled around when he nursed and I was feeling guilty about leaving him so often to attend to legal and other business matters. I was very angry about not seeming to have any other choice because these things had to be taken care of.

I hadn't noticed the anger spilling over to Patrick but as things settled down, he began to nurse regularly again. When he was 15 months old he still nursed two or three times a day.

Nursing Patrick proved to be a good transition for me. I was comforted by his closeness. When my husband

525

died, there was such a void. In a sense, nursing our baby
was a connection with my husband. A baby will sleep in
your arms. He will cuddle, and stroke, and touch, and
unconditionally love you. Nursing helped diminish my
feelings of total loss and loneliness.

Other widowed mothers mention that their babies seem
to sense the loss and react to it in their own ways. Separation
from mother at this time can cause grief reactions in babies—
including nursing strikes. If you have a fussy baby, lots of
"talk therapy" with friends, and contact with other mothers of
fussy nursing babies can help to keep your perspective as you
share the joys, humor, and problems. There is a group specifically geared towards widows, called THEOS (They Help
Each Other Spiritually) which can be helpful, also. See
Appendix: Organizations to Help the Nursing Mother, for
further information on contacting this group.

Divorce or Separation

Many of the same feelings that are experienced by mothers
after the deaths of their husbands are also felt by mothers who
are separated or divorced.

In addition, there is frequently the added factor of tension
in the home preceding the actual separation of the mother and
father. After the separation, that tension is gone, but the child
may fear that mother may also leave him. Breastfeeding provides continuity and literal reassurance of her presence.

Impending loss can create stress. One mother of a three-
year-old boy and a two-month-old girl was stunned when her
husband announced that he wasn't happy in the marriage and
wanted a separation. Before they took that step, they agreed to
spend several sessions with a marriage counselor. This mother
describes her feelings at the time:

I experienced every possible emotion and you can imagine
what happened to my milk. I was like a zombie floating
in and out of the house. I went for three days on coffee
and water. I nursed Mary whenever possible, but there

wasn't much there, and no let-down. At this point, I began using the extra breast milk that I had regularly expressed and frozen since her birth. The babysitter fed her by bottle when I was away from her or too upset to put her to breast. I wish I could say that my mothering saw me through, but I can't. There were times when I was so numb that my baby would cry and I could only look at her. Then there were times when knowing that I had to nurse her helped me hold myself together.

No matter how inevitable or even how welcome divorce is, it is not without painful emotions. Even with relief of tension, there is the grief and mourning that comes with a death . . . the death of a relationship. Mary explains how she dealt with these emotions:

Lisa was four years old and Sharon was six months old when my husband told me he wanted a divorce. Lisa was confused about what was happening, but Sharon seemed happy as long as she was with me and I maintained her routine.

There was an immediate decrease in my milk supply. I had been donating ten ounces of milk a day to a mother's milk bank, and suddenly two or three ounces was all the extra milk I had. However, Sharon nursed as usual and seemed satisfied.

Those first three months of my separation were a very emotional time. I felt confused, and guilty about the failure of my marriage. I was fearful of the future, and torn by self-doubt.

I finally decided that professional counseling would help me. A close friend cared for both girls while I attended six weeks of group therapy and an eight-week divorce workshop which helped me accept the finality of the divorce. The baby was drinking from a cup by this time and easily went the three hours without nursing.*

---

* Private one-to-one therapy with the counselor coming to your home is one way to avoid separation of mother and baby. Also, a therapist who is supportive of breastfeeding will put a mother at ease about bringing her baby to the office.

If You Are an Unmarried Mother

As a single mother who is nursing, you may feel the lack of a partner with whom to share your concerns. If most of your friends are single nonmothers, this can increase the sense of being alone. La Leche League support, information, and help with breastfeeding can be particularly important, by putting you in contact with other nursing mothers.

Suzette was unmarried when her first baby was born. She shares her experience:

> I suppose I had no worse problems than a married mother might have, but not having another person to share my concerns with probably amplified them. Because my baby was fussy and seemingly hungry all the time, I fell into the supplementary bottle routine for the first two months, until I finally had the courage (with help from La Leche League) to kick it. I know every new mother worries about the same type of things I did, but most can discuss them with their husbands or their friends.
>
> Nursing did make my life a lot easier. Since I was usually unable to go out without my baby anyway (no built-in babysister and no babysitter funds) I was better able to tote him around when I went places.

Suzette went back to work when her baby was four months old. She arranged to leave her son with a babysitter, and came home for lunch so she could nurse. When her baby was a year old and beginning to wean, Suzette met and dated a man (whom she eventually married) who didn't mind taking *both* mother and child out on dates!

If Your Husband Is Away

Some mothers alone are women who have loving, supportive husbands, who for various reasons are away a great deal.

When children are aware that their father is no longer with them (even if it's only a temporary absence), they sometimes think he doesn't love them anymore. This is what Kristin found. Twice her husband, who is a senior chief in the Navy, was away for more than six months. During the long separations, Kristin said it seemed that her boys needed the reassurance of being able to see her almost every minute.

This obvious need to be close to mother made Kristin very insistent on being with two-year-old Stevie when he became sick and was going to be hospitalized for diagnostic tests. Because there was no rooming-in policy, she asked to take him home as soon as possible. It took only 45 minutes for the X-rays and blood tests to be completed, and during that time Kristin stayed with Stevie, comforting and reassuring him. When the test results showed nothing requiring hospitalization, she was able to take him home. She says:

> Home again, I breastfed Stevie almost constantly. During the first 24 hours, when he wasn't sleeping or nursing, Stevie kept crying, "I want my Daddy." I felt relief that I could be with him to comfort him. With Daddy gone, sudden abandonment by mother (such as separation during hospitalization) is especially terrifying to a little child.

Following a lengthy separation, fathers and their families have adjustments to make when they are reunited. Maybe your toddler has been sleeping in bed with you and nursing at night. If your husband doesn't realize that breastfeeding is a source of comfort and satisfaction for you and the baby, he may not like this sleeping arrangement. Perhaps you can compromise by nursing your baby to sleep, then putting him in his own bed, which could be right next to yours. You may find it helpful to discuss the ideas from a book such as *The Family Bed: An Age-Old Concept in Child Rearing*. (1)

When Father Objects to Nursing

For various reasons, fathers are sometimes opposed to the idea of breastfeeding. If this is the case, a mother may be "alone" in her desire to breastfeed, although the father is not absent.

A father may have been looking forward to bottlefeeding the baby. He may feel deprived of a special time if you nurse. Talk with him about the benefits of breastfeeding, and the many ways in which he can participate in the baby's care, such as giving him a bath, dressing him and changing diapers, playing with him and feeding him solid foods when that time comes. Having baby sleep with you, besides being convenient for night nursings, allows him the chance to snuggle back under his father's protective arm after a satisfying feeding.

If father insists on giving a bottle, some mothers have expressed breast milk to avoid potential allergy problems. There is always a chance, once you start giving bottles, that your baby will learn to prefer the easier sucking. If father insists on frequent bottle feedings (which usually lead to early weaning), he may be giving you a disguised message that he wants you to pay more attention to him. He may be envious of the little one who is having all his needs met by you, and feel left out. Listen for the real messages, the ones telling you what he needs.

Prior planning is the best way to overcome a husband's objections to nursing. Before the baby arrives, educate yourself and be fully convinced that breastfeeding is best for your baby. Leave some of your reading material around where it is available to your husband and invite him to discuss what you each have read.

Nancy explained how her husband's background influenced his attitude toward nursing. He felt very strongly that nobody but the husband, in the privacy of the bedroom, should see his wife's breasts. She said, "When I'd try to talk to him about breastfeeding and what I'd learned, he'd leave the room." Nancy and the baby eventually demonstrated the value of breastfeeding. Before the baby was born, Nancy read out loud about breastfeeding during car trips. After she was born, the baby herself was a great source of education. In the end, the father became convinced of the advantages of breastfeeding, and supported his wife.

You really have two goals: one, breastfeeding; the other, gaining your husband's support. To do this, one mother suggests you begin with a trial nursing period of two to four weeks. If he is concerned that someone else will see you breastfeeding, assure him that you will practice ways to nurse discreetly. During this period, mention how well things are going, how happy his baby and you are, how healthy the baby is, how convenient it is, and how much you appreciate his being open to something so foreign to him. Hopefully, at the end of a few weeks, your husband will begin to be more appreciative of breastfeeding and more in tune with your feelings about continuing for a longer time. In the beginning, getting your husband's agreement on short-term goals may be easier than trying to gain his approval for breastfeeding until the baby weans.

Some fathers never quite resolve their mixed feelings about breastfeeding. However, it is okay for him to have reservations and it is still possible for you to nurse discreetly. If this is your situation, you may want to find another source of support. Seeing things differently is a part of life . . . and so is working out conflicts. Many an objecting father, after having had an opportunity to express his anxiety and having subsequently found it unwarranted after all, has been "converted" and perhaps even begun to brag to family and friends about the advantages of breastfeeding.

Taking Care of Yourself

When you are alone, you need to examine and set your priorities. Take one day at a time, cope with problems as they actually arise, instead of dreading situations which may not occur. Don't expect too much of yourself.

Don't neglect yourself. It's easy to get in the habit of eating poorly. Some mothers share each other's cooking occasionally for variety.

Try to pamper yourself once in a while, maybe with a new hairdo, or a meal in a restaurant. Planning a chance to get a breath of fresh air is important to you and to the rest of your family. Feelings of suffocation sometimes breed resentment. Some mothers have been urged to wean their babies and get

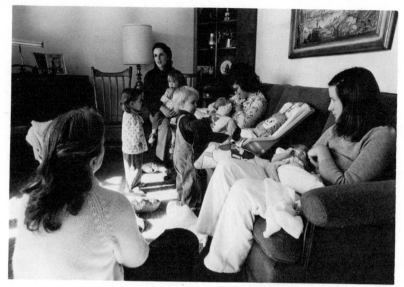

Rodale Press Photography Staff

La Leche League meetings can provide support and reassurance for mothers alone. Besides offering information and help with breastfeeding, La Leche League can be a means of putting you in contact with other nursing mothers.

away for a weekend but have found that weaning really isn't necessary with planning and friendly support. (See Separation for a Few Days, chapter 23, "Nursing and Working.")

Your Cheering Squad

Dana Raphael, in *The Tender Gift: Breastfeeding* (2), refers to the importance of having someone to "mother the mother." Mothers who are not being nurtured by their husbands may need some physical and emotional support from time to time. Just talking with others and knowing that they share common feelings is encouraging. As one mother said, "We all have those guilt feelings that 'maybe my child is doing that because I'm a single parent'. We need to share with a friend and find out that her child is doing some of the same things even though the father is there. It can be a big relief."

Emotional support can be gained from family, friends, church groups and La Leche League. Professional counseling may be beneficial, especially if you can find a counselor who is supportive of breastfeeding. Your local La Leche League group leader or your pediatrician may be able to refer you to such a counselor in your area. For further suggestions on how to locate counselors, see Appendix: Organizations to Help the Nursing Mother.

Appendix

Organizations to Help the Nursing Mother

No matter what special situation you are facing, your breast-feeding experience will be enhanced by sharing experiences and discussing approaches with other mothers. Breastfeeding groups offer personal assistance and encouragement, and may be able to put you in touch with someone who has nursed in a situation similar to yours. Informative literature is often available for loan or may be purchased.

In addition, many support groups organized nationally and locally are ready to help families in special situations, by providing information and/or services. Check your phone book to see if there is a local group. If no group is listed, contact the national office to locate the group nearest you.

Doctors, ministers, social workers, and libraries are sources of possible referrals to organizations in addition to those listed here.

Childbirth

American Society for Psychoprophylaxis in Obstetrics, Inc. (ASPO)
1523 L Street, NW, Suite 410
Washington, DC 20005

> A group of physicians, parents and professionals offering training and certification of prenatal class instructors in the Psychoprophylactic Method of Childbirth Preparation (Lamaze method). ASPO also operates an information and referral service that directs parents to qualified instructors and physicians.

Cesareans/Support, Education, and Concern (C/SEC, Inc.)
15 Maynard Road
Dedham, MA 02026

> An organization which seeks to provide information on many aspects of cesarean childbirth in order to make couples aware of what the procedure involves and what options may be available to them.

International Childbirth Education Association
PO Box 70258
Milwaukee, WI 53220

> A volunteer organization which brings together persons interested in family-centered maternity and infant care. Services include promoting and encouraging preparation for childbearing, breastfeeding, and family-centered maternity care and assistance in the establishment of local groups.

Breastfeeding and Child Care

Breastfeeding Information Services
10952 Templeton Drive
Philadelphia, PA 19154

> An organization which provides information and support through telephone contact, literature and monthly meetings. Also assists the medical profession in supporting the nursing mother.

Children In Hospitals, Inc.
31 Wilshire Park
Needham, MA 02192

> A group of parents and health-care professionals that seeks to educate those concerned about the need for ample contact between children and parents when either is hospitalized. It encourages hospitals to adopt flexible visiting and living-in policies.

Fathers and Mothers Learning through Education and Experience
(FAMLEE)
Box 15
Telford, PA 18969

> A nonprofit organization which supports mothers who wish to breastfeed through informal meetings and 24-hour phone counseling.

Lact-Aid
Division of Resources in Human Nurturing
Box 6861
Denver, CO 80206

> Further information on Lact-Aid nursing supplementers is provided.

Appendix

La Leche League International, Inc.
9616 Minneapolis Avenue
Franklin Park, IL 60131

> An organization devoted to helping and encouraging mothers who want to nurse their babies. Local group leaders are mothers who have nursed their own babies, and who assist others in the art of breastfeeding through monthly meetings and telephone counseling. LLL makes available various publications: a manual, *The Womanly Art of Breastfeeding;* Information Sheets, containing information on many aspects of breastfeeding; and the bimonthly *La Leche League News,* featuring informal stories, reports on medical research, practical suggestions. This material is read and approved by the appropriate professional consultants before publication. A complete list of publications is available upon request. LLL has the advice and support of a Professional Advisory Board, whose members are all qualified professionals.

The Netsy Company
34 Sunrise Avenue
Mill Valley, CA 94941

> This company manufactures the Swedish Milk Cup and Breast Shield.

Nursing Mothers Committee
Family Centered Parents, Inc.
Box 142
Rockland, DE 19732

> This organization provides support and encouragement of a nonmedical nature to breastfeeding mothers.

Nursing Mothers Counsel, Inc.
PO Box 7364
Menlo Park, CA 94025

> A group of mothers which encourages and supports other mothers in successfully breastfeeding their children. The Counsel works closely with local hospitals, providing seminars and counseling to those maternity patients who wish to breastfeed.

Parents Concerned for Hospitalized Children, Inc.
176 North Villa Avenue
Villa Park, IL 60181
> A group of parents and professionals which encourages health care facilities to develop family-oriented pediatric care. Services include support of families and education of parents as to effects of hospitalization on children, and appropriate measures to prevent or lessen trauma.

Milk Banks

California

Mother's Milk Unit—No. Calif. Transplant Bank
Maria Teresa Asquith, Coordinator
751 South Bascom Avenue
San Jose, CA 95128

Mother's Milk Bank of Monterey County
Mary Madruga, R.N., Coordinator
Childbirth Education League of Salinas
PO Box 1423
Salinas, CA 93901

San Diego Mother's Milk Bank—University Hospital
Brian Saunders, M.D., Coordinator
225 West Dickinson Street
San Diego, CA 92103

Mother's Milk Bank, Inc.
Children's Hospital—Suite 110
3700 California Street
San Francisco, CA 94118

Delaware

Wilmington Milk Bank
Elizabeth J. Langerak, Coordinator
Wilmington Medical Center
501 West Fourteenth Street
Wilmington, DE 19899

Hawaii

Nursing Mothers Association, Inc. (Milk Bank)
DeEtta Cunningham, Coordinator
Hilo Hospital
1190 Waianuenue Avenue
Hilo, HI 96720

Hawaii Mother's Milk, Inc.
Randi Silleck, Coordinator
226 North Kuakini Street
Honolulu, HI 96817

Kentucky

Louisville Breast Milk Program
Mrs. Patricia Stiebling
Norton—Children's Hospitals, Inc.
PO Box 655
Louisville, KY 40201

Massachusetts

Central Massachusetts Regional Milk Bank
Miriam Erickson, Coordinator
Hahnemann Hospital
281 Lincoln Street
Worcester, MA 01605

Minnesota

St. Paul Children's Hospital Milk Bank
Sue LaRock, R.N., Coordinator
311 Pleasant Avenue
St. Paul, MN 55102

New Hampshire

Dartmouth Medical School
Laurie Rippe, R.N., Nurse Consultant
Dept. of Maternal and Child Health
Hanover, NH 03755

North Carolina

Piedmont Mother's Milk Bank
Mary Rose Tully, Coordinator
4025 Greenleaf Street
Raleigh, NC 27606

Texas

Providence Memorial Hospital
Mother's Milk Bank
Belinda Brice, R.N.
2001 North Oregon Street
El Paso, TX 79902

Virginia

Children's Hospital of Kings' Daughters
Frederick Wirth, M.D.
609 Colley Avenue
Norfolk, VA 23507

Family Relations

Couple-to-Couple League
PO Box 11084
Cincinnati, OH 45211
>An interfaith organization offering married couples help with the successful practice of natural family planning. CCL teaches ecological breastfeeding and the full sympto-thermal method.

Parents Anonymous
2810 Artesia Boulevard
Redondo Beach, CA 90278
> A nationwide self-help organization dedicated to aiding parents who abuse or neglect their children, or fear that they will do so without help.

Parents without Partners
7910 Woodmont Avenue
Suite 1000
Washington, DC 20014
> Activities conducted by volunteer members make up a well-rounded program to help single parents. Local chapters throughout the United States and Canada offer discussions, lecture series, family-oriented activities and numerous social activities for adults.

They Help Each Other Spiritually (THEOS)
10521 Lindberg Avenue
Pittsburgh, PA 15235
> A national organization with local chapters, featuring a Christian ministry of mutual self-help for young and middle-aged widowed people and their families. Members support each other in coping with grief, loneliness and changed life circumstances.

Diseases, Developmental Conditions, Disabilities

Adrenal Metabolic Research Society of the Hypoglycemia Foundation, Inc.
PO Box 98
Fleetwood
Mount Vernon, NY 10552
> A nonprofit corporation geared toward studying the incidence, causes, and treatment of hypoglycemia. Various publications are available concerning allergies, diet, alcoholism, and glandular functions.

Allergy Foundation of America
801 Second Avenue
New York, NY 10017

A voluntary health agency established to increase knowledge of the causes and best treatment for asthma and diseases related to allergy.

American Foundation for the Blind, Inc.
15 West Sixteenth Street
New York, NY 10011

The Foundation prints a directory of agencies serving the visually handicapped. It also publishes a directory of aids and appliances such as clothing tags and canned food labels, scales, and cooking aids.

The Arthritis Foundation
3400 Peachtree Road, NE
Atlanta, GA 30326

An organization offering information concerning arthritis and available community services. Local chapters distribute literature and sponsor forums and lectures to keep patients and physicians aware of the latest developments in arthritis research and treatment.

Association for Children with Learning Disabilities
5225 Grace Street
Pittsburgh, PA 15236

An association geared toward increasing public understanding of learning disabilities and stimulating improved school and community relationships. ACLD sponsors lectures and meetings and publishes a monthly newsletter.

Better Hearing Institute
1430 K Street, NW, Suite 600
Washington, DC 20005

An educational organization that provides information and encouragement to the hearing- and speech-impaired and their families. The Institute works mainly through television, radio, and magazines, publishes much of its own material, and sponsors lectures.

Appendix

Cleft Parent Guild
c/o Crippled Children's Society
7120 Franklin Avenue
Los Angeles, CA 90046
> This is a source of names and addresses of cleft parent groups throughout the United States.

Closer Look
Box 1492
Washington, DC 20013
> This organization publishes a guide explaining state laws and directs parents of children with emotional, physical, or mental handicaps to services and financial help to which they are legally entitled.

Cystic Fibrosis Foundation
3379 Peachtree Road, NE
Atlanta, GA 30326
> National voluntary health organization offering support for research, clinical care, and educational programs benefiting children with cystic fibrosis and other respiratory diseases.

Epilepsy Foundation of America
1828 L Street, NW, Suite 406
Washington, DC 20036
> A national organization which works with government, industry, and the general public on behalf of people with epilepsy. Local chapters provide members with low-cost prescription drugs, group life insurance plans, and offer counseling and employment help.

Juvenile Diabetes Foundation
23 East Twenty-sixth Street
New York, NY 10010
> An international voluntary health agency devoted to the study of causes, prevention, and the cure of diabetes. It provides information to the general public and offers counseling and services to the diabetic and his family.

Muscular Dystrophy Association, Inc.
810 Seventh Avenue
New York, NY 10019
>A voluntary agency of scientists and citizens working to combat neuromuscular diseases. It maintains a worldwide research program, free clinics and services for patients and their families, and various public and professional education programs.

National Association of the Deaf
814 Thayer Avenue
Silver Spring, MD 20910
>A private consumer organization dedicated to protecting the rights of deaf people. The association provides information on deafness and sign language and refers individuals to legal aid, counseling, and education services.

National Association for Down's Syndrome
PO Box 63
Oak Park, IL 60303
>A group of parents of Down's syndrome children devoted to providing support to new parents and educating its members and the general public about Down's syndrome.

National Association for Retarded Citizens (NARC)
2709 Avenue E, East
Arlington, TX 76011
>A volunteer organization devoted to improving the welfare of all mentally retarded persons. NARC Research and Demonstration Institute is designed to improve the life of the retarded citizen through research, demonstrations and the development of new approach policies. Publications are available.

National Easter Seal Society for Crippled Children and Adults
2023 West Ogden Avenue
Chicago, IL 60612
>The nation's largest voluntary health agency that serves the handicapped. The Society operates treatment, research, and education programs throughout the United States and Puerto Rico.

The National Foundation-March of Dimes
1275 Mamaroneck Avenue
White Plains, NY 10605

An association dedicated to the prevention of birth defects and any life-threatening condition in the newborn. March of Dimes supports a network of research, education, and medical service programs.

National Genetics Foundation, Inc.
9 West Fifty-seventh Street
New York, NY 10019

A group which provides diagnosis, treatment, and genetic counseling to those afflicted with genetic disorders. The foundation operates a nationwide network of genetic counseling and treatment centers.

National Information and Referral Service for Autistic and Autistic-like Persons
306 Thirty-first Street
Huntingdon, WV 25702

A national organization dedicated solely to the autistic citizen. Primary goals are cures for autistic children and providing appropriate services to help them reach their highest potential.

National Society for Autistic Children
169 Tampa Avenue
Albany, NY 12208

A society that works for the education, welfare, and cure of all children with severe communication and behavior disorders.

Pilot Parents (Toronto)
c/o The Metro Toronto Association for the Mentally Retarded
186 Beverley Street
Toronto, Ontario
Canada M5T 1Z2

An organization which offers emotional and practical support for parents who have recently discovered their children are mentally handicapped. New parents are matched one-to-one with experienced parents in a similar situation.

The Premature and High Risk Infant Association, Inc.
PO Box A-3083
c/o West Glen Branch
Peoria, IL 61614

A group geared toward providing emotional and educational assistance to parents of premature and/or high risk infants. The PHRI Association operates a telephone helpline, holds monthly meetings, publishes several guides on such topics as breastfeeding and caring for the high risk infant, and provides members with many special services.

Recordings for the Blind
215 East Fifty-eighth Street
New York, NY 10022

A national agency which provides tape-recorded educational texts and materials on loan at no cost to visually, physically, and perceptually handicapped individuals. Available on tape are the La Leche League manual, *The Womanly Art of Breast-feeding, Nursing Your Baby* by Karen Pryor, and *The Family Book of Child Care* by Niles Newton.

Recovery, Inc., National Headquarters
116 South Michigan Avenue
Chicago, IL 60603

A nonprofit, self-help organization for people wanting to regain and maintain mental health.

Spina Bifida Association
343 South Dearborn
Chicago, IL 60604

An association that provides information on spina bifida to parents, adults with spina bifida, and professionals in the field.

Twins Mothers National Organization
Box 109
Main Post Office
Toledo, OH 43601

Members of local Mothers of Twins clubs swap ideas on twin care, solutions to common problems and sometimes clothing and baby equipment.

United Cerebral Palsy Association
122 East Twenty-third Street
New York, NY 10010

> An organization dedicated to improving the quality of life for persons with cerebral palsy. Provides information, counseling and service programs for the cerebral palsied and their families.

United States Department of Health, Education and Welfare
300 Independence Avenue, SW
Washington, DC 20203

> Three agencies within this department are the source of helpful information, book lists and pamphlets: Developmental Disabilities Office, National Institute of Mental Health, and National Institute of Neurological and Communicative Disorders and Stroke.

Community Resources

The telephone directory is one place to start in order to locate qualified counselors and service agencies in your area. Consult both the white pages and yellow pages for helpful listings.

White Pages

State Department of Human Resources, Mental Health Division. This division can direct you to the Community Mental Health Center nearest you. These federally funded centers serve geographical districts in each state. They are required by law to provide you with service whether or not you are able to pay. The fees are set according to your income and some health insurance plans cover outpatient treatment regardless of your ability to cover the fee. Services available include:

> Inpatient (hospitalization for short-term treatment and psychiatric emergency)
> Outpatient (individual counseling, marriage counseling, family therapy, group therapy)
> Diagnostic
> Rehabilitative
> Training
> Consultation and education for people in the community (schools, businesses, hospitals, nursing homes)

Family and Children's Services
This local agency is a member of the Family Service Association of America. Individual and group counseling by a professionally trained staff are provided.

Visiting Nurse Association
The association sponsors clinics as well as home visits. It can also direct you to other community service agencies that suit your specific need.

Yellow Pages

For professional counseling, check these listings:

Marriage and Family Counselors
Psychiatrists
Psychologists

or contact the local school psychologist for references.

Under the listing, Social Service Organizations, are found organizations involved in counseling and specific areas such as disabilities, mental health, and homemaker services.

Organizations outside the United States

Nursing Mothers' Association of Australia
National Headquarters
PO Box 230
Hawthorn 3122
Victoria, Australia
In addition to local discussion groups and telephone assistance, this organization publishes helpful booklets and leaflets on many aspects of breastfeeding and child care. For a complete list of publications, write for the catalogue.

Hospital Victor do Amaral (Milk Bank)
Nélio Ribas Centa, M.D.
Av. Iguacú, 1953
Curitiba-Paraná, 80.000
Brazil

Instituto da Puericultura e Pediatria Martagao Gesteira (Milk Bank)
Universidade Federal do Rio de Janeiro
Cidade Universitaria
Ilha do Fundao
Rio de Janeiro, Brazil

Instituto Fernandes Figueira (Milk Bank)
Av. Rui Barbosa 716
Batafogo
Rio de Janeiro, Brazil

Banco de Leite do Hospital dos Servidores (Milk Bank)
Publicos de Sao Paulo
Rua Pedro Toledo 1.8000
Sao Paulo, SP, Brazil

Lactario de Santa Casa (Milk Bank)
Rua Marques de Itu 695
Sao Paulo, SP, Brazil

Children's Centre of the Health Sciences Centre (Milk Bank)
Dr. J. C. Hawarth
685 Bannatyne Avenue
Winnipeg, Manitoba
Canada R3E 0W1

KVINDEMAELKSCENTRALEN (Milk Bank)
Dr. Knud E. Petersen
Children's Hospital (Bornehospitalet)
Drosselvej 57.2000F
Copenhagen, Denmark

Kings College Hospital (Milk Bank)
Dr. H. R. Gamsu, Dept. of Child Health
Denmark Hill, S.E.
London SE5 7DG
England

National Association for the Welfare of Children in Hospitals
7 Exton Street
London, S.E.1.
England

Queen Charlotte's Maternity Hospital (Milk Bank)
Dr. David Harvey
Goldhawk Road
London W6 OXG
England

Lactarium des Hospices Civils de Strasbourg (Milk Bank)
Mademoiselle Lauer, Directrice du Lactarium
23 rue de la Porte de L'Hopital
67000, Strasbourg
France

PPPI
Malaysian Group
Mrs. Mary Lee
8 Jalan Klyne
Kuala Lumpur, 01-21
Malaysia

Amnehjelpen
Box 15
Holmen, Oslo 3
Norway

Singapore Breast Feeding Mothers Group
Mrs. J. Tan
Consumers Associates of Singapore
Shenton Way
Singapore, 1

Swedish Breast Feeding Group (Amning Hajelpen)
c/o Professor B. Vahlquist
Department of Pediatrics
University Hospital
Uppsala, Sweden

Bibliography

General Recommended Reading

Child and Family Reprint, "Management of Successful Lactation," 1972.*

La Leche League International. *The Womanly Art of Breastfeeding.* 2d ed. Franklin Park, Ill.: La Leche League International, 1963.

Montagu, Ashley. *Touching: The Human Significance of the Skin.* New York: Columbia University Press, 1971.

Newton, Niles. *The Family Book of Child Care.* New York: Harper & Row, 1957.

Pryor, Karen. *Nursing Your Baby.* New York: Harper & Row, 1973.

Thevenin, Tine. *The Family Bed: An Age-Old Concept in Child Rearing.* Minneapolis: Privately printed, 1976.†

Introduction: The Kindness of Human Milk

Recommended Reading

Bosco, Dominick. "Why Breast Milk Is the Best Milk for Baby." *Prevention,* April 1976, pp. 92-97.

Grohman, Joann. "In 1870." *La Leche League News,* July/August 1976, p. 58.

Jelliffe, D. B., and Jelliffe, E. F. P. " 'Breast Is Best': Modern Meanings." *New England Journal of Medicine,* 27 October 1977.

Jelliffe, D. B., and Jelliffe, E. F. P., eds. "The Uniqueness of Human Milk." *The American Journal of Clinical Nutrition* 24 (1971): 968-1024.

La Leche League International. "Breastfed Is Best Fed." *La Leche League News,* March/April 1973.

"New Concepts of Infant Nutrition." *Current Medical Research and Opinion,* vol. 4, Supplement 1, 1976, Symposium Issue.

"New Evidence Favors Breastfeeding," *Medical World News,* 16 June 1975, pp. 26-28.

Newton, Niles. "Shall I Breastfeed My Baby?" La Leche League International Information Sheet no. 102.

---

* Available from Child and Family Reprint Dept., Box 508, Oak Park, IL 60303.

†Available by writing P.O. Box 16004, Minneapolis, MN 55416.

State of California Department of Public Health. Maternal and Child Health Branch. "Policy Statement: Breastfeeding—Its Role in Infant Growth and Development." March 1977.

Chapter 1 — What's Normal?

(1), (2), (3), Nursing Mothers' Association of Australia. "Breast and Nipple Preparation and Care." *

(4) Pryor, Karen. *Nursing Your Baby.* New York: Harper & Row, 1963.

(5) See reference no. 1.

(6) See reference no. 4.

(7) La Leche League International. "Nipple Care." Information Sheet no. 103.†

(8) See reference no. 1.

(9) Newton, Michael, and Newton, Niles. "The Normal Course and Management of Lactation." *Clinical Obstetrics and Gynecology.* vol. 5, no. 1, March 1962.

(10) Montagu, Ashley. *Touching: The Human Significance of the Skin.* New York: Columbia University Press, 1971.

(11) Holmes, Carl A. "Comforting Advice on Colic." *Parents' Magazine's Baby Care,* Summer 1974.

(12) Bingham, Ellen. "Why Our Double Standard?" *La Leche League News,* July/August 1974, The Canadian Echo.

(13) Eldridge, Eileen. "What Makes a Spoiled Baby?" *Your New Baby,* March 1968.‡

(14) Newton, Niles. "When Baby's Crying Gets Trying." La Leche League International Information Sheet no. 141.

(15), (16) White, Mary K. "The Waiting Game vs. Gaining Weight." La Leche League International Information Sheet no. 104.

(17) Froehlich, Edwina. "Baby's First Solid Food." La Leche League International Information Sheet no. 105.

(18) "Iron Absorption from Breast Milk or Cow's Milk." *Nutrition Reviews,* vol. 35, no. 8, August 1977, p. 203.

(19) White, Mary. "Does Breastfeeding Space Babies?" Reprint, *Marriage,* January 1961.§

---

* Nursing Mothers' Association of Australia publications are available by writing to the address listed in Appendix.

† La Leche League publications are available from La Leche League International, see Appendix for address.

‡ Available from Breastfeeding Information Services, 10952 Templeton Drive, Philadelphia, PA 19154.

§ Available from La Leche League International.

Bibliography

(20) Kippley, John, and Kippley, Sheila. *The Art of Natural Family Planning.* Cincinnati: Couple-to-Couple League, 1977.

(21) Kippley, Sheila. *Breastfeeding and Natural Child Spacing: The Ecology of Natural Mothering.* New York: Harper & Row, 1974.

(22) La Leche League International. "Thoughts about Weaning." Information Sheet no. 125.

Recommended Reading

Bauman, Carolyn. "Variations in Weight Gain." *La Leche League News,* July/August 1971, p. 60.

Countryman, Betty Ann. "How the Nurse Can Help the Breastfeeding Mother." La Leche League International Publication no. 118.

Fraiberg, Selma. "How a Baby Learns to Love." *Redbook,* May 1971. La Leche League International Reprint no. 123.

Hymes, James L. Jr. *The Child Under Six.* Englewood Cliffs, N.J.: Prentice-Hall, 1964.

La Leche League International. "Information, Please! Breastfeeding: First Step toward Preventive Dentistry." *La Leche League News,* July/August 1972, p. 57.

La Leche League International. "The Biological Specificity of Milk." Information Sheet no. 14.

La Leche League International. "The Nursing Couple Is Different." Information Sheet no. 140.

La Leche League International. "White Paper on Infant Feeding Practices." Information Sheet no. 158.

Raphael, Dana. *The Tender Gift: Breast Feeding.* New York: Schocken, 1976.

Chapter 2 — Nursing Techniques

(1) La Leche League International. "Guidelines for Milk Donations." Information Sheet no. 89.

(2) Nursing Mothers' Association of Australia. "Storing and Using Expressed Breast Milk."

(3) La Leche League International. "Reference Information—Aids for Relactation—List of Milk Banks." Information Sheet no. 89b.

(4) La Leche League International. "Nursing Fashions Packet." Information Sheet no. 98.

Recommended Reading

Applebaum, Richard M. "The Modern Management of Successful Breastfeeding." *Pediatric Clinics of North America* 17 (1970):203-25.

Countryman, Betty Ann. "How the Nurse Can Help the Breastfeeding Mother." La Leche League International Publication no. 118.

La Leche League International. "Breastfeeding and the Oral Contraceptive Pill." Information Sheet no. 18.

La Leche League International. "Losing Your Milk?" Information Sheet no. 83.

La Leche League International. "The Pacifier." Information Sheet no. 110.

Nursing Mothers' Association of Australia. "Hand Expressing—A Practical, Illustrated Guide."

Nursing Mothers' Association of Australia. "Increasing Your Supply—Hints on Building Up Your Milk Supply."

Nursing Mothers' Association of Australia. "Inverted Nipples."

Olds, Sally W., and Eiger, Marvin S. *The Complete Book of Breastfeeding.* New York: Workman, 1972.

Chapter 3 — Nutrition for Mother and Baby

(1) Boie, Shirley A. *Cookless Recipes.* Los Angeles: Boie Enterprises, 1968.*

(2) See reference no. 1.

(3) Newton, Michael, and Newton, Niles. "The Normal Course and Management of Lactation." *Clinical Obstetrics and Gynecology,* vol. 5, no. 1, March 1962.

(4) Brewer, Tom. "Prenatal Complications." *New Dynamics of Preventive Medicine,* vol. 2. Leon Pomeroy, ed. Miami: Symposia Specialists, 1974.

(5) Bosco, Dominick. "Why Breast Milk Is the Best Milk for Baby." *Prevention,* April 1976, pp. 92-97.

(6) Mayer, Jean. "Fat Babies Grow into Fat People." *Family Health.*

(7) Coffin, Lewis A. *The Grandmother Conspiracy Exposed.* Out of print.

(8) La Leche League International. *The Basic Concepts of La Leche League.* 1978.

(9) Froehlich, Edwina. "Baby's First Solid Food." La Leche League International Information Sheet no. 105.

(10) White, Mary K. "The Waiting Game vs. Gaining Weight." La Leche League International Information Sheet no. 104.

(11) White, Mary. "Does Breastfeeding Space Babies?" Reprint. *Marriage,* January 1961.

(12) Mackay, H. M. M. "Anemia in Infancy: Its Prevalency and Prevention." *Archives of Diseases in Childhood* 3 (1928):1175.

---

* Available by writing P.O. Box 66235, Los Angeles, CA 90066.

Bibliography

(13) McMillan, Julia A.; Landaw, S. A.; and Oski, F. A. "Iron Sufficiency in Breastfed Infants and the Availability of Iron from Human Milk." *Pediatrics* 58 (1976):5. La Leche League International Information Sheet no. 61.

(14) Kinderlehrer, Jane. *Confessions of a Sneaky Organic Cook.* Emmaus, Pa.: Rodale Press, 1971.

(15) Pryor, Karen. *Nursing Your Baby.* New York: Harper & Row, 1963.

(16) White, Mary. "Information, Please! Fluoride." *La Leche League News,* May/June 1970, pp. 44-45.

Recommended Reading

Applebaum, Richard. "The Modern Management of Successful Breastfeeding." *Pediatric Clinics of North America* 17 (1970):203-25.

Ewald, Ellen. *Recipes for a Small Planet.* New York: Ballantine, 1973.

Goldbeck, Nikki, and Goldbeck, David. *The Supermarket Handbook.* New York: Harper & Row, 1973.

Hauser, Gayelord. *The Gayelord Hauser Cookbook.* New York: Capricorn Books, 1946.

"Iron Absorption from Breast Milk or Cow's Milk." *Nutrition Reviews,* vol. 35, no. 8, August 1977, p. 203.

Jauch, Virginia C. "Maternal Nutrition in the 1970's." *Food and Nutrition News,* vol. 46, no. 3, February 1975.

Johnson, Roberta, ed. *Mother's in the Kitchen. The La Leche League Cookbook.* Franklin Park, Ill.: La Leche League International, 1971.

Kenda, Margaret, and Williams, Phyllis S. *The Natural Baby Food Cookbook.* New York: Avon, 1973.

La Leche League International. "Losing Your Milk?" Information Sheet no. 83.

La Leche League International. "The Care and Feeding of Families." *La Leche League News,* May/June 1975.

La Leche League International. "White Paper on Infant Feeding Practices." Information Sheet no. 158.

Lappé, Frances M. *Diet for a Small Planet.* New York: Ballantine, 1975.

Mayer, Jean. "When You're Eating for Two." *Family Health,* October 1973.

Oliver, Martha H. *Add a Few Sprouts to Eat Better for Less Money.* New Canaan, Conn.: Keats, 1975.

Robertson, Laurel; Flinders, Carol; and Godfrey, Bronwen. *Laurel's Kitchen.* Berkeley, Calif.: Nilgiri Press, 1976.

Shneour, Elie A. "Good Nutrition Should Begin at Conception." *Modern Medicine,* 15 April 1974.

Smith, Esther L. *Good Foods That Go Together.* New Canaan, Conn.: Keats, 1975.

Williams, Phyllis. *Nourishing Your Unborn Child.* New York: Avon, 1975.

Worthington, Bonnie S. *Nutrition in Pregnancy and Lactation.* St. Louis: C. V. Mosby, 1977.

Chapter 4 — Breast and Nipple Problems

(1) Applebaum, Richard M. "The Modern Management of Successful Breastfeeding." *Pediatric Clinics of North America* 17 (1970): 203-25.

(2) Newton, Michael, and Newton, Niles. "The Normal Course and Management of Lactation." *Clinical Obstetrics and Gynecology,* vol. 5, no. 1, March 1962.

(3) Nursing Mothers' Association of Australia. "Inverted Nipples."

(4) *The Womanly Art of Breastfeeding.* 2d ed. Franklin Park, Ill.: La Leche League International, 1963.

(5) Gunther, Mavis. *Infant Feeding.* Chicago: Henry Regnery Company, 1971.

(6) La Leche League International. "Breast Infections." *League Spirit* of Southern California and Nevada, Spring 1975, p. 8.

Recommended Reading

Brischler, Susann. "Sore Nipples? Try This." *La Leche League News,* January/February 1972, p. 14.

Hubbard, Ellen. "How We Solve Breastfeeding Problems." *RN Magazine,* vol. 33, no. 3, March 1970. La Leche League International Reprint no. 133.

La Leche League International. "And Speaking of Sore Nipples." *Leaven,* July/August 1974, p. 21.

La Leche League International. "Ice for Sore Nipples?" *Leaven,* January/February 1974, P. 4.

La Leche League International. "Inverted Nipples." Information Sheet no. 108.

La Leche League International. "Let There Be Light (Not Heat)." *Leaven,* July/August 1974, p. 21.

La Leche League International. "Nipple Care." Information Sheet no. 103.

La Leche League International. "Nursing through Surgery." *La Leche League News,* January/February 1975, p. 11.

La Leche League International. "Sore Breast—What, Why, & What to Do." Information Sheet no. 12.

La Leche League International. "Sore Nipples." *Leaven,* November/December 1974, p. 32.

Bibliography

La Leche League International. "That Ice Treatment." *Leaven,* May/June 1974, p. 21.

La Leche League International. "Thrush." Information Sheet no. 19.

Meltzer, Angela. "Inverted Nipples . . . Persistence Pays Off." *La Leche League News,* November/December 1974, Alabama-Georgia insert.

Nursing Mothers' Association of Australia. "Breast and Nipple Preparation and Care."

Nursing Mothers' Association of Australia. "Breast Problems—First Aid for Blocked Ducts and Breast Infections."

Nursing Mothers' Association of Australia. "Nipple Problems—First Aid for Sore, Cracked, or Blistered Nipples."

Rothenberg, Robert. *Complete Book of Breast Care.* New York: Crown, 1975.

Spock, Benjamin. *Baby and Child Care.* rev. ed. New York: Pocket Books, 1968.

Chapter 5 — Nursing after a Cesarean Childbirth

(1) Donovan, Bonnie. *The Cesarean Birth Experience.* Boston: Beacon Press, 1977.

(2) Cesareans/Support, Education, Concern. "I Would Like to . . ." *C/SEC Newsletter,* vol. I-1, February 1975, p. 2.*

(3) La Leche League International. "Breastfeeding after the Cesarean Section." Information Sheet no. 80.

Recommended Reading

Applebaum, Richard M. "The Modern Management of Successful Breastfeeding." *Pediatric Clinics of North America* 17 (1970): 203-25.

Arena, J. M. "Drugs and Breast Feeding." *Clinical Pediatrics* 5 (1966): 472.

Barnett, C. R. et al. "Neonatal Separation: The Maternal Side of Interactional Deprivation." *Pediatrics* 45 (1970):197-205.

Birth and the Family Journal. Fall 1977. Many articles on cesarean childbirth.

Brody, Jane E. "Cesarean Births." *Woman's Day,* 24 April 1978, p. 68.

Cesareans/Support, Education, Concern. "A Few of Our Philosophies." *C/SEC Newsletter,* vol. I-2, July 1975, p. 2.

---

* C/SEC publications are available by writing to the address listed in Appendix.

Cesareans/Support, Education, Concern. "Childbirth by Cesarean Section."

Cesareans/Support, Education, Concern. "Frankly Speaking. A Pamphlet for Cesarean Couples."

Cesareans/Support, Education, Concern. "Guidelines for Childbirth Instructors."

Cesareans/Support, Education, Concern. (Lown, Mary.) "Mothers Comment." *C/SEC Newsletter*, vol. I-2, July 1975, p. 7.

Frothingham, T. E. "Breastfeeding Contraindications." *Journal of the American Medical Association* 228 (1974):1228.

Hausknecht, Richard, and Ratner, Joan. *Having a Cesarean Baby*. New York: Dutton, 1978.

Knowles, John A. "Excretion of Drugs in Milk, a Review." *Journal of Pediatrics* 66 (1965):1068-82.

Nolan, George H. *Cesarean Childbirth.*°

Vorrheur, Helmuth. "Contraindications to Breast-Feeding." *Journal of the American Medical Association* 227 (1974):676.

White, Mary, and Thornton, Mary Catherine. "Together, and Nursing, from Birth." La Leche League International Information Sheet no. 20.

Chapter 6 — Nursing a Premature Baby

(1) Corner, B. D. "The Premature Infant." *Practitioner* 187 (1961): 165.

(2) Barlow, Barbara et al. "An Experimental Study of Acute Neonatal Enterocolitis—The Importance of Breast Milk." *Journal of Pediatric Surgery* 9 (1974):58.

(3) Berg, Robert B. et al. " 'Early' Discharge of Low Birthweight Infants." *Journal of the American Medical Association* 210 (1969): 1892.

(4) La Leche League International. *La Leche League News*, September/October 1975.

(5) Smallpiece, V., and Davies, P. "Immediate Feeding of Premature Infants with Undiluted Breast Milk." *Lancet* 2 (1964):1349.

(6) Montagu, Ashley. *Touching: The Human Significance of the Skin*. New York: Columbia University Press, 1971.

(7) See reference no. 4.

(8) La Leche League International. "Mandy's Story." *La Leche League News*, July/August 1975, California insert.

° Available at Waldenbooks stores, from Wendy Roe Harvey, 3184 Sing Sing Rd., Horseheads, NY 14845, or from Christine Coleman Wilson, 2491 Pinecrest, Ann Arbor, MI 48104.

Bibliography

Recommended Reading

Bauer, Charles H., and Tinklepaugh, Wendy. "Low Birth Weight Babies in the Hospital: A Survey of Recent Changes in Their Care with Special Emphasis on Early Discharge." *Clinical Pediatrics* 10 (1971):467.

Cook, R. C. M., and Rickham, P. O. "New Syndrome: Intestinal Obstruction Caused by Milk Curds from Early High-Calorie Milk Feeding." *Journal of Pediatric Surgery* 4 (1969):599.

Crosse, F.; Hickmans, B. E.; and Aubrey, Jr. "The Value of Human Milk Compared with Other Foods for Premature Infants." *Archives of Diseases in Childhood* 29 (1964):178.

Dillard, Robert G., and Korones, Sheldon B. "Lower Discharge Weight and Shortened Nursery Stay for Low-Birth-Weight Infants." *New England Journal of Medicine* 288 (1973):131.

Ditchburn, R. K.; Wilkinson, R. H.; Davies, Pamela; and Ainsworth, Patricia. "Plasma Glucose Levels in Infants Weighing 2500 g. and Less Fed Immediately after Birth with Breast Milk." *Biology of the Neonate* 11 (1967):29-35.

Goldman, A. S., and Smith, C. W. "Host Resistance Factors in Human Milk." *Journal of Pediatrics* 82 (1973):1082.

Gordon, H. "Adverse Effects of Prematurity on Growth Re-explained." Paper presented at symposium at Johns Hopkins Hospital, June 1964.

La Leche League International. "Anemia." Information Sheet no. 24.

La Leche League International. "Breastfeeding and the Premature Baby." Information Sheet no. 13.

La Leche League International. *Bridges* no. 14, July 1976.

Mata, Leonardo J., and Wyatt, Richard G. "Host Resistance to Infection." In Jelliffe and Jelliffe, eds., "The Uniqueness of Human Milk." Reprint. *The American Journal of Clinical Nutrition* 24 (1971):968-1024.

Solkoff, Norman et al. Reports in *Medical Tribune* (19 May 1971) and *Medical World News* (March 1971).

Townsend, T. E.; Wirthlin, M. R.; and O'Connor, P. "Use of Stabilization as Basis for Discharge of Premature Infants in a Hospital-Home Care Program." Pine Bluff and Arkansas State Board of Health, 1963.

Wharton, B. A., and Bower, B. D. "Immediate or Later Feeding for Premature Babies?" *Lancet* 2 (1965):969.

Wu, Paul Y. K. et al. " 'Early' versus 'Late' Feeding of Low Birthweight Neonates." *Pediatrics* 39 (1967):733-39.

Chapter 7 — Newborn and Infant Problems

(1) Archavsky, I. A. "Immediate Breast-Feeding of Newborn Infant in the Prophylaxis of the So-Called Physiological Loss of Weight." (Original text in Russian) Abstract in *Courrier* 3 (1953):170.

(2) Klaus, Marshall H., and Kennell, John H. *Maternal-Infant Bonding.* St. Louis: C. V. Mosby, 1976.

(3) La Leche League International. "Protective Role of Mothers' Milk." *La Leche League News,* November/December 1972, p. 89.

(4) White, Mary, and Thornton, Mary Catherine. "Together, and Nursing, from Birth." La Leche League International Information Sheet no. 20.

(5) Coffin, Lewis A. *The Grandmother Conspiracy Exposed.* Out of print.

(6) Brazelton, T. Berry. "What Childbirth Drugs Can Do to Your Child." *Redbook,* February 1971, p. 65.

(7) Brody, Jane E. "Childbirth Drugs and Your Baby." *Redbook,* August 1975.

(8) Fleiss, Paul. "The 'Non-Thriver'—Or Slow Weight Gain in Breast-Fed Infants under Six Months of Age." Unpublished notes, 1976.

(9) Sutherland, Ann. "Fat Babies." *La Leche League News,* March/April 1975, p. 25.

(10) La Leche League International. "Breastfeeding and Jaundice." Information Sheet no. 10.

(11) Arias, Irwin M., and Gartner, Lawrence M. "Jaundice in Breast-Fed Neonates." *Journal of the American Medical Association* 218 (1971)

(12) La Leche League International. "Jaundiced Baby in the Hospital." *La Leche League News,* May/June 1976, California insert.

(13) Gartner, Lawrence M., and Arias, Irwin M. "Studies of Prolonged Neonatal Jaundice in the Breast-Fed Infant." *Journal of Pediatrics* vol. 68, no. 1, pp. 54-56.

Recommended Reading

Apgar, Virginia, and Beck, Joan. *Is My Baby All Right?* New York: Trident Press, 1972.

Graef, John W., and Cone, Thomas E. Jr., eds. *Manual of Pediatric Therapies.* Boston: Children's Hospital Medical Center, 1974.

Holmes, Carl A. "Comforting Advice on Colic." *Parents' Magazine's Baby Care,* Summer 1974.

Jelliffe, D. B., and Jelliffe, E. F. P., eds. "The Uniqueness of Human Milk." *The American Journal of Clinical Nutrition* 24 (1971): 968-1024.

Bibliography

La Leche League International. "Breastfeeding and Drugs in Human Milk." Special Information Sheet.*

La Leche League International. "Breastfeeding and the Oral Contraceptive Pill." Information Sheet no. 18.

La Leche League International. "Medications for the Nursing Mother." Information Sheet no. 21.

Neumann, Charlotte G., and Alpaugh, Melinda. "Birthweight Doubling Time: A Fresh Look." *Pediatrics* 57 (1976): 469-73.

Newton, Michael; Newton, Niles; and Applebaum, Richard M. "Management of Successful Lactation." *Child and Family* Reprint Booklet Series, 1972.

Newton, Niles. "When Baby's Crying Gets Trying." La Leche League International Information Sheet no. 141.

O'Brien, Thomas E. "Excretion of Drugs in Human Milk." *American Journal of Hospital Pharmacy* 31 (1974):844-54.

Chapter 8 — Malformations of Baby's Nose, Mouth, and Digestive Tract

(1) Ross Laboratories. "Cleft Lip and Cleft Palate." Pamphlet. Columbus, Ohio, 1970.

(2) Grady, Edith. Cleft Palate and Cleft Lip Information Packet. Lafayette, Ind.

(3) Spock, Benjamin. *Baby and Child Care*. rev. ed. New York: Pocket Books, 1968.

(4) Silver, Henry K.; Kempe, C. Henry; and Bruyn, Henry B. *Handbook of Pediatrics*. Los Altos, Calif.: Lange Medical Publications, 1975.

Recommended Reading

Berkowitz, Samuel. *Steps in Habilitation for the Cleft Lip and Palate Child*. Evansville, Ind.: Mead Johnson & Co., 1972.

Berkowitz, Samuel. *The Road to Normalcy for the Cleft Lip and Palate Child*. Evansville, Ind.: Mead Johnson & Co., 1972.

Gibbs, Jeanne Marie. "Cleft Palate Babies: One Mother's Experience." *Nursing Care*, January 1973, pp. 19-23.

McDonald, Eugene T. *Bright Promise*. Chicago: National Easter Seal Society for Crippled Children and Adults, 1959.

Nelson, Waldo E., consulting ed.; Vaughan, Victor C., and McKay, R. James, eds. *Textbook of Pediatrics*. Philadelphia: W. B. Saunders, 1975.

---

* Distribution restricted to professional persons.

Ribble, Margaret H. *The Rights of Infants.* New York: New American Library, 1973.

Robertson, James. *Young Children in Hospital.* New York: Barnes & Noble, 1970.

Snyder, Gilbert B.; Berkowitz, Samuel; Bzoch, Kenneth; and Stool, Sylvan. *Your Cleft Lip and Palate Child: A Basic Guide for Parents.* Evansville, Ind.: Mead Johnson Laboratories.

Wicka, Donna, and Falk, Mervyn. *Advice to Parents of a Cleft Palate Child.* Springfield, Ill.: Charles C. Thomas, 1970.

Chapter 9 — Problems Related to Baby's Altered Body Chemistry

(1) Nelson, Waldo E., consulting ed.; Vaughan, Victor C., and McKay, R. James, eds. *Textbook of Pediatrics.* Philadelphia: W. B. Saunders, 1975.

(2) Light, Marilyn Hamilton. "Hypoglycemia and Me." Adrenal Metabolic Research Society of the Hypoglycemia Foundation, Inc.

(3) Smallpiece, V., and Davies, P. "Immediate Feeding of Premature Infants with Undiluted Breast Milk." *Lancet* 2 (1964):1349.

(4) National Cystic Fibrosis Research Foundation. "Your Child and Cystic Fibrosis." May 1973.

(5) Duncan, Lois. "Our Daughter's Double-Diet Problem." *Redbook,* October 1975, p. 51.

(6) Haire, Doris, and Haire, John. *The Medical Value of Breastfeeding.* International Childbirth Education Association, 1974.

(7) La Leche League International. "PKU—Worth Repeating." *La Leche League News,* July/August 1971, p. 57.

(8) State of California Department of Public Health. "The Low Phenylalanine Diet." Bureau of Health Education publication.

Recommended Reading

Eckhert, Curtis D.; Sloan, Martin V.; Hurley, Lucille S.; and Duncan, John R. "Zinc Binding: A Difference between Human and Bovine Milk." *Science,* 195 (1977):789-90.

Johnson, Charles F. "Understanding Phenylketonuria." Child Development Clinic, Department of Pediatrics, University of Iowa.

La Leche League International. "Hastily Jotted Notes." *La Leche League News,* January/February 1968, Michigan insert.

La Leche League International. "Help for Tommy." *La Leche League News,* May/June 1971. pp. 45-47.

Silver, Henry K.; Kempe, C. Henry; and Bruyn, Henry B. *Handbook of Pediatrics.* Los Altos, Calif.: Lange Medical Publications, 1975.

Thomas, Linda L. *Caring and Cooking for the Allergic Child.* New York: Drake, 1974.

Bibliography

Chapter 10 — Nursing a Baby with Special Developmental Conditions

(1) Benda, Clemens E. *Down's Syndrome: Mongolism and Its Management.* New York: Grune & Stratton, 1969.
(2) Jelliffe, D. B., and Jelliffe, E. F. P., eds., "The Uniqueness of Human Milk." *The American Journal of Clinical Nutrition* 24 (1971):968-1024.
(3) Montagu, Ashley. *Touching: The Human Significance of the Skin.* New York: Columbia University Press, 1971.
(4) Newton, Niles. *The Family Book of Child Care.* New York: Harper & Row, 1957.
(5) United States Department of Health, Education and Welfare. "Fact Sheet: Hydrocephalus." DHEW Publication no. (NIH) 75-385.
(6) Marlow, Dorothy R., and Sellew, Gladys. *Textbook of Pediatric Nursing.* Philadelphia: W. B. Saunders, 1962.
(7) See reference no. 5.
(8) Haigh, Lesley. "All Is Calm." *La Leche League News,* November/December 1970, pp. 86-87.
(9) United States Department of Health, Education and Welfare. "Spina Bifida—A Birth Defect." DHEW Publication no. (NIH) 72-309, 1972.
(10), (11) Silver, Henry K.; Kempe, C. Henry; and Bruyn, Henry B. *Handbook of Pediatrics.* Los Altos, Calif.: Lange Medical Publications, 1975.
(12) Scherzer, Alfred L. "Early Diagnosis, Management, and Treatment of Cerebral Palsy." *Rehabilitation Literature,* vol. 35, no. 7, July 1974.
(13) Seaver, Jacqueline. "Cerebral Palsy—More Hope Than Ever." Public Affairs Pamphlet no. 401.
(14) Centerwall, Siegried A., and Centerwall, Willard R. *Down Syndrome.* Department of Pediatrics, School of Medicine, Loma Linda University, California. 1977.
(15) Nelson, Waldo E., consulting ed.; Vaughan, Victor C., and McKay, R. James, eds. *Textbook of Pediatrics.* Philadelphia: W. B. Saunders, 1975.
(16), (17) National Society for Autistic Children. "Could Your Child Be Autistic?"
(18) Wing, Lorna. "Feeding Problems." National Society for Autistic Children.
(19) Handmaker, Stanley D. *My Child Has Down Syndrome.* Charles R. Drew Postgraduate Medical School, 1976.

Recommended Reading*

Braney, Mary Louise. "The Child with Hydrocephalus." *American Journal of Nursing*, vol. 73, no. 5, May 1973.

Brewer, Thomas H. "Nutritionally Speaking." *La Leche League News*, September/October 1974, p. 72.

Bruce, Margaret, and Veigh, Gretchen. *A Practical Manual for Parents of Children with Myelomeningocele.*†

Children's Memorial Hospital, Chicago, Illinois. "The Hydrocephalic Child."

Clark, Dorothy; Dahl, Jane; and Gonzenbach, Lois. *Look at Me, Please, Look at Me.* Elgin Ill.: Cook, 1973.

Dorland's Illustrated Medical Dictionary. 25th ed. Philadelphia: W. B. Saunders, 1974.

"For Parents of Retarded Children." Liguori Publications. Liguori, Missouri.

Fraiberg, Selma. *The Magic Years.* New York: Charles Scribner's Sons, 1959.

Gauchat, Dorothy. *All God's Children.* New York: Hawthorn, 1972.

Gaver, Jessyca R. *Birth Defects and Your Baby.* New York: Lancer Books, 1972.

Gordon, Thomas. *Parent Effectiveness Training.* New York: David McKay, 1970.

Howells, John G., ed. *Modern Perspectives in Psycho-Obstetrics.* New York: Bruner/Mazell, 1972.

Hunt, Nigel. *The World of Nigel Hunt: The Diary of a Mongoloid Youth.* New York: Garrett, 1967.

Hunter, Marvin; Schueman, Helen; and Friedlander, George. *The Retarded Child from Birth to Five.* New York: John Day Co., 1972.

Kaufman, Barry Neil. *Son Rise.* New York: Harper & Row, 1976.

Kaufman, Barry Neil. *To Love Is to Be Happy With.* New York: Coward, 1977.

Kirk, Samuel A.; Karnes, Merle B.; and Kirk, Winifred D. *You and Your Retarded Child.* Palo Alto, Calif.: Pacific Books, 1968.

Koch, Richard, and Dobson, James C., eds. *The Mentally Retarded Child and His Family.* New York: Bruner/Mazell, 1971.

---

* An extensive book list is available from California Association for Neurologically Handicapped Children, Literature Distribution Center, P.O. Box 1526, Vista, CA 92083.

† Available from Gretchen Veigh, 1065 Findley Dr. East, Pittsburgh, PA 15221.

Bibliography

Levine, Melvin, and Evans, Jean. "How to Tell If Your Child Is Hyper-
active—And What to Do about It." *Redbook,* October 1976, p. 24.
Levy, Jenine. *The Baby Exercise Book, First Fifteen Months.* New
York: Pantheon, 1974.
Menolascino, Frank J., ed. *Psychiatric Approaches to Mental Retardation.*
New York: Basic Books, 1970.
Painter, Jenevieve. *Teach Your Baby.* New York: Simon & Schuster,
1971.
Perske, Robert. *New Directions for Parents of Persons Who Are Retarded.*
Nashville, Tenn.: Abingdon Press, 1973.
Ribble, Margaret A. *The Rights of Infants.* New York: New American
Library, 1973.
Salk, Lee, and Kramer, Rita. *How to Raise a Human Being.* New York:
Warner Communications Co., div. of Random House, 1969.
Sharing Our Caring. Magazine for parents of children with Down's
syndrome. *
Smith, David N., and Wilson, Ann A. *The Child with Down's Syndrome
(Mongolism).* Philadelphia: W. B. Saunders, 1973.
Spitz, René A. *The First Year of Life.* New York: International Uni-
versity Press, 1965.
Stedman's Medical Dictionary. Baltimore: Williams & Wilkins, 1972.
Swinyard, Chester. "The Child with Spina Bifida." New York Univer-
sity Medical Center Publication.
United States Department of Health, Education and Welfare. "Cerebral
Palsy." Public Health Service Publication no. 713.
United States Department of Health, Education and Welfare. "Learn-
ing Disabilities Due to Minimal Brain Dysfunction." DHEW Pub-
lication no. (NIH) 71-154.
United States Department of Health, Education and Welfare. "What
Are Developmental Disabilities?" DHEW Publication no. (OHD)
76-29002.

Chapter 11 — Dealing with Allergies

(1) Schachter, Joseph. "Allergy Statistics." National Institute of Allergy and Infectious Diseases, DHEW Publication no. (NIH)
75-757.
(2) Glaser, Jerome; Dreyfuss, Eric; and Logan, Jonathan. "Dietary
Prophylaxis of Atopic Disease." *Practice of Pediatrics,* vol. 2, ch. 72.
Hagerstown, Md.: Medical Dept. of Harper & Row, 1976.
(3) Frazier, Claude A. *Parents' Guide to Allergy in Children.* Garden
City, N.Y.: Doubleday, 1973.

---

* Available by writing Box 196, Milton, WA 98354.

(4) Grulee, C. G., and Sanford, H. N. "The Influence of Breast and Artificial Feeding on Infantile Eczema." *Journal of Pediatrics* 9 (1936):223.

(5) "Breast-Fed Infants Protected from Allergies." *Annals of Allergy,* December 1976.

(6) Gerrard, John W. "Allergy in Infancy." *Pediatric Annals,* October 1974.

(7) Frazier, Claude A. "All about Food Allergies." *Parents' Magazine,* March 1978, p. 16.

(8) See reference no. 2.

(9) White, Mary. "Information, Please! Is It Really Diarrhea? Must I Stop Nursing?" *La Leche League News,* July/August 1973, pp. 57-58.

(10) See reference no. 2.

(11) Mowat, Joy. "Chad." *La Leche League News,* July/August 1974, The Canadian Echo.

(12) White, Mary. "Information, Please!" *La Leche League News,* September/October 1974, p. 75.

(13) Harris, M. Coleman, and Shure, Norman. *All about Allergy.* Englewood Cliffs, N.J.: Prentice-Hall, 1969.

(14) Froehlich, Edwina. "Baby's First Solid Food." La Leche League International Information Sheet no. 105.

Recommended Reading

Aas, Kjell. *The Allergic Child.* Springfield, Ill.: Charles C. Thomas, 1971.

Brazelton, T. Berry. "What You Should Know about Children's Allergies." *Redbook,* January 1976, p. 24.

Conrad, Marion L. *Allergy Cooking.* New York: Thomas Y. Crowell, 1960.

Crook, William G. *Your Allergic Child.* Jackson, Tenn.: Pedicenter Press, 1975.

Dawson, Ann. "Sterling Food for a Sterling Boy." *La Leche League News,* July/August 1968, p. 51.

Feingold, Ben. *Why Your Child Is Hyperactive.* New York: Random House, 1975.

Guthrie, R. A., and Riordan, Jan. "Fact and Fantasy." *Journal of the Kansas Medical Society* 77 (1976):389-92.

Hill, James K. "Gastrointestinal Allergy and Food Allergy." *Allergy for the Practicing Physician.* Methodist Hospital Graduate Medical Center, Indianapolis, Indiana.

Jones, Dorothea Van Gundy. *The Soybean Cookbook.* New York: ARC Books, 1971.

Bibliography

La Leche League International. "Anemia." Information Sheet no. 24.

La Leche League International. "Food Sensitive." *La Leche League News*, July/August 1977, p. 67.

La Leche League International. "How Many Lives Are Touched?" *La Leche League News*, September/October 1970, pp. 68-69.

Little, Billie. *Recipes for Allergics*. New York: Grosset & Dunlap, 1968.

Martin, F. "The Colicky Baby." *Annals of Allergy* 12 (1954):700.

Matsumura, Tatsuo et al. "Egg Sensitivity and Eczematous Manifestations in Breast-Fed Newborns with Particular Reference to Intra-uterine Sensitization." *Annals of Allergy* 35 (1975):221-29.

Rapaport, Howard G., and Linde, Shirley M. *The Complete Allergy Guide*. New York: Simon & Schuster, 1970.

Rapp, Doris J. *Allergies and Your Child*. New York: Holt, Rinehart & Winston, 1972.

Rudolph, Jack, and Rudolph, Burton M. *Allergies*. New York: Pyramid Books, 1973.

Sainsbury, Isobel. *The Milk-Free and Egg-Free Cookbook*. Springfield, Ill.: Charles C. Thomas, 1974.

Schuman, Joan. "Allergy—Still a Mystery." *Science World*, 25 April 1974, pp. 11-13.

Somekh, Emile. *Allergy and Your Child*. New York: Harper & Row, 1974.

Thomas, E. Paul. "Psychosomatic Aspects of Allergy." *Allergy for the Practicing Physician*. Methodist Hospital Graduate Medical Center, Indianapolis, Indiana.

Thomas, Linda L. *Caring and Cooking for the Allergic Child*. New York: Drake, 1974.

Wade, Carlson. *The Complete Rice Cookbook*. New York: Pyramid Books, 1973.

White, Mary. "Information, Please! Fluoride." *La Leche League News*, May/June 1970, pp. 44-45.

White, Mary. "Optimal Infant Nutrition. Avoiding Allergies and Other Problems." La Leche League International Information Sheet no. 16.

Wood, Marion. *Gourmet Food on a Wheat-Free Diet*. Springfield, Ill.: Charles C. Thomas, 1967.

Chapter 12 — When Baby Is Sick or Hospitalized

(1) Gerrard, John. "Breastfeeding: Second Thoughts." *Pediatrics*, vol. 54, no. 6, December 1974.

(2) Cunningham, Allan S. "Morbidity in Breast-Fed and Artificially Fed Infants." *The Journal of Pediatrics*, vol. 90, no. 5, May 1977, pp. 726-29.

(3) La Leche League International. "Diarrhea in Infancy." Information Sheet no. 15.
(4) Thevenin, Tine. *The Family Bed: An Age-Old Concept in Child Rearing.* Minneapolis: Privately printed, 1976.
(5) Nursing Mothers' Association of Australia. "Plastered Kids."
(6) La Leche League International. "I Just Took It for Granted." Reprint no. 54 (Twins).

Recommended Reading

Annas, George J. *The Rights of Hospital Patients.* New York: Avon Books, 1975.
Countryman, Betty Ann. "In Hospital: The Child and the Family." La Leche League International Publication no. 143.
Jelliffe, D. B., and Jelliffe, E. F. P., eds. "The Uniqueness of Human Milk." *The American Journal of Clinical Nutrition* 24 (1971): 968-1024.
La Leche League International. "Nursing a Baby in Traction." *La Leche League News,* September/October 1973, p. 69.
Robertson, James. *Young Children in Hospital.* New York: Barnes & Noble, 1970.
White, Mary. "Information, Please! Is It Really Diarrhea? Must I Stop Nursing?" *La Leche League News,* July/August 1973, pp. 57-58.

Chapter 13 — When Mother Is Sick or Hospitalized

(1) La Leche League International. "The Biological Specificity of Milk." Information Sheet no. 14.
(2) Remington, M. D., and Klein, Jerome O. *Infectious Diseases of the Fetus and Newborn Infant.* Philadelphia: W. B. Saunders, 1976.
(3) La Leche League International. "A Nursing Mother Recovering from Infectious Hepatitis." Information Sheet no. 23.
(4) Battaglia, Frederick C. "Hepatitis Doesn't Hinder Mothering!" *La Leche League News,* July/August 1967, p. 13.
(5) James, Linda. "The Greatest Comfort." *La Leche League News,* November/December 1968, p. 84.
(6) Magill, Barbara. "Persistence Pays." *La Leche League News,* July/August 1970, p. 53.
(7) Muszalski, Mary. "Breastfeeding and Poison Oak." *La Leche League News,* July/August 1975, California insert.
(8) La Leche League International. "Breastfeeding and Drugs in Human Milk." Special Information Sheet.*

---

* Distribution restricted to professional persons.

Bibliography

(9) Stutler, Gail. "This Mountain of Mine." *La Leche League News,* July/August 1972, p. 58.

(10) Althoff, Evelyn. "Nursing and How! With a Broken Collar Bone." *La Leche League News,* January/February 1966, p. 11.

(11) La Leche League International. "A Letter to the Editor." *Bridges,* no. 14, July 1976, p. 4.

(12) La Leche League International. "Medications for the Nursing Mother." Information Sheet no. 21.

(13) See reference no. 11.

(14) Knowles, John A. "Effects on the Infant of Drug Therapy in Nursing Mothers." *Drug Therapy,* May 1973, p. 65.

(15) Fomon, S., and Wei, S. H. Y. *Nutritional Disorders of Children— Prevention, Screening and Followup.* U.S. Department of Health, Education and Welfare. Washington, D.C.: U.S. Government Printing Office, 1976.

(16) La Leche League International. "Breastfeeding and the Oral Contraceptive Pill." Information Sheet no. 18.

(17) La Leche League International. *The Womanly Art of Breastfeeding* 2d ed. Franklin Park, Ill.: La Leche League International, 1963.

(18) See reference no. 8.

(19) Vorrheur, Helmuth. "Drug Excretion In Breast Milk." *Postgraduate Medicine* 56 (1974):102.

(20) Harlap, Susan, and Davies, A. Michael. "Infant Admissions to Hospital and Maternal Smoking." *Lancet,* 30 March 1974, p. 529.

(21) Pryor, Karen. *Nursing Your Baby.* New York: Harper & Row, 1973.

(22) Chun, George. "Marijuana: A Realistic Approach." *California Medicine,* April 1971, pp. 7-13.

(23) Linden, Marcia. "It Can Be Done—If You Want to!" *La Leche League News,* May/June 1968, Maryland-Virginia insert.

(24) Zola, Ann. "All Things Are Possible." *La Leche League News,* September/October 1970, California insert.

(25) James, Dorothy. "I Nursed Another Mother's Baby." O'Neill, Jean. "I Left My Baby with Another Mother." *La Leche League News,* May/June 1966, p. 3.

(26) Robertson, James, and Robertson, Joyce. "Quality of Substitute Care as an Influence in Separation Responses." *Children in Hospitals* Newsletter, Winter 1976.

(27) La Leche League International. "A Story from Alaska." *La Leche League News,* March/April 1968, Northwest Corner insert.

(28) Farrell, Linda. "Women Who Give." *La Leche League News,* July/August 1974, p. 50.

Recommended Reading

Kippley, John, and Kippley, Sheila. *The Art of Natural Family Planning.* Cincinnati: Couple-to-Couple League, 1977.

Kippley, Sheila. *Breastfeeding and Natural Child Spacing: The Ecology of Natural Mothering.* New York: Harper and Row, 1974.

Knowles, John A. "Drugs Excreted into Breast Milk." *Pediatric Therapy,* 1968-69.

La Leche League International. "A Note on Drug Calls." *League Spirit,* Spring 1976, p. 10.

La Leche League International. "Pneumonia and Drugs." *La Leche League News,* May/June 1966, California insert.

La Leche League International. "When Mother Is Ill." *La Leche League News,* July/August 1965, pp. 8-10.

La Leche League International. "Where There's a Will . . ." *La Leche League News,* March/April 1968, Arizona insert.

La Leche League International. "You Do the Best You Can." *La Leche League News,* July/August 1969, p. 52.

McQueen, Mary. "In Perspective." *La Leche League News,* July/August 1972, p. 59.

Milam, Betty. "Courage!" *La Leche League News,* July/August 1967, p. 10.

Moen, Lynn. "A California Mother's Success Story." *La Leche League News,* July/August 1968, California insert.

Shearer, Lloyd. "Women and Alcohol." *Parade Magazine,* 22 February 1976.

Sullivan, Judi. "A Very Special Guest." *La Leche League News,* November/December 1970, p. 92.

University Hospital, San Diego, Calif. "Transmission of Drugs in Human Milk." *Perinatal Medicine Newsletter.*

Chapter 14 — Working Together: Doctor, Hospital, Parents

(1) Garrison, Webb. "The Care-by-Parent Ward." *Parents' Magazine* 46 (1971):34.

(2) Brazelton, T. Berry. "If Your Child Goes to the Hospital." *Redbook,* April 1974.

(3) Bowlby, John. *Child Care and The Growth of Love.* 2d ed. Baltimore: Penguin Books, 1965.

(4) Bowlby, John. *Attachment and Loss.* vol. 1 *Attachment* (1969), vol. 2 *Separation* (1973). New York: Basic Books.

(5) Robertson, James. *Hospitals and Children: A Parents' Eye View.* New York: International Universities Press, 1963.

Bibliography

(6) Robertson, James. *Young Children in Hospital.* 2d ed. New York: Barnes & Noble, 1970.

(7) See reference no. 1.

(8) La Leche League International. *The Womanly Art of Breastfeeding.* 2d ed. Franklin Park, Ill.: La Leche League International, 1963.

(9) White, Mary, and Thornton, Mary Catherine. "Together, and Nursing, from Birth." La Leche League Information Sheet no. 20.

(10) La Leche League International. "White Paper on Infant Feeding Practices." Information Sheet no. 158.

(11) La Leche League International. *La Leche League News,* July/August 1975, California insert.

(12) Doan, Marlyn S. "Visiting Hours Are Over." *Parents' Magazine,* January 1976, p. 24.

(13), (14) Countryman, Betty Ann. "In Hospital: The Child and the Family." La Leche League International Publication no. 143.

(15) Annas, George J. *The Rights of Hospital Patients.* New York: Avon Books, 1975.

(16), (17) See reference no. 2.

(18) Gregg, Elizabeth M., and Boston Children's Medical Center Staff, eds. *What to Do When There's Nothing to Do.* New York: Dell, 1970.

(19) See reference no. 13.

(20) See reference no. 1.

(21) See reference no. 13.

Chapter 15 — Inducing or Reestablishing Your Milk Supply: For Natural Born or Adopted Baby

(1) Newton, Michael, and Newton, Niles. "The Normal Course and Management of Lactation." *Clinical Obstetrics and Gynecology,* vol. 5, no. 1, March 1962.

(2) Carlson, Regina. "Why Nursing a Baby Means Love to Me." *Redbook,* December 1973, p. 59.

(3) Hormann, Elizabeth. "Relactation: A Guide to Breastfeeding the Adopted Baby." La Leche League International Information Sheet no. 159.

(4) Pryor, Karen. *Nursing Your Baby.* New York: Harper & Row, 1973.

(5) Newton, Niles. "Breastfeeding." *Psychology Today,* June 1968. La Leche League International Reprint no. 130.

(6) Raphael, Dana. *The Tender Gift: Breast Feeding.* New York: Schocken, 1976.

(7) See reference no. 5.

Recommended Reading

Bumgarner, Norma Jane. *Helping Love Grow: Some Hints for Mothering Your Adopted Baby.* Norman, Okla.: Privately printed, 1972.°

Mowat, Joy. "Chad." *La Leche League News,* July/August 1974. The Canadian Echo.

Welch, Martha McKeen. *Just Like Puppies.* New York: Coward-McCann, 1969.

Chapter 16 — Nursing While Pregnant

(1) White, Mary. "Does Breastfeeding Space Babies?" Reprint, *Marriage,* January 1961.

(2) Gioiosa, Rose. "Breast Feeding and Child Spacing." La Leche League International Information Sheet no. 121.

(3) Horne, Ann E. "Observations and Reflections on Nursing Siblings Who Are Not Twins." La Leche League International Information Sheet no. 75.

(4) La Leche League International. "Information, Please! Colostrum." *La Leche League News,* March/April 1975, p. 25.

(5) See reference no. 3.

(6) La Leche League International. *The Womanly Art of Breastfeeding.* 2d ed. Franklin Park, Ill.: La Leche League International, 1963.

(7) See reference no. 3.

(8) McClelland, Vicki. "Big Mommies, and Little Girls, Too, Can Change Their Minds." *La Leche League News,* January/February 1976, California insert.

Chapter 17 — Nursing Siblings

(1) Horne, Ann E. "Observations and Reflections on Nursing Siblings Who Are Not Twins." La Leche League International Information Sheet no. 75.

(2) Baldwin, Dorothy. *Understanding Your Baby; A Course in Child Development 0-3 Years.* London: Ebury Press, 1975.

(3) Ilg, Frances L., and Ames, Louise B. *The Gesell Institute's Child Behavior.* Perennial Library. New York: Harper & Row, 1976.

(4) Newton, Niles. *The Family Book of Child Care.* New York: Harper & Row, 1957.

(5) Thevenin, Tine. *The Family Bed: An Age-Old Concept in Child Rearing.* Minneapolis: Privately printed, 1976.

(6) See reference no. 4.

° Available from N. J. Bumgarner, 1712 Lenox Drive, Norman, OK 73069.

Bibliography

(7) Montagu, Ashley. *Touching: The Human Significance of the Skin.* New York: Columbia University Press, 1971.

(8) Bricklin, Alice G. *Mother Love: The Book of Natural Child Rearing.* Philadelphia: Running Press, 1975.

(9) Bumgarner, Norma Jane. "Nursing Siblings: If You Want to, You Can." Paper presented at the state meeting of the La Leche League of Oklahoma, 1972.

Recommended Reading

Horbinski, Brigid. "Sleeping in That Family Bed." *La Leche League News,* January/February 1975, p. 10.

Koestler, Maureen. "Two Is More Than One." Paper by the president of Breastfeeding Information Services, Nursing Mothers' Committee, Childbirth Education Association of Greater Philadelphia.

La Leche League International. "Sleeping in That Family Bed." *La Leche League News,* March/April 1975, p. 22.

La Leche League International. "Unusual Breastfeeding Situations." *La Leche League News,* September/October 1968, p. 76.

McClelland, Beth. "More about the 'Family Bed.'" *La Leche League News,* May/June 1975, p. 44.

Chapter 18 — Nursing Twins

(1) Pandey, Jenny. "Two for the Price of One? The Care and Breast Feeding of Twins." Nursing Mothers' Association of Australia.

(2) Bedeski, Shirley. "A Star to Reach For." *La Leche League News,* March/April 1972, p. 21.

Recommended Reading

Gehman, Betsy Holland. *Twins: Twice the Trouble, Twice the Fun.* Philadelphia & New York: J. B. Lippincott, 1965.

Jeske, Ilze. "Pam's Twins." *La Leche League News,* January/February 1977, p. 16.

Johnson, Carolyn. "Twins." La Leche League International Information Sheet no. 54.

Mitchell, Marilyn. "What's It Like Having Twins?" *Baby Talk,* September 1967, pp. 4-5.

"No Two Alike. Diapers to Dating." Ohio Federation of Mothers of Twins, 1961.

Scheinfeld, Amram. *Twins and Supertwins.* Philadelphia & New York: J. B. Lippincott, 1967.

Spock, Benjamin. *Baby and Child Care.* rev. ed. New York: Pocket Books, 1968.

Twin Mothers Club of Bergen County, New Jersey, 1971. "And Then
    There Were Two."
Warta, Gail. "A Struggle for Life." *La Leche League News,* November/
    December 1977, p. 103.
Weisman, Lorraine. "Nursing Twins." *La Leche League News,* Janu-
    ary/February 1977, p. 5.

Chapter 19 — Nursing an Older Baby

(1) Wood, Elizabeth. "Who Is 'An Older Nursing Baby'?" *La Leche
    League News,* November/December 1970, p. 86.
(2) Bricklin, Alice G. *Mother Love: The Book of Natural Child Rearing.*
    Philadelphia: Running Press, 1975.
(3) Harris, Thomas A. *I'm O.K.—You're O.K.* New York: Harper &
    Row, 1973.
(4) Ilg, Frances L., and Ames, Louise B. *The Gesell Institute's Child
    Behavior.* Perennial Library. New York: Harper & Row, 1976.
(5) Edwards, Ralph. "The Physical Aspects of Maleness and Female-
    ness." *Child and Family,* Winter 1969.
(6) Montagu, Ashley. *Touching: The Human Significance of the Skin.*
    New York: Columbia University Press, 1971.
(7) Thevenin, Tine. *The Family Bed: An Age-Old Concept in Child
    Rearing.* Minneapolis: Privately printed, 1976.
(8) La Leche League International. "Needs and Priorities: Babies . . .
    Toddlers . . . Parents." Information Sheet no. 77.

Recommended Reading

Bird, Lois. *How to Make Your Husband Your Lover.* New York: Ban-
    tam, 1974.
Bird, Lois. *How to Make Your Wife Your Mistress.* New York: Double-
    day, 1972.
Dunn, Marena. *La Leche League News,* July/August 1973, California
    insert.
Entwistle, Lois. "He's a Big Boy Now." *La Leche League News,* March/
    April 1975, pp. 20-21.
Froehlich, Edwina. "Thoughts about Weaning." La Leche League In-
    ternational Reprint no. 125.
Hymes, James L. Jr. *The Child Under Six.* Englewood Cliffs, N.J.:
    Prentice-Hall, 1964.
Inkeles, Gordon. *The Art of Sensual Massage.* San Francisco: Straight
    Arrow Press, 1972.
King, Lee, and Falatovics, Sharon. "On Weaning." *La Leche League
    News,* January/February 1974, p. 5.

Bibliography

La Leche League International. "And/or: Important and/or Interesting Bits of Information." *La Leche League News,* January/February 1974, p. 15.

La Leche League International. *La Leche League News,* March/April 1977, Florida insert.

La Leche League International. *La Leche League News.* March/April 1977, Virginia-West Virginia insert.

La Leche League International. Section V, Transcripts, Fourth International Convention.

Masters, William H., and Johnson, Virginia E. *Human Sexual Response.* Boston: Little, Brown, 1966.

Masters, William H., and Johnson, Virginia E. *The Pleasure Bond.* Boston: Little, Brown, 1975.

Moldover, Edwina. "The Late Evening Nursing." *La Leche League News,* January/February 1976, p. 4.

Newton, Michael, and Newton, Niles. "The Normal Course and Management of Lactation." *Clinical Obstetrics and Gynecology* vol. 5, no. 1, March 1962.

Wilke, Richard B. *Tell Me Again, I'm Listening. How to Make Your Marriage Work.* Nashville: Abingdon Press, 1973.

Chapter 20 — Nursing Strikes and One-Sided Nursing

(1) La Leche League International. "And/or. Important and/or Interesting Bits of Information." *La Leche League News,* November/December 1973, p. 91.

(2) Nursing Mothers' Association of Australia. "Coping with Breast Refusal."

(3) Newton, Niles. *The Family Book of Child Care.* New York: Harper & Row, 1957.

(4) See reference no. 2.

(5) Gray, Laman A. Sr. "Breastfeeding after Cancer." *The Consultant,* August 1976, p. 170.

(6) Rogers, Lynn. "Breastfeeding after a Mastectomy." *La Leche League News,* March/April 1978, pp. 23-24.

Recommended Reading

Kushner, Rose. *Breast Cancer. A Personal History and an Investigative Report.* New York: Harcourt Brace Jovanovich, 1975.

La Leche League International. "Ever Hear of a Nursing Strike?" Information Sheet no. 57.

Muszalski, Mary. "Breastfeeding and Poison Oak." *La Leche League News,* July/August 1975, California insert.

Chapter 21 — Nursing during Stressful Times

(1) Newton, Niles, and Newton, Michael. "Mothers' Reactions to Their Newborn Babies." *Journal of the American Medical Association* 181 (1962):206-10.

(2) Ladas, A. "How to Help Mothers Breastfeed." *Clinical Pediatrics* 9 (1970):702-5.

(3) Shaw, J. Unpublished survey. Atlanta, Georgia, 1976.

(4) Bardon, D. "Puerperal Depression." In *Psychosomatic Medicine in Obstetrics and Gynecology.* Third International Congress. London: S. Karger, 1971. pp. 335-37.

(5) Sullivan, H. S. *The Interpersonal Theory of Psychiatry.* New York: W. W. Norton, 1953.

(6) Maslow, A. H., and Szilagyi-Kessler, I. "Security and Breastfeeding." *Journal of Abnormal Psychology* 41 (1946):83-85.

Recommended Reading

Aguilera, D. C., and Messick, J. M. *Crisis Intervention: Theory and Methodology.* St. Louis: C. V. Mosby, 1970.

Bowlby, John. *Attachment and Loss.* vol. 1. New York: Basic Books, 1969.

Caplan, G. *Principles of Preventive Psychiatry.* New York: Basic Books, 1964.

Coleman, A., and Coleman, L. *Pregnancy: The Psychological Experience.* New York: Seabury Press, 1973.

Cullberg, J. "Mental Reactions of Women to Perinatal Death." In *Psychosomatic Medicine in Obstetrics and Gynecology.* Third International Congress. London: S. Karger, 1971. pp. 326-29.

Forbes, R. "The Father's Role." In *Psychosomatic Medicine in Obstetrics and Gynecology.* Third International Congress. London: S. Karger, 1971. pp. 281-83.

Gopalan, C. "Studies on Lactation in Poor Communities." *Journal of Topical Pediatrics* 4 (1958):87-97.

Gunther, John. *Death Be Not Proud.* New York: Harper & Row, 1949.

James, Muriel, and Jongeward, Dorothy. *Born to Win.* Reading, Mass.: Addison-Wesley, 1971.

Kubler-Ross, E. *On Death and Dying.* New York: MacMillan, 1969.

La Leche League International. "Losing Your Milk?" Information Sheet no. 83.

Newton, Niles. "When Baby's Crying Gets Trying." La Leche League International Information Sheet no. 141.

Newton, Niles, and Newton, Michael. "Psychologic Aspects of Lactation." *New England Journal of Medicine* 277 (1967):1179-88.

Bibliography

Parad, H. J., ed. *Crisis Intervention. Selected Readings.* New York: Family Service Association of America, 1965.

Pitt, B. "Neurotic (or Atypical) Depression Following Childbirth." In *Psychosomatic Medicine in Obstetrics and Gynecology.* Third International Congress. London: S. Karger, 1971. pp. 347-49.

Reusch, J. *Therapeutic Communication.* New York: W. W. Norton, 1961.

Ribble, Margaret. *The Rights of Infants.* New York: New American Library, 1973.

Rose, J. A. "The Prevention of Mothering Breakdown Associated with Physical Abnormality of the Infant." In G. Kaplan, ed., *Prevention of Mental Disorders in Children.* New York: Basic Books, 1961. pp. 265-82.

Satir, Virginia. *Peoplemaking.* Palo Alto, Calif.: Science and Behavior Books, 1972.

Chapter 22 — Mothers with Special Physical Problems

(1) La Leche League International. "Diabetes and the Nursing Mother." Information Sheet no. 17.

(2) Miller, Diane Linda. "Birth and Long-Term Unsupplemented Breastfeeding in 17 Insulin-Dependent Diabetic Mothers." *Birth and the Family Journal,* 1977.

(3) O'Brien, T. E. "Excretion of Drugs in Human Milk." *American Journal of Hospital Pharmacy* 31 (1974):853.

(4) Miller, Diane Linda. "Diabetic Mother Advocates Breastfeeding for Mutual Health, Happiness, and Satisfaction." *Diabetes in the News,* Juvenile Diabetes Special, June 1974.

(5) La Leche League International. *La Leche League News,* July/August 1963, p. 2.

(6) La Leche League International. "Out of the Tunnel." "Thyroid Problem." *La Leche League News,* September/October 1976, pp. 69-70; p. 75.

(7) The Medical Letter, Inc. *The Medical Letter on Drugs and Therapeutics,* vol. 16, no. 6 (Issue 396).*

(8) La Leche League International. "Drugs for Epilepsy." *La Leche League News,* November/December 1971, p. 89.

(9) United States Department of Health, Education and Welfare. "Muscular Dystrophy: Hope through Research." Public Health Service Publication no. 996.†

---

* Available from The Medical Letter, Inc., 56 Harrison St., New Rochelle, NY 10801.

† Available from National Institutes of Health, Bethesda, MD 20014.

Recommended Reading

"Diabetics Should Breast-feed to Improve Mother-Infant Bonding." *Ob-Gyn News*, vol. 13, no. 6. 15 March 1978, p. 21.

Graber, Alan L. *Diabetes and Pregnancy: A Guide for the Prospective Mother with Diabetes.* Nashville: Vanderbilt University Press, 1973.

Hiland, Mary W. "My Special Fear of Becoming a Mother." *Redbook*, December 1974, p. 58.

Klaus, Marshall H., and Kennell, John H. *Maternal-Infant Bonding.* St. Louis: C. V. Mosby, 1976.

La Leche League International. "Letter to an Expectant (Blind) Mother." *La Leche League News*, November/December 1976, pp. 86-87.

O'Donovan, Pat. "My Fight for the Right to be a Mother." *Redbook*, April 1976, p. 46.

Salmon, M. B. "Diabetes and Breastfeeding." *The Joy of Breastfeeding.* part V, ch. 1. Demarest, N.J.: Techkits, Inc., 1977.

Chapter 23 — Nursing and Working

(1) Cahill, Mary Ann. "Breastfeeding and Working." La Leche League International Publication no. 58.

(2) Newton, Niles. "They Say." *La Leche League News*, March/April 1974, p. 22.

(3) Princess Grace of Monaco. "Why Mothers Should Breast-Feed Their Babies." *Ladies Home Journal*, August 1971, p. 56.

(4) See reference no. 1.

Recommended Reading

Athanas, Kathy. "Mommy Was a Part-Time Soldier." *La Leche League News*, July/August 1977, p. 62.

Cogan, Rosemary. "For the Working Mother-to-Be: Nursing Your Baby." Reprint.*

Evans, Pamela M. "They Say." *La Leche League News*, March/April 1977, p. 32.

Klaus, Marshall H., and Kennell, John H. *Maternal-Infant Bonding.* St. Louis: C. V. Mosby, 1976.

---

* Available from Childbirth Without Pain Education League, Inc. 3940 Eleventh St., Riverside, CA 92501.

Bibliography

La Leche League International. "An Actress Who Believes in Life." *La Leche League News,* September/October 1974, p. 69.

LeClair, Dee. "In a College Classroom." *La Leche League News,* July/August 1971, pp. 51-52.

Phillips, Janette. "To Work or Not to Work." *La Leche League News,* January/February 1978, pp. 13-14.

Platt, Shirley. "It Didn't Work." *La Leche League News,* July/August 1977, p. 62.

Rhea, Martha. "She Took Baby Along." *La Leche League News,* January/February 1977, p. 7.

Ribble, Margaret A. *The Rights of Infants.* New York: New American Library, 1973.

Stratton, Dolly. "Breastfeeding and the Working Mother." *La Leche League News,* July/August 1977, p. 64.

Zigler, Cissy. "A Flight Attendant." *La Leche League News,* July/August 1977, p. 63.

Chapter 24 — Traveling with a Nursing Baby

(1) Richards, Kit. "Backpacking with Baby." *La Leche League News,* July/August 1971, pp. 49-50.

(2) Hickey, Mary Jeanne. "Herbert James Went to the Fair." *La Leche League News,* May/June 1966, p. 11.

(3) Benecke, Sheila. "How to Simplify Air Travel with a Breast-fed Baby." *La Leche League News,* July/August 1976, Illinois insert.

Recommended Reading

Gregg, Elizabeth M.; and Boston Children's Medical Center Staff, eds. *What to Do When There's Nothing to Do.* New York: Dell, 1968.

Hadley, Leila. *Fielding's Guide to Traveling with Children in Europe.* New York: Fielding Publications, 1972.

Johnson, June. *838 Ways to Amuse a Child.* New York: Gramercy, 1962.

Kast, Claire M.; Smith, Ellen; and Wilson, Mary. "Traveling with Toddlers." *La Leche League News,* May/June 1968, pp. 42-43.

La Leche League International. "Take Baby with You." *La Leche League News,* September/October 1974, pp. 67-68.

La Leche League International. "The Portable Baby." *La Leche League News,* September/October 1965, p. 10.

World Book Encyclopedia. Childcraft Encyclopedia vol. II. "Make and Do." Chicago: Field Enterprises.

Chapter 25 — When You Go It Alone

(1) Thevenin, Tine. *The Family Bed: An Age-Old Concept in Child Rearing.* Minneapolis: Privately printed, 1976.

(2) Raphael, Dana. *The Tender Gift: Breast Feeding.* New York: Schocken, 1976.

Recommended Reading

Akmakjian, Hiag. *The Natural Way to Raise a Healthy Child.* New York: Praeger, 1975.

Briggs, Dorothy C. *Celebrate Yourself.* Garden City, N.Y.: Doubleday, 1976.

Briggs, Dorothy C. *Your Child's Self-Esteem.* Garden City, N.Y.: Doubleday, 1970.

Eagle, Genevieve. "My Fight to Become the Fullest Full-Time Mother." *Redbook,* June 1976, p. 47.

Faber, Adele, and Mazlish, Elaine. *Liberated Parents, Liberated Children.* New York: Grosset & Dunlap, 1974.

Friday, Nancy. *My Mother/My Self.* New York: Delacorte Press, 1977.

Ginott, Haim. *Between Parent and Child.* New York: MacMillan, 1965.

Ginott, Haim. *Between Parent and Teenager.* New York: MacMillan, 1969.

Gordon, Thomas. *Parent Effectiveness Training.* New York: David McKay, 1970.

Hazell, Lester Dessez. *Commonsense Childbirth.* New York: Putnam, 1969.

Hope, Karol, and Young, Nancy. *Momma Handbook: The Sourcebook for Single Mothers.* New York: New American Library, 1976.

Ilg, Frances L., and Ames, Louise B. *The Gesell Institute's Child Behavior.* Perennial Library. New York: Harper & Row, 1976.

James, Muriel, and Jongeward, Dorothy. *Born to Win.* Reading, Mass.: Addison-Wesley, 1971.

Kassorla, Irene. *Putting It All Together.* New York: Brut Productions, 1973.

Klein, Carole. *The Single Parent Experience.* New York: Avon, 1973.

Krantzler, Mel. *Creative Divorce.* New York: M. Evans, 1975.

La Leche League International. "Meeting the Needs of the Child in the Single Parent Family." Session 108, La Leche League Conference, Toronto, Canada, 1977.

La Leche League International. "On Discipline: A Symposium." Publication no. 164.

Bibliography

Missildine, W. Hugh. *Your Inner Child of the Past.* New York: Simon & Schuster, 1963.

Salk, Lee, and Kramer, Rita. *How to Raise a Human Being.* New York: Warner Communications Co. div. of Random House, 1969.

Satir, Virginia. *Peoplemaking.* Palo Alto, Calif.: Science and Behavior Books, 1972.

About the Major Assistants and Consultants

Assistants

The women mentioned here have all made valuable contributions to this book. They have generously given their time and shared their experiences so that what they learned about breastfeeding can benefit others. Some of these mothers collaborated with me on certain chapters, as indicated, while others provided stories and advice throughout the book.

REGINA CARLSON—"Inducing or Reestablishing Your Milk Supply: For Natural Born or Adopted Baby"
Regina and her husband, Kenneth, live in New Jersey and are the parents of Ben (adopted as a toddler), Anna (born to them), and Nora (adopted as a baby and breastfed by Regina). Ben is half Sikh (from India), Anna is a blue-eyed blond like her parents, and Nora is half Negro, half Caucasian. Regina's interests focus on individual rights and health education.

JUSTINE CLEGG—"When Mother Is Sick or Hospitalized"
As a La Leche League leader and assistant to the regional coordinator of leader applicants, Justine has come in contact with many mothers who have breastfed during sickness or hospitalization. Justine delivered all three of her children by cesarean section and had hepatitis, the flu, breast infections, colds, food poisoning, and heart problems during periods when she was nursing. She and her husband, Bill, live in Florida with their children, Roger, Elizabeth, and Sarah.

NANCY COHEN—"Nursing after a Cesarean Childbirth"
Nancy is a co-founder and current coordinator of C/SEC (Cesareans/Support, Education and Concern). She is also a La Leche

League leader and former area professional liaison person for La Leche League. Her husband, Paul, is a dentist and is recognized as a medical associate by La Leche League International. Nancy and Paul have two children, Eric and Elissa, and they live in Massachusetts.

ELIZABETH CROFTS
Elizabeth is a nurse and former obstetrical instructor. A member of the Board of Directors of La Leche League International and Director of the Professional Liaison Department of La Leche League International, she has assisted with most of the chapters in the book. Elizabeth and her husband, Lyman, are the parents of Anne, Eileen, Lenore, and Jimmie. The family resides in Connecticut.

PHYLLIS DAHL, R.N.—"Breast and Nipple Problems"
Phyllis is a chapter professional liaison person for La Leche League. She has a B.S. degree in nursing and worked in obstetrics and public health nursing. She and her husband, David, have three sons: Mark, Peter, and Daniel. Because of a nipple problem, she gave up on her attempts to nurse Mark, but with information and support was able to nurse Peter and Daniel. The family lives in Minnesota.

SHERI HANSEN
Sheri is a former La Leche League leader and is currently chairperson of the professional liaison committee of the Cleft Parent Guild of Los Angeles. She has organized a unique training program for parents to assist in lay counseling of other parents of newborns with clefts. Sheri and her husband, Pat, are the parents of Molly, Lisa (who was born with a cleft lip and palate), and Jenny. Sheri has assisted with many of the chapters in the book.

NANCY HIETA—"Dealing with Allergies"
Nancy is a La Leche League leader in California and the mother of Erik, Stephen, and Karin. Both she and her husband, Richard, are allergic and although their children were breastfed, each has food allergies. This makes cooking a challenge for Nancy since members of the family react to different allergens. While nursing Karin, Nancy was on a limited diet to help Karin avoid even trace amounts of foods to which she was allergic.

MARGARET HOWIE, R.N.—"Nursing a Baby with Special Developmental Conditions"
Margaret was a nurse before she had children and is now a La
Leche League leader in Ontario, Canada. Her family includes
husband Douglas, and children Peter, Christopher, Michelle, and
Kathleen. Michelle, who is hypotonic, did not start walking until
three years of age. At that time, her hypotonia was diagnosed as a
symptom of mild cerebral palsy.

LINDA LEHRER—"Nutrition for Mother and Baby"
Linda was the mother of two sons, Kevin and Adam. She was also
the state librarian for La Leche League of Massachusetts. It was
while attending La Leche League meetings that she became interested in nutrition. She read extensively on the subject and gave talks
on nutrition. Her husband Harvey says, "Helping others was always
an important part of Linda's life. Her desire to help nursing
mothers with problems, through this book, became a focal point in
her life before she died."

JODY NATHANSON
Jody is the mother of four boys, David, Geoffrey, Bennett, and Joel.
She has been active in La Leche League of Southern California
since 1962, and is a member of the Board of Directors of La Leche
League International. She is also an International Instructor in
Human Relations. With her husband, Sherman, she pioneered the
use of Happy Baby Carriers in 1964, paving the way for babies to
accompany their mothers wherever they go. Jody has assisted with
most of the chapters in the book.

JEANNE SHAW, R.N., M.N.—"Nursing during Stressful Times"
Jeanne is a former La Leche League leader and contact for mothers
of twins. She is now a clinical specialist in Psychiatric-Mental
Health Nursing in Atlanta, Georgia. Jeanne and her husband,
Allen, are the parents of Billy, Liz, and twins Sheila and Joseph.

KAROLYN SIMON, R.N.—"Nursing after a Cesarean Childbirth"
Karolyn is the mother of Nathaniel, and twins Joshua and Gabriel
(the second twin, Gabriel, was born by cesarean). She is a regis-
tered nurse and worked three years on orthopedics. She has a B.S.
and M.S. in biology and taught zoology for 2½ years at Southern

Connecticut State College. Karolyn, husband Gerald and children now live in Sacramento, California.

ROSE SODERGREN—"Nursing Siblings"
—"Nursing an Older Baby"
Rose is a La Leche League leader and a letter writer for La Leche League International. She and husband, Len, have four children, Mary, Cliff, Eric, and Andy. Rose's breastfeeding experience includes nursing her daughter until she was four years old and nursing siblings.

PEGGY TEETER, R.N.
Peggy and her husband, Paul, are the parents of three sons, Dan, John, and Brian. She has been a La Leche League leader since 1969 and area professional liaison person for La Leche League of California since 1975. Peggy worked for several years in pediatric and newborn/obstetric nursing. She has assisted with many of the chapters in the book.

Medical Consultants

MARGARET H. DAVIDSON, M.D.
Margaret H. Davidson is an Adjunct Assistant Professor in the Department of Pediatrics, Harbor General Hospital, University of California at Los Angeles School of Medicine, Torrance, California. She is also coordinator of the Child Health and Disability Prevention Program for the Coastal Region of the Los Angeles County Department of Health Services and director of a Pediatric Nurse Practitioner Program. Dr. Davidson's administrative, clinical and teaching activities all relate to providing primary health care for the children of medically underserved families. Dr. Davidson and her husband have three children.

PAUL M. FLEISS, M.D., M.P.H.
Paul Fleiss is an Assistant Clinical Professor at the University of Southern California and Lecturer in the School of Public Health at the University of California at Los Angeles. He is a La Leche League medical associate and is in private practice in Hollywood. About 80 percent of his patients start out being breastfed and after six months, 80 per cent are *still* breastfed. Dr. Fleiss and his wife, Elissa, have six children.

DERRICK B. JELLIFFE, M.D., F.R.C.P., F.A.A.P.
Derrick B. Jelliffe has written numerous articles, papers and books and has been a participant in professional meetings in many countries. His professional experience has been in England, Nigeria, Jamaica, India, Uganda, and the United States. Since 1971 he has been head of the Division of Population, Family and International Health and Professor of Public Health, School of Public Health, and Professor of Pediatrics, School of Medicine, University of California at Los Angeles. He is on many advisory boards, including the Professional Advisory Board of La Leche League International. Dr. Jelliffe has co-authored many articles and books with his wife, E. F. Patrice Jelliffe.

HAROLD M. MALLER, M.D.
Harold M. Maller is a Clinical Associate Professor of Pediatrics, University of Southern California School of Medicine; Attending Pediatrician, Children's Hospital of Los Angeles; Chairman of the Pediatric Department, Valley Presbyterian Hospital, Van Nuys, California, and is a La Leche League medical associate. He has a remarkable practice in that over 90 percent of his patients are breastfeeding. He and his wife, Judy, and their four children live in Encino, California.

JOHN D. MICHAEL, M.D.
John D. Michael is a pediatrician in private practice at the Ross Valley Medical Clinic, Greenbrae and Novato, California. He is a medical associate of La Leche League International; a Fellow of the American Academy of Pediatrics; Board Certified by American Board of Pediatrics; a Clinical Instructor, Department of Pediatrics, University of California Medical School, San Francisco; and Clinical Instructor, Department of Pediatrics, Children's Hospital and Medical Center, San Francisco. Dr. Michael and his wife Harriett (who is a La Leche League leader in Novato), have three children.

MARK THOMAN, M.D., F.A.A.P., A.B.M.T.
Mark Thoman is a pediatrician member of the Professional Advisory Board of La Leche League International; Director of the Cystic Fibrosis Clinic in Des Moines, Iowa; editor-in-chief of AACTION (publication of the American Academy of Clinical Toxicology) and medical advisor to the Des Moines chapter of the International Childbirth Education Association. Dr. Thoman lives in Des Moines and is the father of seven children.

Index